W9-BWS-478

THE ULTIMATE
Women's Guide to
Beating Disease
AND LIVING A HAPPY, ACTIVE LIFE
2016

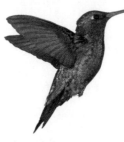

FROM THE EDITORS OF BOTTOM LINE HEALTH

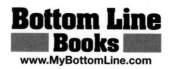

Bottom Line
Books
www.MyBottomLine.com

CONTENTS

Contents

Contents

Contents

11 • UNDOING PAIN AND AUTOIMMUNE DISEASE

12 • ALLEVIATE DEPRESSION AND EMOTIONAL UPSET

APPENDICES

APPENDIX 1

FOOD AND FITNESS FOR ULTIMATE HEALTH

APPENDIX 2

MEDICAL MISCONCEPTIONS THAT HARM YOUR HEALTH

APPENDIX 3

OPTIMUM AGING

PREFACE

We are proud to bring to you *The Ultimate Women's Guide to Beating Disease and Living a Happy, Active Life 2016*. This essential volume features trustworthy and actionable life-saving information from the best health experts in the world—information that will help women beat the conditions that are most deadly to them.* In the following chapters you'll find the latest discoveries, best treatments and scientifically proven remedies to keep you living a long, happy and active life.

Whether it's heart care, the latest on stroke, breast cancer prevention and treatment, breakthrough fibroid treatments or cutting-edge nutritional advice, the editors of *Bottom Line Health* talk to the experts—from top women's health doctors to research scientists to leading alternative care practitioners—who are creating the true innovations in health care.

In this 2016 Edition, we've gone beyond diseases and have included two chapters and an appendix of life-enhancing health information on pain, depression, fitness, diet, medical misconceptions and aging...all of which are essential to living a happy, active life. And it's all backed by breaking studies and top health experts.

Over the past four decades, we have built a network of literally thousands of leading physicians in both alternative and conventional medicine. They are affiliated with the premier medical and research institutions throughout the world. We read the important medical journals and follow the latest research that is reported at medical conferences. And we regularly talk to our advisors in major teaching hospitals, private practices and government health agencies for their insider perspective.

The Ultimate Women's Guide to Beating Disease and Living a Happy, Active Life 2016 is a result of our ongoing research and connection with these experts, and is a distillation of their latest findings and advice. We trust that you will glean new, helpful and affordable information about the health topics that concern you most...and find vital topics of interest to family and friends as well.

As a reader of a Bottom Line book, please be assured that you are receiving well-researched information from a trusted source. But, please use prudence in health matters. Always speak to your physician before taking vitamins, supplements or over-the-counter medication...stopping a medication...changing your diet...or beginning an exercise program. If you experience side effects from any regimen, contact your doctor immediately.

Be well,
The Editors, *Bottom Line Health*
Stamford, Connecticut

*"Leading Causes of Death in Females," Centers for Disease Control and Prevention (*http://www.cdc.gov/women lcod/2010/index.htm*).

Chapter 1

HEART HELP FOR WOMEN

Early Onset Hot Flashes May Point to Raised Heart Disease Risk

Women who start having hot flashes at a younger age may be at increased risk for heart disease, according to two studies conducted by the same team of researchers.

One of the studies also found that women who have more frequent hot flashes during a typical day may be at raised risk for cardiovascular conditions.

Led by Rebecca Thurston, PhD, of the University of Pittsburgh, the studies found that women who begin experiencing hot flashes earlier in life appear to have poorer function of the lining of the blood vessels than those who have hot flashes at a later age, or not at all.

Impaired function in the blood vessel's walls—called reduced endothelial function —is the earliest sign of heart disease, the researchers noted.

Study #1

In one study, 189 women either in or just out of menopause wore a special monitor for 24 hours to track the frequency of their hot flashes. Their blood vessel health was checked via ultrasound tests to arteries in the forearm.

The study found that more hot flashes in that 24-hour period were linked to worse blood flow in younger women—those aged 52 or younger.

The number of hot flashes per day also seemed key. Women who experienced 10 or more episodes per day had a 50% reduction in how well their vessels expanded during normal blood flow, compared to women without any hot flashes, the researchers said.

Study #2

The second study drew on questionnaires given to 104 older women in the postmenopausal stage who already had signs of heart disease. It found that women who said they experienced their first hot flash when young (age 42 or below) had significantly worse blood vessel health than those whose hot

Rebecca Thurston, PhD, associate professor of psychiatry, epidemiology, psychology and clinical and translational science, University of Pittsburgh.

Suzanne Steinbaum, MD, director, women and heart disease, Lenox Hill Hospital, New York City.

Vijayapraveena Paruchuri, MD, director, Center for Adult Congenital Heart Disease, Winthrop-University Hospital, Mineola, New York.

American College of Cardiology, news release.

flashes started later in life. The finding held even after the researchers accounted for age, hormone use and history of heart disease, the team said.

The studies were presented at the annual meeting of the American College of Cardiology in San Diego.

Implication

"Hot flashes occur at a time in a woman's life when her risk for heart disease increases," said Dr. Thurston, who is an associate professor of psychiatry, psychology and epidemiology at the university. The new findings suggest that earlier onset of hot flashes may help doctors spot women who are at greater risk for heart disease, she said.

According to the researchers, more than 70% of women have hot flashes and night sweats at some point during menopause.

Expert Commentary

Women with early onset hot flashes may be "a group for whom early prevention and aggressive preventive strategies should be implemented," said Suzanne Steinbaum, MD, director of women and heart disease at Lenox Hill Hospital in New York City.

"As we learn more about these unique risk factors for women, it is imperative that we target a prevention strategy, as we know that the outcomes for heart disease in women are worse," she said.

Vijayapraveena Paruchuri, MD, directs the Center for Adult Congenital Heart Disease at Winthrop-University Hospital in Mineola, New York. She believes the new study "builds on recent findings that the hormonal profile and changes unique to women are important considerations that physicians need to be aware of."

More Research Needed

Further research is needed to pinpoint the precise age at which hot flashes seem to be most strongly linked with poor endothelial function, to determine if the severity of hot flashes plays a role, and to identify any

shared mechanisms between hot flashes and endothelial function, the research team said.

The U.S. National Institute on Aging website has more about hot flashes and other menopausal symptoms at *nia.nih.gov.* Search "Menopause."

---

6 Secrets to Holistic Heart Care

Joel K. Kahn, MD, clinical professor of medicine at Wayne State University School of Medicine in Detroit and director of Cardiac Wellness at Michigan Healthcare Professionals. He is a founding member of the International Society of Integrative, Metabolic and Functional Cardiovascular Medicine and the author of *The Whole Heart Solution. DrJoelKahn.com*

You don't smoke, your cholesterol levels look good and your blood pressure is under control.

This means that you're off the hook when it comes to having a heart attack or developing heart disease, right? Maybe not.

Surprising statistic: About 20% of people with heart disease do not have any of the classic risk factors, such as those described above.

The missing link: While most conventional medical doctors prescribe medications and other treatments to help patients control the "big" risk factors for heart disease, holistic cardiologists also suggest small lifestyle changes that over time make a significant difference in heart disease risk.* *My secrets for preventing heart disease…*

Secret #1: Stand up! You may not think of standing as a form of exercise. However, it's more effective than most people realize.

Think about what you're doing when you're not standing. Unless you're asleep, you're probably sitting. While sitting, your body's metabolism slows…your insulin becomes less effective…and you're likely to experience a gradual drop in HDL "good" cholesterol.

*To find a holistic cardiologist, go to the website of the American Board of Integrative Holistic Medicine, *ABIHM.org*, and search the database of certified integrative physicians.

A study that tracked the long-term health of more than 123,000 Americans found that those who sat for six hours or more a day had an overall death rate that was higher—a whopping 37% for women (18% higher for men)—than those who sat for less than three hours.

What's so great about standing? When you're on your feet, you move more. You pace…fidget…move your arms…and walk from room to room. This type of activity improves metabolism and can easily burn hundreds of extra calories a day. Standing also increases your insulin sensitivity to help prevent diabetes. So stand up and move around when talking on the phone, checking e-mail and watching television.

Secret #2: Count your breaths. Slow, deep breathing is an effective way to help prevent high blood pressure—one of the leading causes of heart disease. For people who already have high blood pressure, doing this technique a few times a day has been shown to lower blood pressure by five to 10 points within five minutes. And the pressure may stay lower for up to 24 hours.

During a breathing exercise, you want to slow your breathing down from the usual 12 to 16 breaths a minute that most people take to about three breaths. I use the "4-7-8 sequence" whenever I feel stressed.

What to do: Inhale through your nose for four seconds…hold the breath in for seven seconds…then exhale through the mouth for eight seconds.

Also helpful: A HeartMath software package, which you can load on your computer or smartphone, includes breathing exercises to help lower your heart rate and levels of stress hormones.

Cost: $129 and up, at *HeartMath.org*. You can also sign up for some free tools on this website.

Secret #3: Practice "loving kindness." This is an easy form of meditation that reduces stress, thus allowing you to keep your heart rate and blood pressure at healthy levels.

Research has shown that people who meditate regularly are 48% less likely to have a heart attack or stroke than those who don't meditate. "Loving kindness" meditation is particularly effective at promoting relaxation—it lowers levels of the stress hormones adrenaline and cortisol while raising levels of the healing hormone oxytocin.

What to do: Sit quietly, with your eyes closed. For a few minutes, focus on just your breathing. Then imagine one person in your life whom you find exceptionally easy to love. Imagine this person in front of you. Fill your heart with a warm, loving feeling…think about how you both want to be happy and avoid suffering…and imagine that a feeling of peace travels from your heart to that person's heart in the form of white light. Dwell on the image for a few minutes. This meditation will also help you practice small acts of kindness in your daily life—for example, giving a hand to someone who needs help crossing the street.

Secret #4: Don't neglect sex. Men who have sex at least two times a week have a 50% lower risk for a heart attack than those who abstain. Similar research hasn't been done on women, but it's likely that they get a comparable benefit.

Why does sex help keep your heart healthy? It probably has more to do with intimacy than with the physical activity itself. Couples who continue to have sex tend to be the ones with more intimacy in their marriages. Happy people who bond with others have fewer heart attacks—and recover more quickly if they've had one—than those without close relationships.

Secret #5: Be happy! People who are happy and who feel a sense of purpose and connection with others tend to have lower blood pressure and live longer than those who are isolated. Research shows that two keys to happiness are to help others be happy—for example, by being a volunteer—and to reach out to friends and neighbors. Actually, any shared activity, such as going to church or doing group hobbies, can increase survival among heart patients by about 50%.

Secret #6: Try Waon (pronounced Wa-own) therapy. With this Japanese form of "warmth therapy," you sit in an infrared (dry) sauna for 15 minutes then retreat to a resting area for half an hour, where you wrap yourself in towels and drink plenty of water. Studies show that vascular function improves after such therapy due to the extra release of nitric oxide, the master molecule in blood vessels that helps them relax.

Some health clubs offer Waon treatments, but the dry saunas at many gyms should offer similar benefits. I do not recommend steam rooms—moist heat places extra demands on the heart and can be dangerous for some people.

Step Out in the Sun

Avoiding the sun can be deadly. According to a recent finding, women who said that they did not sunbathe and avoided the sun in other ways were twice as likely to die over a 20-year period as women with the greatest sun exposure.

Possible reason: Sunlight is necessary for vitamin D production—and low vitamin D levels are associated with increased risk for death from cardiovascular disease and other causes.

Pelle G. Lindqvist, MD, PhD, associate professor of obstetrics and gynecology and director of education at Karolinska University Hospital, Stockholm, Sweden. He is lead author of a study published in *Journal of Internal Medicine*.

The Hidden Heart Disease Doctors Miss in Women

Holly S. Andersen, MD, attending cardiologist and director of Education and Outreach at the Ronald O. Perelman Heart Institute of New York-Presbyterian Hospital in New York City and medical adviser to the Women's Heart Alliance. She is an expert in the field of heart disease in women.

It's hard to imagine, with all the technology available today, that heart disease could be completely missed. But that's exactly what's frequently occurring with a tricky heart condition known as small vessel disease or coronary microvascular disease (MVD).

Here's what happens: Patients, most often women, have chest pain, other symptoms that suggest heart disease or even heart attacks. But when doctors examine their coronary arteries, they find no evidence of blockage and often rule out heart disease.

Result: Patients go without the vital treatment they need.

Mystery solved: The problem in these cases, researchers have recently discovered, often lies in the tiny blood vessels—which can't be seen with the naked eye or conventional heart disease testing—that branch off the larger coronary arteries in the heart.

Researchers still have much to learn about MVD, but here's what's known now and what you can do to protect yourself…

A Different Kind of Heart Disease

The most common variety of coronary heart disease (CHD) is caused by atherosclerotic plaques—cholesterol-containing deposits that pile up and narrow one or more of the large arteries that carry blood to the heart, restricting flow. When the heart gets too little blood to meet its needs—during exertion, for example—people with CHD have chest pain (angina). And if blood flow is restricted even further—usually due to a clot lodged in the narrowed artery—a heart attack and death may occur.

Plaque is often involved in MVD, too. But instead of accumulating in clumps that block off segments of specific coronary arteries, cholesterol is deposited more evenly inside whole areas of microscopic circulation. Additionally, in MVD the walls of the tiny arteries are injured or diseased—instead of opening wider to allow more blood to reach the heart during exercise or at times of emotional stress, they tighten up, constricting blood flow when it's needed most.

The reason for this is unclear, but it seems that at least some of the time, it's due to malfunction of the endothelial cells that line the blood vessels. The resulting symptoms can be indistinguishable from garden-variety CHD—and the risk for heart attack may be just as real.

Do You Have Microvascular Disease?

Diabetes and high blood pressure raise one's risk for MVD, as does CHD. High cholesterol, obesity, smoking and a lack of physical activity are risk factors, too, and like CHD, MVD becomes more common with advancing age.

Symptoms of MVD can be identical to the classic signs of CHD—pain, a squeezing sensation or pressure in the chest, usually during activity or emotional stress. The discomfort can also occur in the shoulders, arms, neck or jaw.

MVD tip-off: Painful episodes of MVD usually last longer—more than 10 minutes, and sometimes longer than 30 minutes—than those of classic CHD.

Other symptoms of MVD: Fatigue or lack of energy, trouble sleeping and shortness of breath. Women are particularly likely to have these vague manifestations rather than the kind of distinct chest pain that we usually associate with heart disease. Forty percent of women don't have chest pain even while having a heart attack, whether it's caused by CHD or MVD.

Another clue: With MVD, patients often notice symptoms during daily activities and/ or during times of mental stress rather than during times of physical exertion as is more often the case with CHD.

Getting a Diagnosis

The standard tests for heart disease may not uncover MVD. If you suspect you have the condition, be sure to see a cardiologist with significant experience in treating MVD. An academic medical center is the best place to find such a doctor. *He/she may be able to diagnose it from your symptoms, medical history and earlier test results, or he may order additional tests...*

•**Nuclear imaging,** which uses a radioactive compound injected into the bloodstream to reveal a detailed image of the heart and blood flow through the arteries, including microcirculation.

•**Magnetic resonance imaging (MRI)** to produce a picture of the heart and its circulation without subjecting the patient to dye or radiation.

•**Positron emission tomography (PET),** which provides information on metabolism in the heart. This can uncover certain areas that aren't getting enough fuel and oxygen, suggesting MVD.

If You Have MVD

If MVD is diagnosed, the goal is to keep it from progressing and to prevent heart attack and stroke. *Key strategies...*

•**Tweak your diet, and punch up your exercise routine.** A healthy eating plan, such as the Mediterranean diet, emphasizes fruits, vegetables, legumes, whole grains and nuts and fish, which contain healthy fats. Weight control and exercise reduce heart disease risk overall and also reduce blood pressure and help prevent diabetes, which are additional MVD risk factors. Beyond its general cardiovascular benefits, regular exercise appears to improve the function of the endothelial cells that line blood vessels and function poorly in MVD.

•**Get help from medication.** Doctors prescribe the same medications to treat MVD as for CHD—to reduce blood pressure and cholesterol. Aspirin or other drugs to reduce clotting risk are recommended as well.

Some evidence suggests that statins may be particularly useful because they not only reduce cholesterol but also improve endothelial function and relax the muscles around tiny blood vessels.

Similarly, calcium channel blockers, such as *amlodipine* (Norvasc), and ACE inhibitors, like *enalapril* (Vasotec), may be good choices for lowering blood pressure because they too help keep arteries open.

●**Get treated for anemia if you have it.** Anemia (low red blood cell count) may slow the growth of cells that help repair artery walls. This condition is treated with iron or B-12 supplements.

Note: If you have CHD and MVD (it's possible to have both) and have had angioplasty, a stent or bypass surgery, be aware that these procedures do not help MVD.

Do You Have a Heart Attack Gene? Finding Out Could Save Your Life!

Bradley F. Bale, MD, cofounder of the Heart Attack & Stroke Prevention Center, Nashville, and medical director of the Heart Health Program, Grace Clinic, Lubbock, Texas. He is coauthor, with Amy Doneen, ARNP, and Lisa Collier Cool, of *Beat the Heart Attack Gene: The Revolutionary Plan to Prevent Heart Disease, Stroke, and Diabetes.*

Even if you do everything right—you don't smoke, you're not overweight and you manage your cholesterol and blood pressure—your odds of having a heart attack might be higher than you think.

An eye-opening case: One of our patients, a 44-year-old executive whom we nicknamed "Superwoman," looked very healthy. Her Framingham Risk Score—a standard measure of heart disease risk predicted that she had only a 1% risk of having a heart attack over the next 10 years. That should have been good news—except that other tests we did, which most doctors do not routinely give, showed that her real risk was about 40 times higher.

The Tests You Need

Many of the tests that are used to detect heart disease are decades old. Some look for risk factors (such as arterial narrowing) that have less to do with the actual risk of having a

heart attack than most people think. Many of the tests that can make a difference still aren't used by most doctors.

Most cardiologists routinely recommend angiography, an imaging test that looks for large blockages in the coronary arteries. If a blockage of 70% or more is found, a patient might be advised to receive a stent or undergo a bypass, surgical procedures that don't always help and can have a high rate of complications.

Severely blocked arteries can be a problem, but a more common, and typically overlooked, threat is from small deposits inside artery walls. A patient might have dozens or even hundreds of deposits that are too small to be detected with angiography.

The risk: When these "hidden" deposits are exposed to inflammation—triggered by insulin resistance, smoking, a poor diet or stress, for example—they can rupture, tear the blood vessel lining and trigger a clot, the cause of most heart attacks.

New approaches: Doctors can now predict the risk for a heart attack with far more accuracy than in the past—if you know which tests to ask for. *Tests I recommend…*

●**Carotid intima-media thickness (CIMT).** This is an effective way to measure atherosclerosis inside an artery wall (between the intima and media layers). The FDA-approved test uses an ultrasound wand to look for the thickening of the carotid arteries that occurs when plaque between the two layers accumulates and pushes outward.

An isolated area of thickness measuring 1.3 mm or greater indicates plaque—and an increased risk for a heart attack or stroke.

Most patients who have excessive arterial thickening will be advised by their doctors to exercise more, eat a healthier diet and take a daily baby aspirin to reduce the risk for clots. A cholesterol-lowering statin drug also may be prescribed.

●**Genetic tests.** More than half of all Americans have one or more gene variations that increase the risk for a heart attack and a stroke. According to research published in *Circulation,* up to 70% of patients who are given the genetic tests described below will be reclassified as having a higher heart attack risk than their doctors originally thought. The cost of testing has dropped to about $100 per gene. Your insurance may cover the cost. *Important gene tests…*

•9P21. If you inherit two copies of this "heart attack gene" (one from each parent), your risk of developing heart disease or having a heart attack at an early age (in men, under age 45…in women, under age 55) is 102% higher than that of someone without the gene. And increased risk continues if you are already past these ages.

You'll also have a 74% increased risk for an abdominal aortic aneurysm, a dangerous weakening in the heart's largest blood vessel. If you test positive, your doctor will advise earlier and more frequent abdominal aortic ultrasounds. If you smoke, stop now. Most aortic aneurysms occur in smokers.

You should also exercise for at least 22 minutes daily (the amount found in research to be protective) and maintain healthy cholesterol and blood pressure levels.

Important: Patients with the 9P21 gene often are advised to have an ankle-brachial index test, which involves measuring blood pressure in the arms and ankles. It's used to diagnose peripheral artery disease (PAD), plaque build-ups in the legs that quadruple or even quintuple the risk for a heart attack or stroke.

•Apo E. This gene affects how your body metabolizes nutrients. There are different types of Apo E. The 3/3 genotype—64% of Americans have it—increases cardiovascular disease, but not as much as the 3/4 or 4/4 types. Those with 3/4 or 4/4 need to eat a very low-fat diet (with no more than 20% of calories from fat). Those with the 3/3 genotype are advised to eat a Mediterranean-style diet—focusing mainly on plant foods…fish… and olive oil.

•KIF6. Patients with the so-called arginine gene variant have up to a 55% increased risk for cardiovascular disease. There are no particular lifestyle changes known to be especially helpful for these patients. It's also useful to know if you're a noncarrier of

KIF6—as such, you won't receive significant risk reduction if you are prescribed either *atorvastatin* (Lipitor) or *pravastatin* (Pravachol), two of the most popular statin drugs. Instead, you'll need a different statin, such as *lovastatin* (Mevacor).

Another Crucial Test

An oral glucose tolerance test can detect insulin resistance years or even decades before it progresses to diabetes. But many doctors still use the simpler A1C test. It's more convenient—it doesn't require fasting—but it often fails to detect insulin resistance, one of the main causes of heart attacks and strokes. Insulin resistance leads to inflammation that can trigger plaques to rupture and form clots.

With an oral glucose tolerance test, your blood sugar is measured. Then you drink a sweet solution, and your blood sugar is measured again two hours later. A level of 100 mg/dL to 139 mg/dL could indicate insulin resistance. Higher levels may indicate prediabetes—or, if they're high enough, full-blown diabetes.

Next steps: Regular exercise is critical if you have insulin resistance or diabetes.

Also helpful: Weight loss, if needed, reduced intake of sugary beverages and foods, and a diet rich in fruits, vegetables and grains.

Artery Inflammation: Six Simple, Lifesaving Tests

Bradley Bale, MD, medical director, Grace Clinic Heart Health Program, Lubbock, Texas, and cofounder, Heart Attack & Stroke Prevention Center, Spokane. He is coauthor, with Amy Doneen, ARNP, and Lisa Collier Cool, of *Beat the Heart Attack Gene: The Revolutionary Plan to Prevent Heart Disease, Stroke and Diabetes.*

A fire could be smoldering inside your arteries…a type of fire that could erupt at any moment, triggering a heart attack or stroke. In fact, the fire could be building right this minute and you wouldn't even know it. That's because the usual things doctors look at when gauging cardiovascular risk—cholesterol, blood pressure, blood sugar, weight—can all appear to be fine even when your arteries are dangerously hot.

What does work to detect hot arteries? A set of six simple, inexpensive and readily available blood and urine tests.

Problem: Few doctors order these tests, and few patients know enough to ask for them. Without the warnings these tests provide, patients often have no way of knowing just how great their risk is for heart attack or stroke and whether or not their preventive treatments are working—until it's too late. *Here's how to protect yourself...*

The Body's Army on Attack

Hot arteries are not actually hot (as in very warm)—instead, in this case "hot" refers to the effects of chronic inflammation. Why call them hot, then? Chronic arterial inflammation can put you on the fast track to developing vascular disease by speeding up the aging of your arteries. It's so dangerous to the arterial lining that it's worse than having high LDL cholesterol. And if your arteries are already clogged with plaque—which acts as kindling for a heart attack or stroke—inflammation is what lights the match.

Inflammation in the body isn't always bad, of course. In fact, it's an important aspect of healing. When something in your body is under attack, the immune system sends in troops of white blood cells to repair and fight off the attacker, and temporary inflammation results. That's why when you cut yourself, for example, you'll see swelling at the site of the injury—it's a sign that your white blood cells are at work for your benefit.

But: When an attack against your body persists (for instance, as occurs when you have an ongoing infection of the gums), your white blood cells continue to drive inflammation. When it turns chronic, inflammation becomes highly damaging to many tissues, including the arteries.

Normally, the endothelium (lining of the arteries) serves as a protective barrier between blood and the deeper layers of the arterial wall. However, when that lining is inflamed, it can't function well and it gets sticky, almost like flypaper, trapping white blood cells on their way through the body. The inflamed endothelium becomes leaky, too, allowing LDL "bad" cholesterol to penetrate into the wall of the artery. The white blood cells then gobble up the cholesterol, forming fatty streaks that ultimately turn into plaque, a condition called atherosclerosis. Then when the plaque itself becomes inflamed, it can rupture, tearing through the endothelium into the channel of the artery where blood flows. This material triggers the formation of a blood clot—a clot that could end up blocking blood flow to the heart or brain.

The 6-Part Fire Panel

Just as firefighters have ways of determining whether a blaze is hiding within the walls of a building, certain tests can reveal whether inflammation is lurking within the walls of your arteries. I use a set of six tests that I call the "fire panel." Each reveals different risk factors and, for several of the tests, too-high scores can have more than one cause—so it's important to get all six tests, not just one or two.

The fire panel can identify people at risk for developing atherosclerosis...reveal whether patients who already have atherosclerosis have dangerously hot arteries that could lead to a heart attack or stroke...and evaluate patients who have survived a heart attack or stroke to see whether their current treatments are working to reduce the inflammation that threatens their lives. Your individual test results will help determine your most appropriate course of treatment.

I recommend that all adults have this panel of tests done at least every 12 months—or every three to six months for patients at high risk for heart attack or stroke. All of these tests are readily available...are inexpensive and usually covered by insurance...and can be ordered by your regular doctor. *Here are the six tests...*

•**F2 Isoprostanes.** My nickname for this blood test is the "lifestyle lie detector" because it reveals whether or not patients are practicing heart-healthy habits. The test, which measures a biomarker of oxidative stress, helps determine how fast your body's cells are oxidizing, or breaking down. According to one study, people who have the highest levels of F2 isoprostanes are nine times more likely to have blockages in their coronary arteries than people with the lowest levels.

The score you want: A normal score is less than 0.86 ng/L...an optimal score is less than 0.25 ng/L.

•**Fibrinogen.** An abnormally high level of this sticky, fibrous protein in your blood can contribute to the formation of clots...it's also a marker of inflammation. One study divided people into four groups (quartiles) based on their fibrinogen levels and found that stroke risk rose by nearly 50% for each quartile. High fibrinogen is particularly dangerous for people who also have high blood pressure because both conditions damage the blood vessel lining and make it easier for plaque to burrow inside.

Normal range: 440 mg/dL or lower.

•**High-Sensitivity C-Reactive Protein (hs-CRP).** Your liver produces C-reactive protein, and the amount of it in your blood rises when there is inflammation in your body—so an elevated hs-CRP level generally is considered a precursor to cardiovascular disease. The large-scale Harvard Women's Health Study cited this test as being more accurate than cholesterol in predicting risk for cardiovascular disease...while another study of women found that those with high scores were up to four times more likely to have a heart attack or stroke than women with lower scores. A high hs-CRP score is especially worrisome for a person with a large waist. Excess belly fat often is a sign of insulin resistance (in which cells don't readily accept insulin), a condition that further magnifies heart attack and stroke risk.

The score you're aiming for: Under 1.0 mg/L is normal...0.5 mg/L is optimal.

•**Microalbumin/Creatinine Urine Ratio (MACR).** This test looks for albumin in the urine. Albumin is a large protein molecule that circulates in the blood and shouldn't spill from capillaries in the kidneys into the urine, so its presence suggests dysfunction of the endothelium. Though this test provides valuable information about arterial wall health, doctors rarely use it for this purpose.

Important: New evidence shows that MACR levels that have traditionally been considered "normal" can signal increased risk for cardiovascular events.

Optimal ratios, according to the latest research: 7.5 or lower for women and 4.0 or lower for men.

•**Lipoprotein-Associated Phospholipase A-2 (Lp-PLA2).** This enzyme in the blood is attached to LDL cholesterol and rises when artery walls become inflamed. Recent research suggests that it plays a key role in the atherosclerosis disease process, contributing to the formation of plaque as well as to the plaque's vulnerability to rupture, Dr. Bale said. People with periodontal (gum) disease are especially likely to have elevated Lp-PLA2 scores—chronic inflammation can start in unhealthy gums and, from there, spread to the arteries.

Normal range: Less than 200 ng/mL.

•**Myeloperoxidase (MPO).** This immune system enzyme normally is found at elevated levels only at the site of an infection. When it is elevated in the bloodstream, it must be assumed that it's due to significant inflammation in the artery walls and leaking through the endothelium. This is a very bad sign. "MPO produces numerous oxidants that make all cholesterol compounds, including HDL 'good' cholesterol, more inflammatory. If your blood levels of MPO are high, HDL goes rogue and joins the gang of inflammatory thugs. It also interacts with another substance in the bloodstream to produce an acid that can eat holes in blood vessel walls. Smokers are particularly prone to high MPO levels.

Normal range: Less than 420 pmol/L.

9

How to Put Out the Fires

While the "fire panel" tests above may seem exotic, the solution to the hot artery problem, for most of us, is not. That's because the best way to combat chronic inflammation is simply to maintain a healthful lifestyle. You just have to do it! *Key factors include…*

●**Following a heart-healthy Mediterranean-style diet.**

●**Managing stress.**

●**Getting plenty of exercise.**

●**Guarding against insulin resistance.**

●**Taking good care of your teeth and gums.**

●**Not smoking.**

In some cases, lifestyle changes alone are enough to quell the flames of chronic inflammation and to put your arteries on the road to recovery. In other cases, patients also need medication such as statins and/or dietary supplements such as niacin and fish oil. Either way, the good news is that once you shut the inflammation off, the body has a chance to heal whatever disease and damage has occurred—so you're no longer on the fast track to a heart attack or stroke.

Niacin and Statins Don't Mix

Niacin has few benefits for people taking statins and significant risks. Niacin is prescribed with statins to lower LDL (bad cholesterol) and triglycerides and to raise HDL (good cholesterol). But statins by themselves are just as good at preventing heart attack and stroke. Niacin increases patients' risk for gastrointestinal, musculoskeletal, infectious, bleeding-related and diabetes-related side effects—and even death, according to a new study of more than 25,000 people.

Robert H. Eckel, MD, is professor of medicine…professor of physiology and biophysics…and Charles A. Boettcher II Chair in Atherosclerosis at University of Colorado Anschutz Medical Campus, Aurora. He also is past president of the American Heart Association.

Ask Your Doctor About This Drug

Combination drug prevents heart attack and stroke better than a statin alone, says Robert M. Califf, MD. Vytorin, which contains the statin simvastatin plus ezetimibe, a drug that prevents the body from absorbing cholesterol, brought down levels of LDL (bad) cholesterol more than simvastatin did on its own. Vytorin had no more side effects than taking a statin alone. Patients who took Vytorin had 6.4% reduced risk for cardiac events. Vytorin should be considered when a statin alone leaves the patient with LDL greater than 70 mg/dL or when the patient cannot take a full dose of a statin because of a side effect.

Robert M. Califf, MD, vice-chancellor for clinical and translational research and director of the Duke Translational Medicine Institute, Durham, North Carolina. He led a study presented at a recent meeting of the American Heart Association.

Painful Hand Osteoarthritis Could Mean Heart Disease

Study titled "Hand osteoarthritis in relation to mortality and incidence of cardiovascular disease: data from the Framingham Heart Study," by researchers from section of preventive medicine and epidemiology, Boston University School of Medicine, and department of rheumatology, Diakonhjemmet Hospital, Oslo, Norway, published in *Annals of the Rheumatic Diseases*.

You may feel little, if any, pain, stiffness or weakness if you have osteoarthritis. In fact, you may not even know you have it at all. But when pain does set in—if you wince every time you grab a bag of groceries or turn a key…or if you simply have gnawing achiness or stiffness in your hands—your osteoarthritis is more alarming. It might be a sign that you're at risk for a life-

Do This Before Starting a Statin

Before starting a statin, have a coronary artery calcium (CAC) test, advises Khurram Nasir, MD, MPH. The CAC test more accurately predicts cardiovascular risk than factors such as cholesterol, blood pressure, current smoking and diabetes. In 35% of people considered high risk according to those factors, a CAC test showed that risk was relatively low and could be managed by lifestyle modifications instead of medication. The test is widely available…takes about three minutes…and costs $75 to $100, which may be covered by insurance.

Khurram Nasir, MD, MPH, is a cardiovascular disease specialist and director of wellness and prevention research at Baptist Health South Florida, Miami Beach. He is senior author of a study published in *European Heart Journal*.

threatening disease that has nothing to do with your bones—heart disease.

Studies have already shown that rheumatoid arthritis is associated with atherosclerosis (hardening of arteries). Now, researchers from Norway and Boston University School of Medicine have shown a heart disease link with osteoarthritis, too.

To better rule out whether heart disease in patients with osteoarthritis was simply linked to being immobile too much of the time—as happens with people who have osteoarthritis of the spine, hip and knee—the researchers focused only on hand osteoarthritis. Specifically, they wanted to see if there was a link between osteoarthritis of the hands and coronary heart disease, congestive heart failure and a type of stroke called atherothrombotic brain infarction.

"Coronary heart disease" describes heart attack as well as a painful condition called coronary insufficiency syndrome, in which blood flow to the heart's arteries is decreased because of narrowing of the arteries caused by plaque buildup. Congestive heart failure,

also caused by narrowing of the arteries, is a condition in which the heart can't pump adequately to supply the body with enough oxygenated blood.

For a study population, the researchers went to the renowned Framingham Heart Study database. The researchers were looking to identify people whose MRIs proved that they had osteoarthritis of the hands—some with symptoms, some without—and compare them against each other and people who did not have osteoarthritis. In all, the researchers studied 1,348 people who were between the ages of 50 to 75. Of these, 540 had symptom-free hand osteoarthritis and 186 had symptoms. The rest were osteoarthritis-free.

The Hand-Heart Link

Researchers found no association between hand osteoarthritis and congestive heart failure, atherothrombotic stroke or a higher risk of death due to heart disease. They did, however, find an association between coronary heart disease and hand osteoarthritis. In fact, if you have symptomatic hand osteoarthritis, you are more than twice as likely to have a heart attack and coronary insufficiency as someone who does not have it. Even the people with symptomless hand osteoarthritis had an increased risk, although the increase was so slight that it couldn't scientifically be considered strong evidence. Researchers believe that the connection between arthritis and heart disease is likely rooted in inflammation (a factor in both conditions). Note that the researchers did account for other risk factors, such as smoking, age, gender and weight, to make sure that their findings were not linked to these instead of osteoarthritis.

What this means for you. Hand osteoarthritis is mainly caused by normal wear and tear, so the older you get, the more likely that you have it. Sixty percent of Americans over the age of 60 have hand osteoarthritis. Of these, 8% have symptoms (pain and stiffness). Eight percent might not seem like much, but it amounts to about three million people. Although pain and stiffness may be an indication that the osteoarthritis is at a

Watch Out for These Heart Disease Risks...

●**Angry outbursts increase risk for heart attack fivefold**—and risk for stroke fourfold. The higher risk disappears in about two hours but is significant. Risk is highest among people who often get angry and have existing risk factors, such as prior heart problems.

Probable reason: Anger causes a stress response in the body that raises heart rate and blood pressure.

Analysis of case studies conducted between 1966 and 2013 led by researchers at Harvard Medical School and Beth Israel Deaconess Medical Center, both in Boston, published online in *European Heart Journal.*

●**A woman's past can affect heart health.** Women who suffered childhood sexual abuse (not just physical abuse) are more likely to develop atherosclerosis. Doctors should consider it when assessing cardiovascular risks.

Stroke.

●**Marriage can hurt your heart.** Longtime married couples who have mixed feelings toward each other had the highest rate of coronary artery calcification (a predictor of coronary artery disease), according to a new study of 136 couples married for an average of 36 years.

Reason: Constant ambivalent feelings create stress, which can raise blood pressure.

Bert Uchino, PhD, professor of psychology, The University of Utah, Salt Lake City.

●**Stay away from exhaust.** Women who lived within 164 feet of a major roadway were 38% more likely to suffer sudden cardiac death than those who lived farther away, according to a new study.

Possible reason: Increased air pollution.

Circulation.

more severe stage, how and why are not yet completely known.

As for how to know if you have hand osteoarthritis if the condition is pain-free, there are signs to watch out for. For one, you may not be able to move the hand as agilely as you once did. Also, you may notice swelling and bony knobs or bumps near the affected joints.

Physical exercise, such as tai chi and yoga, can help keep a lid on osteoarthritis, and while various treatments can help manage the pain, you may want to monitor your heart health more closely, given the findings of this study. A visit to a cardiologist to find out if you have signs of heart disease may be worth your while.

Nighttime Heart Risk for People with Diabetes

According to a recent finding, hypoglycemia (low blood sugar levels) at night can cause life-threatening changes in heart rate in people with type 2 diabetes. Risk for slow heart rate was eight times higher when blood sugar levels dropped at night. Low blood sugar also increased risk for arrhythmias and other heart-rate abnormalities.

Self-defense for people with diabetes: Check with your doctor to ensure that your glycemic goals are personalized for you. Consider using a glucose monitor that will alert you when blood sugar levels are low, especially if you also have or are at risk for heart disease.

Study of people with type 2 diabetes who had been on insulin for at least four years by researchers at University of Sheffield, England, published in *Diabetes.*

Red Wine or White Wine: Does It Matter to Your Heart?

Study titled "In Vino Veritas," presented at the annual meeting of the European Society of Cardiology in Barcelona, Spain.

One of the most satisfying and simplest pleasures in life is enjoying a great glass of wine in the evening. And we've been told that having a glass of red wine with meals is one of the best things for heart, health and longevity. It's touted as one of the magic ingredients in the Mediterranean diet. Or is it? Researchers are now re-exploring the role of wine in heart health—and whether red wine is all that it is cracked up to be. You may have more options.

In Wine, There Is Truth

A recent Czech study, dubbed the In Vino Veritas ("in wine, there is truth") study, sought to discover the truth about the role of red wine and cardiovascular health. The study is the first long-term trial to compare the effects of red and white wine on HDL ("good") cholesterol and LDL ("bad") cholesterol.

The researchers had 146 men and women who were at risk for heart disease drink red or white wine for one year. The wines were grown on the same vineyard and were from the same vintage, and their components were compared, with the red wine (a pinot noir) containing much higher flavonol and polyphenol content and antioxidant potential than the white wine (a chardonnay-pinot). How much wine the participants were to drink was decided by the World Health Organization's definition of moderate alcohol consumption—seven ounces per day for women and 10 ounces for men up to five times per week. The study participants were not asked to make any changes to their usual diets. (Czech food is traditionally very much unlike the Mediterranean diet, by the way…heavy on

meat, potatoes, dumplings, rich sauces and sweets.) However, the dietary and exercise habits, weight, cholesterol and blood sugar levels and liver enzymes of the participants were monitored, as was how well they kept to their wine-drinking regimens.

The results: The researchers found that subjects' LDL cholesterol levels were lower at the end of the study compared to their base levels at the beginning—whether they drank red or white wine. Great! It's what everyone's doctor likes to see. However, although red wine has long been thought to increase HDL cholesterol levels, no significant change was seen, on average, in this study. No change was seen in triglyceride (blood fat), blood sugar levels or liver enzymes either after one year of daily wine drinking.

Bottom line on this study: Wine may not impact your good-cholesterol levels—but it can improve bad-cholesterol levels. And there's no need for you to merely tolerate a glass of red "for health reasons" if you really prefer white. A toast to your health!

Eat an Avocado to Lower Your Cholesterol

Adults who ate a small avocado every day for five weeks instead of a sugary dessert or beverage had significantly lower cholesterol than those who didn't eat one.

Explanation: Avocados contain mono-unsaturated fat, fiber, phytosterols and other nutrients believed to lower the amount of cholesterol in the blood.

Tip: Add avocado to salads, sandwiches or lean protein, such as chicken or fish dishes, and eat guacamole with fresh veggies—not high-sodium chips.

Penny Kris-Etherton, PhD, RD, distinguished professor of nutrition, The Pennsylvania State University, University Park.

The Right Way to Take Calcium to Protect Your Heart

Calcium supplements can be dangerous if not taken with magnesium. On its own, calcium causes contraction of heart cells—one study found that it doubles heart attack risk. Magnesium counters calcium's contracting effect and also stops calcium from forming plaque and causing atherosclerosis (hardening of the arteries). The ratio of calcium to magnesium should be 2:1 or lower—that is, 1,000 mg of calcium to 500 mg or more of magnesium. Use magnesium dimalate so that the supplement does not cause diarrhea. Jigsaw is a good slow-release formula available through *Amazon.com*.

Dennis Goodman, MD, board-certified cardiologist and director of integrative medicine, New York University School of Medicine, New York City. He is author of *Magnificent Magnesium: Your Essential Key to a Healthy Heart & More.*

Better Milk for Heart Health

When the nutritional content of 384 samples of organic and conventional whole milk from around the country was analyzed, the organic milk had 62% more healthful omega-3 fatty acids and 25% less harmful omega-6s than conventional milk.

Reason: Organic-fed dairy cows spend more time grazing on pasture grasses that contain omega-3s than do cows used to produce conventional milk. A balance of omega-3s and omega-6s is essential for heart health.

Note: Organic milk is more expensive than conventional brands.

Charles Benbrook, PhD, research professor, Center for Sustaining Agriculture and Natural Resources, Washington State University, Puyallup.

How Breast Cancer Patients Can Avoid Heart Disease

Study titled "Active breathing coordinator reduces radiation dose to the heart and preserves local control in patients with left breast cancer: Report of a prospective trial," from researchers in the department of radiation oncology at Thomas Jefferson University, Philadelphia, published in *Practical Radiation Oncology.*

For patients with cancer of the left breast, radiation therapy can be a cure that kills because it exposes a woman's healthy heart and lungs to unnecessary radiation—which increases a woman's risk of ischemic heart disease (blockage of heart vessels that ultimately result in heart attack). But good news! Researchers have found an ingenious solution that is remarkably simple. It's based on something you naturally do every day—breathe.

But this heart-saving technique is not just any kind of breathing.

The technique involves holding your breath. By filling your lungs and holding your breath during radiation therapy, your lungs, heart and other organs are pushed out of the way of the radiation beam.

Patients using this technique aren't expected to hold their breaths perfectly during radiotherapy. A machine called the Active Breathing Coordinator (ABC for short) helps them. The patient breathes through a mouthpiece connected to the ABC device, which monitors lung volume. When lung volume is just right and has pushed the heart and other organs out of the way of the radiation beam, the technician operating the machine closes a valve on its mouth piece to create a breath hold and instructs the patient to stay right there. The breath is held for about 20 seconds.

Also, instead of radiation being given all at once, it is given in pulses in lower doses than usual to also reduce the amount of radiation that might hit the heart, lungs or other organs. The pulses are coordinated with the breath holds.

Previous research has shown that this breathing technique does help protect the heart and lungs from radiation, but no one could say exactly how well it did so and especially whether lower doses of radiation were effective at efficiently beating the breast cancer until a research team from Thomas Jefferson University Department of Radiation Oncology in Philadelphia put it to the test.

They recruited 81 women with cancer of the left breast who had more than 5 cubic centimeters of their hearts located where a radiotherapy beam needed to be directed. Radiation was shot into breast tissue in pulses while patients held their breaths with the aid of the ABC machine. When measuring results, researchers accounted for age, tumor stage and conditions that contribute to heart disease such as high cholesterol and high blood pressure.

And the results were stellar. After an eight-year follow-up period in which patients received regular health checkups, the survival rate was 96%. Not only were the patients' hearts kept safer and healthier in the aftermath of breast cancer radiotherapy, but 88% of the patients got the same cancer-fighting benefit with the lower doses of pulsed radiation as they would have gotten with the regular dose.

Not everyone will feel comfortable with the machine or qualify for it. You have to be able to hold your breath for up to 20 seconds, and it's only for patients whose hearts are "in the line of fire" of a radiotherapy beam. But if you're receiving radiotherapy for cancer of the left breast, it makes sense to ask your doctor if ABC is right for you and can be included in your treatment.

Walking 2,000 Extra Steps a Day Lowers Heart Attack Risk by 10%

This is the equivalent of a 20-minute walk. Over the course of a six-year study, each time a person increased his/her activity by another 2,000 steps, his risk for heart attack went down by another 8%.

Study of 9,306 adults from 40 countries for six years by researchers at University of Leicester, UK, published in *The Lancet*.

Irregular Heartbeat May Be Caused by Your Pain Reliever

Bruno H. Stricker, MB, PhD, professor of pharmaco-epidemiology, department of epidemiology, Erasmus Medical Center, Rotterdam, The Netherlands. His study was published in *BMJ Open*.

If you've ever filled a prescription for a nonsteroidal anti-inflammatory drug (NSAID), such as *meloxicam* (Mobic) or *celecoxib* (Celebrex), your pharmacist probably handed you a long printout listing all the side effects associated with the drug. And you may already be aware that long-term use of NSAIDs can put you at risk for gastric bleeding, heart attack, stroke and heart failure. But in the latest research, another danger becomes clear.

Prescription NSAIDs are also linked to atrial fibrillation, an electrocardio glitch that makes the heart beat fast or irregularly—and this dangerous side effect can emerge within mere days of starting an NSAID.

The latest study was of 8,423 older adults (people whose average age was about 69). None of the people participating had atrial fibrillation at the study's start, but, over the course of 13 years, it developed in 10% of them. Although previous research had shown a link between NSAID use and atrial fibrillation, this study showed that, after just 15 days of using a prescription NSAID, a person had a 76% higher risk of having atrial fibrillation than a person who had never ever used an NSAID.

Are You In Danger?

Of course, lots of different health conditions can cause atrial fibrillation, including existing cardiovascular disease, lung disease, hyperthyroidism and sleep apnea. Use of tobacco or alcohol as well as use of certain drugs, such as albuterol or theophylline, which are prescribed for asthma, bronchitis and chronic obstructive pulmonary disease, also can set off atrial fibrillation. So you can't necessarily blame the NSAIDs for the high rate of atrial fibrillation in this study—but the increase in risk suggested in this study was so great that it can't be ignored.

Atrial fibrillation is not always a sign of danger, according to the National Heart, Blood, and Drug Institute. An episode might be a brief and rare occurrence that is of little consequence to your well-being. But if episodes happen a few times within a week and then go away, it is likely that they will eventually happen again and increasingly more often. When atrial fibrillation becomes frequent, you need to take action...because you may be at risk for stroke or heart attack.

More alarming, atrial fibrillation can be silent—that is, you may not have any of the typical symptoms such as dizziness, fatigue and shortness of breath—but it can still increase your risk for heart disease and stroke. All the more reason to do what you can to avoid atrial fibrillation from happening at all.

To Protect Yourself

Scientists need to do more digging to find out whether NSAIDs can set off risky frequent episodes of atrial fibrillation. In the meantime, if you need a pain reliever, talk to your doctor about how certain pain drugs may affect heart health and voice your concerns about NSAID use. You might even seek out a pain specialist skilled in nondrug approaches to pain management. *Also, remember that there are some proven alternatives to NSAIDs for pain relief...*

• **Glucosamine sulfate is an alternative treatment for osteoarthritis pain.** Although glucosamine sulfate supplements are not anti-inflammatory or pain-relieving drugs per se, they can reduce inflammation and ease pain over time because they help the body repair damaged joints. In fact, many studies have shown that over time, glucosamine sulfate provides better relief of osteoarthritis symptoms than do NSAIDs.

• **Ginger,** which has anti-inflammatory properties similar to those of some NSAIDs, can relieve some muscle pain. What's more, unlike NSAIDs, ginger desensitizes peripheral nerves to pain and reduces the body's production of certain chemicals, called cytokines, which contribute to inflammation.

Puzzling Palpitations

Robert Stark, MD, internist and cardiologist, medical director of the Cardiovascular Prevention Program at Greenwich Hospital/Yale New Haven Health and a clinical faculty member at New York Medical College in Valhalla. *RobertStarkMD.com*

Chances are, you hardly ever notice the steady rhythm of your heart, even though it beats approximately 100,000 times a day. But there may be times when you can feel your heart beating. Perhaps it's racing, even though you haven't done anything strenuous. Or maybe you notice a fluttering sensation...an abrupt thump...or a flip-flop feeling.

Is this a sign that something is seriously wrong with your heart or just a harmless "glitch" in your normal heartbeat?

Listening to Your Heart

Most people think of heart palpitations as a racing or pounding sensation in the heart, but the term actually applies whenever you have any unpleasant awareness of your own heartbeat. Palpitations can be normal—when you exercise, for example, you'll feel your heart pounding.

Heart palpitations also can be caused by arrhythmias, heartbeat irregularities that may (or may not) be harmless. For example, if you're under a lot of stress, drink too much coffee or use a cold medicine with a stimulating ingredient (such as pseudoephedrine), you may experience arrhythmias.

When there may be a problem: If palpitations are repetitive or recurrent over the course of a day, this could be a sign of heart damage or disease. So could palpitations that last more than a few seconds or are accompanied by dizziness, shortness of breath or other symptoms. These palpitations should always be checked by a physician (in some cases, on an emergency basis). You might need tests—including blood work and an electrocardiogram (EKG or ECG)—to analyze the heartbeat and identify likely problems. *Unusual heart sensations—and what they could mean…*

• **Sensation. Skipped beats.**

What it could be: Premature atrial contractions (PACs), which occur in the heart's upper chambers, or atria…or premature ventricular contractions (PVCs), which affect the lower chambers, or ventricles. These are the most common types of palpitations—and usually the least serious.

With these palpitations, the heart simply beats earlier than it should. You might feel a "pause" in your heartbeat, followed by a strong "thump" as the heart compensates for the delayed beat.

Most individuals have occasional PVCs. PACs are also common. If you don't have a history of heart disease (including atherosclerosis), your doctor will probably tell you not to worry.

Exception: When PVCs are repetitive, with one following right after the other for seconds or minutes. This pattern increases the risk for a more serious arrhythmia called ventricular tachycardia.

Treatment options: For frequent premature heartbeats, you may need an antiarrhythmic medication. There are many such drugs, including *disopyramide* (Norpace), *propranolol* (Inderal) and *sotalol* (Betapace).

Helpful: Cutting back or avoiding alcohol, caffeine, smoking and emotional stress often can reduce the frequency of PVCs and PACs and may prevent the need for medication.

• **Sensation. Racing** (as with a very fast pulse) and/or fluttering.

What it could be: Atrial fibrillation. It's a serious arrhythmia that you may or may not feel—and it might occur with sudden sweating or chest pain that feels like a heart attack. It also can cause dizziness, weakness and/or shortness of breath. With atrial fibrillation, the heart's upper chambers beat too erratically to efficiently pump blood to the lower chambers.

Result: Blood pools in the atria and may form clots. Each year, about 8% of people with untreated atrial fibrillation have a stroke.

If you have racing and/or fluttering sensations in your heart, go to a hospital emergency department. If your heart turns out to be healthy, you might have had lone atrial fibrillation, a onetime event that's unlikely to be dangerous. But if you keep having these sensations, or they last a long time (or never go away), you're going to need treatment.

Treatment options: If you are experiencing atrial fibrillation, your doctor will try to convert the heartbeat back to a normal rhythm. This can sometimes be done with anti-arrhythmic drugs or with electrical cardioversion, in which an electrical shock is delivered to restore the heart's normal rhythm.

If this treatment doesn't work, you might be given a prescription for a beta-blocker, a calcium channel blocker or other drugs that prevent the heart from racing or fluttering, along with blood-thinning medications to prevent clots. You'll probably need to take the drugs for life. Another approach, known as radiofrequency ablation, uses electricity to permanently damage (ablate) the cells in the heart that are causing abnormal rhythms. This is usually done only when medications and other approaches haven't helped.

• **Sensation. A sudden burst of rapid beats** lasting seconds to hours.

What it could be: Ventricular tachycardia (V tach). Get to an emergency department! V tach usually occurs in people with a history of heart disease. The lower chambers of the heart can start beating faster than 170 times a minute. It can lead to ventricular fibrillation, a dangerous arrhythmia that causes the heart to quiver instead of pump. It's the main

AFib Danger

Widely prescribed heart drug is dangerous for patients with atrial fibrillation (abnormal heart rhythm). There is increasing evidence that those patients taking digoxin are at increased risk for death, compared with patients treated with beta-blockers and calcium channel blockers such as diltiazem and verapamil. About one-quarter of people with atrial fibrillation still are prescribed digoxin, partly because it has been used for so long. But do not stop taking it until you see your doctor.

Samy Claude Elayi, MD, associate professor of medicine at Gill Heart Institute of University of Kentucky, Lexington.

Probably not. A heart murmur is an extra sound made during a heartbeat, often caused by a heart valve that doesn't fully close. Most lifelong heart murmurs do not raise risk for heart disease or need treatment.

However, a heart murmur that begins in older age (over age 60) can indicate progressive changes in the heart such as narrowing of a valve due to calcium buildup. If your doctor hears a murmur that was not present before, you may want to have an ultrasound of the heart (echocardiogram) to evaluate your heart valves and function in order to better estimate your risk for heart disease.

Michael Miller, MD, professor of cardiovascular medicine, University of Maryland School of Medicine, Baltimore, and the author of *Heal Your Heart*.

cause of sudden cardiac arrest, which is usually fatal.

How can you distinguish a racing heart from V tach? You can't. You must be treated at a hospital emergency department, particularly if you're dizzy or have actually lost consciousness—both symptoms of insufficient blood flow.

Treatment options: People with V tach are often treated in an emergency department with antiarrhythmic medications. They might be given a strong electrical shock to restore the heart's normal rhythm.

Once the heart has stabilized, you might need long-term care to prevent future attacks.

Possibilities: An implantable cardioverter defibrillator (ICD), a surgically implanted device that analyzes the heartbeat and administers shocks to prevent ventricular fibrillation…or radiofrequency ablation, which, as mentioned above, purposely damages the parts of the heart that cause abnormal beats.

Heart Murmur Concern

If you have a heart murmur, are you at higher risk for heart disease?

Do You Have a Funny Pulse in Your Abdomen?

Christopher J. Abularrage, MD, assistant professor of surgery, division of vascular surgery and endovascular therapy, The Johns Hopkins Hospital, Baltimore. He has published several articles on aortic aneurysms in the *Journal of Vascular Surgery*, *Annals of Vascular Surgery* and other medical journals.

A pulsating sensation in the abdomen can be a sign of many health problems, such as a hernia or an enlarged spleen. However, the most serious cause is an abdominal aortic aneurysm.

This type of aneurysm is an enlargement of the abdominal aorta, the large blood vessel that extends from the heart to the legs. As the aneurysm enlarges, there is a greater risk for rupture, which is often fatal.

Aneurysms usually develop slowly over many years and often have no symptoms. Signs that an aneurysm may be starting to rupture include severe, sudden, persistent pain in the abdomen or back…dizziness… nausea…and a rapid heart rate. If you have any of these symptoms, get to a hospital emergency department. If your only symptom is a pulsating sensation in the abdomen, your doctor can screen for an aneurysm with an ultrasound (this procedure should be covered by insurance).

Depending on the size of the aneurysm and your overall health, the aneurysm may need to be repaired with traditional open surgery or with a minimally invasive procedure that uses a stent.

Turn On the Air

Car air-conditioning is better for your heart than driving with the windows open. Heart-rate variability—a measure of cardiovascular health—was 32% better in people who ran air-conditioning during a two-hour commute than in people who drove with open windows.

Possible reason: Air-conditioning filters exhaust particles and pollutants that cause internal inflammation and disrupt the heart's electrical signals.

Study of 60 people by researchers at Taipei Medical University, School of Medicine, Taiwan, published in *Science of the Total Environment.*

Cut Heart Disease Risk Without Losing Weight

If overweight people control blood pressure, cholesterol and blood sugar through lifestyle changes and medication, the increased heart disease risk associated with being overweight can be reduced by 50%...and stroke risk can be lowered by 75%. But overweight and obese people still have higher risks for heart disease than people of normal weight.

Study of 1.8 million people by researchers at Harvard School of Public Health, Boston, Imperial College London and University of Sydney, Australia, published in *The Lancet.*

6 Dangerous Myths About Your Blood Pressure

Mark C. Houston, MD, an associate clinical professor of medicine at Vanderbilt University School of Medicine in Nashville and director of the Hypertension Institute of Nashville at Saint Thomas Hospital. He is the author of *What Your Doctor May Not Tell You About Hypertension* and *What Your Doctor May Not Tell You About Heart Disease.*

About one of every three adults in the US has high blood pressure (hypertension). But only about half of these people have it under control. This unfortunate statistic is due, in part, to some common misconceptions about hypertension.

Six myths—and the facts...

Myth #1: In-office blood pressure tests are the gold standard. The automated devices in most doctors' offices are convenient, but they're not as precise as the manual (mercury) blood pressure kits. It's common for automated office blood pressure machines to give readings that are off by several points. The old-fashioned monitors tend to give more precise measurements, since doctors use a stethoscope to listen to the sound of blood flowing.

To get an accurate blood pressure reading, the patient should have rested in a seated position for at least five minutes, and his/her arm should be supported on a table or held by the person giving the test.

Important: Both types of monitors can give a skewed reading due to "white-coat hypertension," higher readings that result from anxious feelings during a doctor's visit.

Fact: You can get accurate blood pressure readings at home as long as you use an automatic, cuff-style monitor that properly fits over your upper arm (not over your wrist or finger) and follow the instructions. The device should be approved by the Association for the Advancement of Medical Instrumentation (AAMI). This ensures that the device has undergone extensive studies to validate its accuracy. To tell if a monitor has AAMI approval, check the label on the device's package.

Myth #2: It's fine to check your blood pressure now and then. Checking your blood pressure every few days or just once a week is fine for maintaining good blood pressure readings but not for achieving good control in the beginning.

New approach: 24-hour ambulatory blood pressure monitoring (ABPM). It's done routinely in the UK but is still a novelty in the US. That's likely to change because studies show that it's the most effective way to measure blood pressure.

With ABPM, patients wear a device (usually around the waist) that controls a blood pressure cuff that measures brachial pressure (inside the arm at the elbow crease). ABPM, which takes readings every 15 to 60 minutes over a 24-hour period, allows your doctor to choose medications and doses more precisely. The test costs $100 to $350, but it is usually covered by insurance with proper diagnostic coding (such as labile, or "episodic," hypertension or resistant hypertension).

My advice: Have the test once when diagnosed with hypertension, and repeat it once or twice a year to see how treatment is working.

Myth #3: It's OK to take blood pressure medication at your convenience. Blood pressure normally drops 10% to 20% during sleep. But about 25% of blood pressure patients (known as nondippers) don't experience this nighttime drop. Their blood pressure is always elevated, and they need to time their medications accordingly.

If a 24-hour test shows that you're a nondipper, your doctor will probably advise you to take medications at night. Taking medications at night—say, at about 9 pm—can reduce the risk for cardiovascular events (such as a heart attack) by 61% compared with taking them in the morning. Nighttime medica-

tions can also help lower the surge in blood pressure that occurs in the morning.

Myth #4: Sodium isn't a big deal for everyone. Much of what we hear or read about blood pressure these days includes references to "salt sensitivity." For people who are salt-sensitive, even small amounts of sodium can cause a rapid rise in blood pressure. But don't assume that you're safe just because your blood pressure doesn't seem to rise when you consume sodium.

Fact: Excessive salt causes vascular damage even in people without hypertension… and it increases the risk that you'll eventually develop high blood pressure.

The recommended daily limit for sodium is 1,500 mg for adults age 51 and over. People who are salt-sensitive should get even less. People who cut back on salt usually see a drop in systolic (top number) blood pressure of six to seven points and a drop in diastolic (bottom number) pressure of three to four points.

Also: Don't assume that sea salt is safe. It has only slightly less sodium chloride than table salt.

Myth #5: You need drugs to control blood pressure. If your blood pressure is 140/90 or higher, your doctor will probably prescribe one or more medications.

But certain nutritional supplements can help boost the effectiveness of those drugs. One study found that 62% of patients who used the DASH 2 diet, exercised, lost weight and took specific supplements for six months were able to reduce or stop their use of blood pressure medications.* *Supplements to discuss with your doctor…*

• **Coenzyme Q10 (CoQ10)** reduces blood pressure by an average of 15/10 points. About half of people who take it can eventually discontinue blood pressure medications.

Typical dose: 120 mg to 225 mg daily.

• **Taurine,** an amino acid, can lower blood pressure by 9/4.1 points.

*For more details on the DASH 2 diet, go to *hypertension institute.com* and search under "National Services."

Typical dose: 2 g to 3 g daily. Larger doses may be needed in some cases.

• **Lycopene is an antioxidant in tomatoes,** grapefruit and other fruits. It reduces blood pressure, blood fats and inflammatory markers such as C-reactive protein. Consider taking this supplement if you don't eat a lot of lycopene-rich foods.

Typical dose: 10 mg to 20 mg daily.

Myth #6: Food won't help your blood pressure. Foods rich in potassium can reduce blood pressure. Try to get at least two-and-a-half times more potassium than sodium in your diet—the ratio that blocks sodium's negative effects.

Good high-potassium foods: A medium-sized potato with skin has 926 mg of potassium, and a medium-sized banana has 422 mg.

Get a Grip to Lower Blood Pressure

People taking medication for high blood pressure lowered their systolic (top number) blood pressure by five points by squeezing a handgrip exerciser three times a week for eight weeks. Participants squeezed the exerciser a total of four times at each session. Researchers speculate that using a handgrip exerciser may produce small changes in pathways that affect the autonomic nervous system, which controls heart rate, blood pressure and blood vessel function.

Study by researchers at McMaster University, Hamilton, Ontario, published in *Scandanavian Journal of Medicine & Science in Sports*.

How Low to Go for Blood Pressure Control

Study titled "Pharmacotherapy for Hypertension in Older Adults: A Systematic Review" by department of pharmacy practice, Oregon State University College of Pharmacy, published in *Drugs & Aging*.

Many of you in your 60s or older who have been fit and health-conscious may be worried—or aggravated—about what your doctor is telling you about your blood pressure. It's up a little. In fact, it has been creeping upward to the point where now the doctor wants to put you on meds, even though research says that most people with mild high blood pressure don't need medication.

Or maybe you're already on a blood pressure–lowering drug because your pressure really was quite high—and it has stayed somewhat high even with medication. Your doctor is still scaring you with factoids about heart attack and stroke and wants to increase your medication dose.

Before you become a victim of your doctor's prescription pad, here's important news that puts a new light on blood pressure control in older people. The treatment, and the blood pressure goals, that make sense for people who are middle age and younger are not necessarily right for more mature folks.

In any case, your doctor is probably harping about upping your medication because he or she is simply following guidelines—professional standards issued by medical societies such as the American Heart Association. The problem is that guidelines are generally based on information from a broad population that mostly includes people in their prime. As people age, their blood pressure naturally tends to increase, and older bodies metabolize drugs differently than younger ones. Given these facts, it does not make sense to treat high blood pressure in older people based on information gathered from younger people. It might even be harmful.

A recent study showed that, if you are on an antihypertensive drug, you'll probably be just fine without upping your medication dosage or switching to a stronger drug as long as your treatment keeps your systolic blood pressure (the first number on your blood pressure readings) at about 150 mmHg (in the range of mild high blood pressure). So, take a deep breath, relax and read on.

More Meds Don't Equal More Benefit

To learn more about cardiovascular disease and medication-related risks in hypertensive people age 65 and older, a team of researchers from the Oregon State University College of Pharmacy analyzed a group of well-designed published studies on the topic. The studies compared different types of antihypertensive drugs against either each other or placebo and/or looked at the benefits and risks of using drugs to achieve different blood pressure targets as recommended by different sets of guidelines and/or evaluated the risks and benefits of antihypertensive drugs.

The results: Whereas antihypertensive drugs were more beneficial than no treatment for older people in terms of lowered incidence of heart attack and stroke, strict control of systolic blood pressure (getting it down to 140 mmHg or lower) was no better than mild control (getting it to 150 mmHg). As for diastolic blood pressure, most of the studies reviewed didn't emphasize or report the findings.

As for the risks and benefits of antihypertensive drugs, some studies showed no age-related side effects and some showed that, compared with younger people, older people were more likely to experience dizziness and weakness, possibly due to orthostatic hypotension (a condition in which blood pressure suddenly drops when you stand up), and bradycardia (slowed heart rate), which itself causes faintness, weakness, shortness of breath, chest pains and mental confusion.

What Does This Mean for You?

The study authors note that more research is needed to determine the best methods for managing high blood pressure in older people. So the take-home from this study is that, if you're a mature adult and need medication to control high blood pressure, discuss these recent findings with your physician and ask if your current treatment goals are the right ones for you.

Another View on Revised Guidelines

Samuel Mann, MD, hypertension specialist at NewYork-Presbyterian Hospital and author of *Hypertension and You*.

For decades, we've been told to keep our blood pressure below 140/90.

Now: New expert guidelines have plenty of doctors crying foul. According to these relaxed recommendations, people over age 60 don't need treatment until systolic (top number) blood pressure rises to 150 or higher (no change was recommended for diastolic pressure). For people under age 60, 140/90 still is the cutoff.

Why the change? The committee that created the guidelines concluded that there isn't enough evidence that the additional blood pressure–lowering prevents heart attacks and strokes. In the absence of benefit, the risk for side effects from medication is not justified. Samuel Mann, MD, disagrees. *He says…*

Most of the studies analyzed by the committee followed patients for only three to five years—not long enough to observe the benefits of lowering systolic pressure to 140 versus 150.

Blood pressure reduction also has other long-term benefits that would not be evident in a three-to-five-year study, such as lower risk for dementia, erectile dysfunction and other vascular-related conditions.

With the many excellent medications available today, we usually can get the systolic pressure under 140 without side effects.

Dr. Mann's takeaway: A target below 140/90 still is best for most adults.

One exception: Adults age 80 and older may do better with systolic pressure of up to 160.

Note: Particularly as we get older, the upper number (systolic) is considered more important. Why? The risk for cardiovascular events, such as heart attack and stroke, has been linked to a high systolic number. A big gap

Better Blood Pressure Monitoring

•**Take your own blood pressure.** Monitoring blood pressure at home instead of only in the doctor's office is more effective for diagnosing and treating hypertension.

Bonus: A new study found that patients using home blood pressure–monitoring kits saved insurance companies up to $1,364 over 10 years, which could translate into lower premiums. Home blood pressure monitoring is also helpful for those at risk for hypertension.

Alejandro Arrieta, PhD, assistant professor of health policy and management, Florida International University, Miami.

•**Report home blood pressure readings to your doctor.** If you take your blood pressure at home, be sure to report these readings to your doctor for a more accurate picture of your heart attack risk.

New finding: An analysis of 5,008 people followed over eight years found that those whose blood pressure readings were high at home but normal in a physician's office (a condition known as masked hypertension) had at least 1.5 times more risk for heart attack and death compared with those whose BP was normal in both settings.

Jan A. Staessen, MD, PhD, head of Hypertension and Cardiovascular Epidemiology, Catholic University of Leuven, Belgium.

•**Different blood pressure readings in each arm indicate cardiac risk.** A difference in pressure of more than 10 points in systolic pressure (the top number) indicates 38% higher risk for a cardiac event.

Study of 3,390 people without cardiovascular disease, age 40 or older, over an average of 13 years, by researchers at Massachusetts General Hospital, Boston, published in *The American Journal of Medicine.*

between the systolic and diastolic (bottom) numbers is also telling because it indicates increased arterial stiffness. For that reason, a blood pressure reading of 160/70 could indicate a problem, but 112/90 would not.

5 Foods That Fight High Blood Pressure

Janet Bond Brill, PhD, RD, nationally recognized nutrition, health and fitness expert who specializes in cardiovascular disease prevention. She has authored three books on the topic, including *Blood Pressure DOWN, Prevent a Second Heart Attack* and *Cholesterol DOWN. DrJanet.com*

Is your blood pressure on the high side? Your doctor might write a prescription when it creeps above 140/90—but you may be able to forgo medication. Lifestyle changes still are considered the best starting treatment for mild hypertension. These include not smoking, regular exercise and a healthy diet. *In addition to eating less salt, you want to include potent pressure-lowering foods, including…*

Raisins

Raisins are basically dehydrated grapes, but they provide a much more concentrated dose of nutrients and fiber. They are high in potassium, with 220 milligrams (mg) in a small box (1.5 ounces). Potassium helps counteract the blood pressure–raising effects of salt. The more potassium we consume, the more sodium our bodies excrete. Researchers also speculate that the fiber and antioxidants in raisins change the biochemistry of blood vessels, making them more pliable—important for healthy blood pressure. Opt for dark raisins over light-colored ones because dark raisins have more catechins, a powerful type of antioxidant that can increase blood flow.

Researchers at Louisville Metabolic and Atherosclerosis Research Center compared people who snacked on raisins with those who ate other packaged snacks. Those in the raisin group had drops in systolic pressure (the top number) ranging from 4.8 points (after four weeks) to 10.2 points (after 12 weeks). Blood pressure barely budged in the no-raisin group. Some people worry about the sugar in raisins, but it is natural sugar (not added sugar) and will not adversely affect your health (though people with diabetes need to be cautious with portion sizes).

My advice: Aim to consume a few ounces of raisins every day. Prunes are an alternative.

Beets

Beets, too, are high in potassium, with about 519 mg per cup. They're delicious, easy to cook (see the tasty recipe on page 25) and very effective for lowering blood pressure.

A study at The London Medical School found that people who drank about eight ounces of beet juice averaged a 10-point drop in blood pressure during the next 24 hours. The blood pressure–lowering effect was most pronounced at three to six hours past drinking but remained lower for the entire 24 hours. Eating whole beets might be even better because you will get extra fiber.

Along with fiber and potassium, beets also are high in nitrate. The nitrate is converted first to nitrite in the blood, then to nitric oxide. Nitric oxide is a gas that relaxes blood vessel walls and lowers blood pressure.

My advice: Eat beets several times a week. Look for beets that are dark red. They contain more protective phytochemicals than the gold or white beets. Cooked spinach and kale are alternatives.

Dairy

In research involving nearly 45,000 people, researchers found that those who consumed low-fat "fluid" dairy foods, such as yogurt and low-fat milk, were 16% less likely to develop high blood pressure. Higher-fat forms of dairy, such as cheese and ice cream, had no blood pressure benefits. The study was published in *Journal of Human Hypertension.*

In another study, published in *The New England Journal of Medicine*, researchers found that people who included low-fat or fat-free dairy in a diet high in fruits and vegetables had double the blood pressure–lowering benefits of those who just ate the fruits and veggies.

Low-fat dairy is high in calcium, another blood pressure–lowering mineral that should be included in your diet. When you don't have enough calcium in your diet, a "calcium leak" occurs in your kidneys. This means that the kidneys excrete more calcium in the urine, disturbing the balance of mineral metabolism involved in blood pressure regulation.

My advice: Aim for at least one serving of low-fat or nonfat milk or yogurt every day. If you don't care for cow's milk or can't drink it, switch to fortified soy milk. It has just as much calcium and protein and also contains phytoestrogens, compounds that are good for the heart.

Flaxseed

Flaxseed contains alpha-linolenic acid (ALA), an omega-3 fatty acid that helps prevent heart and vascular disease. Flaxseed also contains magnesium. A shortage of magnesium in our diet throws off the balance of sodium, potassium and calcium, which causes the blood vessels to constrict.

Flaxseed also is high in flavonoids, the same antioxidants that have boosted the popularity of dark chocolate, kale and red wine. Flavonoids are bioactive chemicals that reduce inflammation throughout the body, including in the arteries. Arterial inflammation is thought to be the "trigger" that leads to high blood pressure, blood clots and heart attacks.

In a large-scale observational study linking dietary magnesium intake with better heart health and longevity, nearly 59,000 healthy Japanese people were followed for 15 years. The scientists found that the people with the highest dietary intake of magnesium had a 50% reduced risk for death from heart disease (heart attack and stroke). According to the researchers, magnesium's heart-healthy benefit is linked to its ability to improve blood pressure, suppress irregular heartbeats and inhibit inflammation.

My advice: Add one or two tablespoons of ground flaxseed to breakfast cereals. You also can sprinkle flaxseed on yogurt or whip it into a breakfast smoothie. Or try chia seeds.

Walnuts

Yale researchers found that people who ate two ounces of walnuts a day had improved blood flow and drops in blood pressure (a 3.5-point drop in systolic blood pressure and a 2.8-point drop in diastolic blood pressure). The mechanisms through which walnuts elicit a blood pressure–lowering response are believed to involve their high content of monounsaturated fatty acids, omega-3 ALA, magnesium and fiber, and their low levels of sodium and saturated fatty acids. Bonus: Despite the reputation of nuts as a "fat snack," the people who ate them didn't gain weight.

The magnesium in walnuts is particularly important. It limits the amount of calcium that enters muscle cells inside artery walls. Ingesting the right amount of calcium (not too much and not too little) on a daily basis is essential for optimal blood pressure regulation. Magnesium regulates calcium's movement across the membranes of the smooth muscle cells, deep within the artery walls.

If your body doesn't have enough magnesium, too much calcium will enter the smooth muscle cells, which causes the arterial muscles to tighten, putting a squeeze on the arteries and raising blood pressure. Magnesium works like the popular calcium channel blockers, drugs that block entry of calcium into arterial walls, lowering blood pressure.

My advice: Eat two ounces of walnuts every day. Or choose other nuts such as almonds and pecans.

Dr. Janet's Roasted Red Beets with Lemon Vinaigrette

Beets are a delicious side dish when roasted, peeled and topped with a lemony vinaigrette and fresh parsley. This recipe is from my book *Prevent a Second Heart Attack*.

- 6 medium-sized beets, washed and trimmed of greens and roots
- 2 Tablespoons extra-virgin olive oil
- 2 teaspoons fresh lemon juice
- 1 garlic clove, peeled and minced
- 1 teaspoon Dijon mustard
- ¼ teaspoon kosher salt
- ¼ teaspoon freshly ground black pepper
- ¼ cup chopped fresh flat-leaf Italian parsley

Preheat the oven to 400°F. Spray a baking dish with nonstick cooking spray. Place the beets in the dish, and cover tightly with foil. Bake the beets for about one hour or until they are tender when pierced with a fork or thin knife. Remove from the oven, and allow to cool to the touch.

Meanwhile, in a small bowl, whisk together the olive oil, lemon juice, garlic, mustard, salt and pepper for the dressing. When the beets are cool enough to handle, peel and slice the beets, arranging the slices on a platter. Drizzle with vinaigrette, and garnish with parsley. Serves six.

Probiotics Help Reduce Blood Pressure

A recent Australian study found that people who regularly ate dairy products containing live probiotic bacteria had a modest but significant reduction in blood pressure. They lowered systolic (top) pressure by 3.56 millimeters of mercury and diastolic (bottom) pressure by 2.38 millimeters.

Best: Aim for one serving of yogurt with live probiotic cultures every day.

Janet Bond Brill, PhD, RD, LDN, nutrition, health and fitness expert in Valley Forge, Pennsylvania, and author of *Blood Pressure Down*.

Don't Let Them Drug You for Mild High Blood Pressure

Stephen A. Martin, MD, assistant professor, University of Massachusetts Medical School, Barre, Massachusetts. His article appeared in *The BMJ*.

Americans are in agreement. We're being overmedicated. Whatever the ailment, there's a supposed quick-cure pill to save the day. Although we are very fortunate to have access to certain lifesaving drugs, we must resist the pharmaceutical-industry onslaught with its risks and side effects!

Latest case in point: Blood pressure control. The latest research shows clearly that many physicians are way too quick to break out their prescription pads when simple lifestyle changes may do the trick to control high blood pressure without the risk of side effects. You might very well be taking unneeded blood pressure medication. *Here's how to know...*

One Size Doesn't Fit All

Of all the people the world over who have high blood pressure, more than 60% have a mild form of it. Although evidence doesn't show that treating mild high blood pressure with drugs changes the risk of a first heart attack or stroke (except for people with diabetes or chronic kidney disease), most patients with mild high blood pressure are treated with medication anyway. Some health organizations want to change the guidelines, but most are resisting. This got Stephen A. Martin, MD, an assistant professor from the University of Massachusetts Medical School, along with a team of American and Canadian doctors, to argue in a recent article in the medical journal *The BMJ* that things have got to change.

For one, they point out, guidelines to treat everyone with mild high blood pressure with drugs are not based on evidence but on "expert opinion." Evidence, on the other hand, tells us that deciding who should be treated with drugs is a little more complicated and should depend not on a number on a blood pressure monitor, but on age, sex and specific risk factors such as diabetes or kidney disease.

In other words, one size does not fit all—despite what the drug companies or even some lackadaisical doctors might want!

According to the American Heart Association, you have mild high blood pressure (also called hypertension) once your blood pressure hits 140/90. The first number represents systolic blood pressure—the maximum pressure when your heart muscle is contracting. The second number represents diastolic pressure—the lowest pressure when your heart is relaxed. Before we go further, here's a quick reference on blood pressure readings:

Desired range: Systolic 90–119/diastolic 60–79.

Prehypertension: Systolic 120-139/diastolic 80-89.

Mild hypertension: Systolic 140–159/diastolic 90–99.

Hypertension: Systolic 160 and higher/diastolic 100 and higher.

The definition of mild hypertension was decided back in 1977 (based on expert opinion, not clinical evidence). Doctors didn't prescribe drugs for it then, but now they virtually all do, so that 94% of people age 65 and older who have any type of hypertension are on a drug, according to Dr. Martin. But an analysis conducted by a team of researchers and published as a Cochrane Review showed that antihypertensive drugs do not reduce risk of heart attack or stroke any better than placebo in people with mild hypertension. The analysis from *The BMJ* also noted that studies that show the benefit of antihypertensive drugs in people with severe hypertension are deceptively used to justify use of these drugs in people with milder forms of it.

Why? Follow the money. The estimated cost of treating mild hypertension in the United States is $32.1 billion per year!

A Better Approach

Dr. Martin and his colleagues pointed out that medicating people with mild hypertension is often an incentive for them (and their doctors) not to make necessary lifestyle changes. Why bother when you can just take a pill? Rather than overdiagnosing hypertension and overprescribing antihypertensive drugs, Dr. Martin says, much more effort needs to be put into encouraging healthy lifestyle changes, while reserving drug treatment for people who really need it—those who are known to be truly at risk for heart disease, such as people with diabetes, chronic kidney disease, metabolic syndrome and blood pressure that is 160/100 or higher.

Besides that, Dr. Martin and his coauthors point out that blood pressure readings by doctors are often inaccurate. Doctors often do not consider, for example, whether a patient has just smoked a cigarette (taken nicotine) or plied him- or herself with caffeine, which can affect blood pressure readings. And then there's "white-coat syndrome," in which anxiety over being examined temporarily increases blood pressure exactly at a time when an accurate reading is needed—while at the doctor's office! Considering that 20% of people with any level of high blood pressure also have white-coat syndrome, there are almost certainly legions of people out there who have been misdiagnosed with mild hypertension and told to take drugs.

What You Can Do

To better ensure that you get an accurate blood pressure reading, do it yourself at home. Yes, home blood pressure monitoring is preferred, according to Dr. Martin, because it removes white-coat syndrome from the picture and also allows a person to take multiple readings instead of just one. Multiple readings give a better sense of what is really happening.

Blood pressure–monitoring devices are widely available. The AHA recommends cuff-style monitors that fit over the upper arm because they are more accurate than wrist and finger monitors. *The AHA gives this guidance for blood pressure monitoring…*

- **Take two.** Measure your blood pressure twice per day at the same times each day, such as morning and evening. And each time you measure it, take two or three readings one minute apart. (Some home monitors will automatically perform three readings in a row and average the results—all you have to do is sit patiently for a few minutes.)

- **Relax.** Don't drink caffeinated beverages or exercise (or smoke) within the 30 minutes before measuring your blood pressure.

- **Keep a log.** Accurately document the date and time of each of your blood pressure readings, and keep that log for presentation to your doctor. (Some monitors have built-in memory to store readings or apps to download the reading to a website for later access.)

If you are told by your doctor that you have mild hypertension and should go on medication, question why and whether lifestyle changes would be the better alternative.

Do Good…to Lower Blood Pressure

People who volunteered an average of four hours a week reduced their risk for hypertension by 40%, a new four-year study of adults over age 50 has found. Volunteers also reported being more satisfied with their lives and having greater self-esteem and fewer symptoms of depression than those who didn't volunteer.

Possible explanation: Volunteering helps improve ties to the community, which can reduce stress. So choose a volunteer commitment you enjoy!

Rodlescia Sneed, MPH, researcher, department of psychology, Carnegie Mellon University, Pittsburgh.

Replace Salt with Herbs and Spices for a Win-Win

Study titled "Effects of a behavioral intervention that emphasizes spices and herbs on adherence to recommended sodium intake," presented at the American Heart Association's Epidemiology and Prevention/Nutrition, Physical Activity and Metabolism 2014 Scientific Sessions meeting.

Do you know why so much processed food in America is so heavily salted? It's because when products are taste-tested, the tasters, who are regular folks like you, prefer salty versions over low-sodium versions without fail. But it's a catch-22. Our taste buds prefer the salty versions not because saltiness is such a thrilling flavor or because our bodies need that much salt (in fact, it hurts us)—but because we have simply grown too accustomed to salty flavors. Food companies love using lots of salt because it's a cheap ingredient and gives food a longer shelf life. And they've trained us to swallow it.

This is one reason why you can't trust "health" studies sponsored by food companies—because they often are poorly designed as studies and really are about marketing, not health. But there is a new study that deserves your attention. It was paid for by the giant spice company McCormick. The results of this study are eye-opening, and they do show a legitimate and healthful way that lots of us can stop eating so much salt.

The study basically pitted spices against salt and asked the question, If people simply used more spices (which are in fact good for you), would they find it easier to cut back on salt—and by exactly how much?

Preparing Your Taste Buds

The McCormick people know that Americans have been trained to think salty food is normal food, so the first thing they attempted to do was to get the 40 participants to overcome their learned taste for lots of salt. They were put on a salt-restricted diet for four weeks. In fact, they couldn't eat or drink anything except what the research team gave them to ensure that they were eating less than 1,500 mg of sodium per day, the maximum recommended by the American Heart Association for people over 50.

To give you an idea of just how dramatic the 1,500-mg limit per day must have seemed, consider that a single can of soup or one freezer-to-microwave prepared entrée can easily contain up to 1,200 mg of sodium.

To confirm what was happening in participants' bodies, researchers tested their urine for sodium levels. An analysis of urine samples collected before starting this phase of the study and again at the end of it showed that the average amount of sodium excreted in urine was slashed in half...from 150 millimoles per day (mmol/d) to 72 mmol/d.

Spicing It Up a Bit

In the next phase of the study, half of the participants were instructed to keep their salt intake low, as they had in the first part of the study, but to do it on their own. The remaining half participated in a behavior-intervention program based on cognitive behavioral science. They attended cooking demonstrations (using lots of spices, of course) and shared mind-broadening information with each other about spices used in their cultural and family recipes. They were encouraged to create and share adaptations of their traditional family recipes that replaced salt with spice. Sounds like a lot of fun, doesn't it? They also learned how to monitor their diets and to wisely choose and order foods when dining out and were encouraged to make a low-sodium diet an ongoing lifestyle choice.

After 20 weeks, the telltale level of sodium in urine for participants who had simply been asked to follow a low-sodium diet was nearly as high as it had been before they ever went on a low-sodium diet...around 150 mmol/d. These people just could not maintain a low-sodium diet out in the "real world" beyond the rigid confines of a highly controlled study.

In contrast, the level of sodium in the urine of the participants who learned how to swap salt for herbs and spices was about 27% lower, at around 110 mmol/d—not as low as the result from the rigid laboratory diet, but easily enough of an improvement for better health!

A Tip from This Study

Why not make a plan with friends and family to try this two-step program and see how it works for you? Go low-sodium for a month—just a mere month. It won't be that hard—in fact, it will be fun if you can swing a group project with this. Be diligent about reading food labels on packaged foods and beverages. Find out just how much salt is in your food with a quick at-a-glance chart from the University of North Carolina School of Medicine found at *www.med.unc.edu/gi/im/staff/clinic/nutrition-files-sodium-chart*.

As you go through your salt-restricted month (that is going to change your life for the better), keep a log of your daily sodium intake to get it consistently below 1,500 mg. Then, when the next month begins, so will the real fun. Plan get-togethers at least weekly with your allies in this going-low-sodium project to brainstorm and share new and delicious ways to prepare recipes with spices instead of salt. You might even find a Meetup group in your area that is doing just this—or start your own and become a dietary innovator in your own community!

Nutritional Benefits of Spices

Seasoning food with spices and herbs has extended benefits. Many spices contain antioxidants and other healthful compounds. For example, cinnamon has been shown to aid in glucose control, which can help protect you against diabetes. Ginger may reduce nausea and inflammation. Allspice has antioxidant, antibacterial and pain-relieving qualities, and black pepper has been shown, in animal experiments, to block fat production. Capsaicin, which comes from red peppers, may, like cinnamon, help regulate blood sugar, and turmeric has been found to be as safe and effective as nonsteroidal anti-inflammatory medicines (such as ibuprofen)

for treatment of arthritis of the knee. So spice it up, people. Eat well and learn how to really enjoy being salt-free.

Aspirin for Blood Clot Prevention

Aspirin for blood clot prevention may be an alternative to warfarin for deep vein thrombosis (DVT) patients. DVT often is treated with the anticoagulant drug warfarin.

But: Long-term use of warfarin to prevent clots may require frequent blood tests and dosage adjustments, and it may cause bleeding in some patients. Newer drugs such as *dabigatran* (Pradaxa) and *rivaroxaban* (Xarelto) are effective, but they can be expensive and some patients cannot tolerate them. An inexpensive daily aspirin reduces risk for clots by 42% without causing excessive bleeding.

Caution: Do not switch from warfarin to aspirin unless you speak to your doctor first.

Study of 1,224 people by researchers at University of Sydney, Australia, published in *Circulation*.

A Charley Horse...or a Deadly Blood Clot?

Daniella Kadian-Dodov, MD, assistant professor of medicine in the department of vascular medicine at the Zena and Michael A. Wiener Cardiovascular Institute and the Marie-Josée and Henry R. Kravis Center for Cardiovascular Health at the Icahn School of Medicine at Mount Sinai Hospital in New York City.

If you've ever been stopped cold by a charley horse, you know just how excruciating these muscle spasms can be. But are you sure it's just a muscle spasm? Or is that leg pain due to something far more serious?

What can cause leg pain...

Peripheral Arterial Disease (PAD)

This is one to worry about. Even though the pain usually isn't intense, it can triple your risk of dying from a heart attack or stroke.

What it feels like: About 10% of people with PAD suffer leg cramps, leg aching and leg fatigue that occur only during physical activity involving the legs (any type of activity can trigger it—even just walking). When you rest your legs, the discomfort goes away, usually in 10 minutes or less. As PAD becomes more severe and blood circulation worsens, pain can occur during rest and result in leg ulcers and even gangrene.

What to do: See a doctor. PAD is usually caused by atherosclerosis, the same condition that leads to most heart attacks. Your doctor will compare the blood pressure in your arms to the pressure at your ankles. If there's a significant difference, that could mean that you have PAD and you'll need an ultrasound of the legs to determine the extent and location of arterial obstructions.

Next steps: The same practices that protect your heart—such as not smoking, controlling diabetes, maintaining healthy blood pressure and getting plenty of exercise—will help stop PAD from worsening and could even reverse it.

Important: You must walk—even when it hurts. Walking ultimately reduces pain and improves circulation by stimulating the growth of blood vessels that bypass the damaged ones. With your doctor's OK, walk five times a week, for 30 to 45 minutes each time. I usually advise my patients to walk fast for two blocks or until they feel moderate pain, then rest a moment and walk fast for two blocks again, repeating until the end of their workout.

Deep Vein Thrombosis (DVT)

It doesn't always cause leg pain, but if pain occurs, this warning could save your life. DVT means that you have a blood clot—most often deep in a leg vein. It can be fatal.

What it feels like: You might notice a sudden, pulsating or aching pain deep in your calf or thigh, sometimes accompanied by redness and/or swelling. DVT usually occurs after you've been immobile for a long time—you're laid up in bed after surgery, for example, or following a long car or plane trip.

What to do: Get to an emergency department or a physician's office where you can get an immediate ultrasound. The clot could break free, travel to the lungs and cause pulmonary embolism, a clot in the lungs that's fatal in up to 30% of cases.

If you have a DVT, your doctor will probably give intravenous or injectable heparin, a blood-thinning drug that prevents the clot from growing. After a day or two, you'll be switched to oral blood-thinning medication, such as *warfarin* (Coumadin) or *dabigatran* (Pradaxa). You'll need to take the medication for about six months. If the clot is not entirely dissolved after treatment, it should be monitored with ultrasound—and if you have had one clot, you might get another one. Prevention is critical.

Everyone—whether you've had a DVT or not—should flex the ankle and calf muscles for about 30 seconds every 20 or 30 minutes when sitting for longer than four hours. Stand up and move around at least every hour or so.

If you have risk factors for blood clots—you're over age 40, obese, have a family history of blood clots or use hormone replacement therapy—ask your doctor about such precautions as taking aspirin before travel and/or wearing compression stockings while you're immobile.

Sciatica

This back condition is typically caused by a herniated spinal disk. The legs become involved because the disk exerts painful pressure on the sciatic nerve, which runs down the backs of the legs.

What it feels like: Intense, shooting and/or knifelike pains may extend through the buttocks and into one leg. Sciatica also can cause leg and/or ankle weakness.

What to do: See your doctor. If you do have sciatica, you may get better within eight weeks by doing physical therapy and using a nonsteroidal anti-inflammatory medication such as *ibuprofen* (Motrin)—90% of sciatica patients do.

Next steps: Consider surgery for a herniated disk/sciatica only when the pain is too intense to handle…you have responsibilities that don't permit extended downtime…or you're having additional symptoms such as muscle weakness or a loss of bowel/bladder control.

When It Really Is a Charley Horse

A muscle spasm, including the infamous "charley horse" of the leg, believed to have been named after a lame horse, can occur after hard exercise or for no obvious reason. It can cause sudden, localized pain (usually with sharp contractions) that often hits the calves.

If you're getting muscle spasms with any sort of regularity, see your doctor. Muscle spasms have a variety of causes—for example, you may have overworked your legs by doing yard work…you may be dehydrated (without enough water, muscle cells can spasm)…or a medication you're taking, such as a diuretic, may be the culprit.

Helpful: Because most muscle spasms are caused, in part, by tight hamstrings (the muscles in the backs of your upper legs), I recommend doing a standing hamstring stretch on a regular basis. Start in a standing position with your knees straight…bend at the waist…and reach for your toes or the floor until you feel a stretch in your hamstrings. Hold for a few seconds, and repeat a few times a day.

Tasty Treat Helps PAD

Dark chocolate may improve walking in people with peripheral artery disease. In a recent study, patients ages 60 to 78 with PAD who ate about 1.5 ounces of chocolate with at least 85% cocoa walked 11% farther and for 15% longer than they walked before eating it.

Possible reason: Dark chocolate's high concentration of polyphenols, antioxidants that appear to improve blood flow to the legs.

Mark Creager, MD, director of the Vascular Center at Brigham and Women's Hospital, Boston.

Can You Survive When Your Heart Just Stops?

Norman S. Abramson, MD, chair of the board of directors of the Sudden Cardiac Arrest Foundation, *SCA-Aware.org*, based in Pittsburgh and a former professor of emergency medicine at the University of Pittsburgh. His research focuses on improving neurological outcomes among survivors of cardiac arrest.

Sudden chest pain isn't something you're likely to ignore. This symptom—along with breathlessness, cold sweats and other classic heart attack symptoms—is a clear sign that you need to call 911.

While a possible heart attack is scary enough, the reality actually could be even worse. With sudden cardiac arrest (SCA), brain damage is almost certain unless you are treated within just a few minutes. And unlike a heart attack, which many people survive, SCA is almost always fatal. But what if that grim picture could be improved?

A chance of survival: New research suggests that paying close attention to early signs that may precede SCA—as well as being prepared in your home, where this killer condition most often strikes—could mean the difference between life and death.

What you need to know…

When the Heart Just Stops

A heart attack occurs when a blood clot interrupts blood flow to a section of the heart. In contrast, with SCA, an electrical malfunction in the heart triggers a dangerous abnormality in the heart rhythm (arrhythmia) that disrupts blood flow to the brain and other organs.

Only about 10% of people who suffer SCA live long enough to get to a hospital. Most—such as newsman Tim Russert who succumbed to SCA in 2008—collapse and then die within minutes.

Are You At Risk?

More than 400,000 Americans (not including hospitalized patients) suffer SCA each year. If your doctor has warned you about elevated cholesterol, high blood pressure or other cardiovascular risk factors, you know that you could be setting yourself up for a heart attack. But the same conditions also mean that you're at risk for SCA.

For certain other people, SCA is truly a stealth killer. It sometimes occurs in those who have "silent" (often congenital) cardiovascular disease. Abusing drugs or alcohol also increases risk for SCA.

Know the Signs

When someone suffers cardiac arrest, the only symptoms that occur simultaneously tend to be sudden collapse and a loss of consciousness. The victim also will have stopped breathing and won't have a detectable pulse.

What's new: Many individuals do have advance warning of SCA—even if they choose to ignore it.

In fact, when researchers recently looked into this, they found that 53% of SCA patients had prior symptoms, including chest pain, shortness of breath, heart palpitations and/or fainting. The symptoms—identical to those that often accompany heart attacks—occurred anywhere from one hour to four weeks before the SCA. Since SCA is so closely tied to heart disease, it makes sense that many victims will have heart disease symptoms before they suffer from SCA. If you have any of these symptoms, consult a doctor!

Protect Yourself

Most of the same approaches that will protect you from a heart attack—such as maintaining a healthy weight and not smoking—will help you avoid SCA. *Also useful for people concerned about SCA...*

• **Consider buying an automated external defibrillator (AED).** It can triple the likelihood of survival when used within the first minute or two of SCA. An AED is about the size of a laptop computer. The cost ranges from $1,200 to $2,500 but might be covered by insurance or Medicare if you have a high-risk arrhythmia or another heart condition. The device is easy to operate. Once it's turned on, a voice and screen explain where to attach the electrodes and when to push the buttons.

Be sure to act quickly: If someone collapses, use the device immediately. It won't prompt you to deliver a shock unless the person is experiencing SCA. For each one-minute delay, the chance of survival from SCA drops about 10%.

Important: I advise everyone who has heart disease or heart disease risk factors to talk to his/her doctor about owning one of these devices (or sharing one with close neighbors)—and to watch an online video or take an in-person class on how to use it. AEDs are available online.

• **Chest compressions.** Even if an AED is available, give chest compressions until it is ready to be placed on the victim's chest. If the heartbeat hasn't started after following AED voice prompts, do chest compressions for two minutes and use the AED again. Or if there's no AED, do chest compressions alone. Don't waste time checking for a pulse or giving mouth-to-mouth breathing—it's the chest compressions that are needed to restart the victim's heart. If someone collapses and is unresponsive and you suspect it's SCA, call 911 first. Then give the compressions, and don't stop (it's hard work, so you may need help from a bystander) until the emergency medical service arrives.

How to do compressions: Put the heel of one hand on the center of the chest (between the nipples)...place the heel of your other hand on top of the first hand for strength...position your body over your hands...and press hard about two inches into the chest.

Try to give at least 100 compressions per minute (almost two per second).

For a hands-only CPR video: Go to Heart.org/HandsOnlyCPR. For more detailed instruction, sign up for in-person training at your local hospital or fire department.

Hospital Care

If you suffer SCA in the hospital (or if you get to an ER in time), you'll be given treatments to restart the heart and re-establish heart, brain and lung functions.

Induced hypothermia, a promising therapy to reduce the damage from SCA, is available at many hospitals. This therapy involves rapid cooling of the body to about 89°F for about 24 hours. Cooling the body as soon as the heart has been restarted lowers the metabolic requirements of the brain and reduces the risk for long-term neurological problems, such as coma.

People who survive SCA may need additional treatments to prevent a second cardiac arrest.

Examples: Some are given an implantable cardioverter defibrillator (ICD), a surgically implanted device that analyzes the heartbeat and administers shocks to treat ventricular fibrillation. Another approach, radio-frequency ablation, uses radio-frequency energy to destroy abnormal heart cells that can cause irregular rhythms.

Women Take Longer to Reach Hospital After Heart Attack

Raffaele Bugiardini, MD, professor of cardiology, University of Bologna, Italy.
American College of Cardiology, news release.

Women having heart attacks get to the hospital for treatment later than men and are more likely to die, a new study finds.

Study Details

Researchers analyzed data from more than 7,400 heart attack patients in Europe. They found that 70% of women took longer than an hour to get to a hospital that could treat them. Only 30% of men with heart attack symptoms took that long. The time to the hospital ranged from as few as five minutes to as long as three days, according to the researchers.

A major reason why women took longer to receive care was that they waited longer than men to call emergency medical services. Women waited an average of one hour to call for help versus 45 minutes for men, according to the study.

"Our findings should set off an alarm for women, who may not understand their personal risk of heart disease and may take more time to realize they are having a heart attack and need urgent medical help," said study author Raffaele Bugiardini, a professor of cardiology at the University of Bologna in Italy.

But even after calling for help, women "seem to disappear somewhere in the health care system," Dr. Bugiardini said.

Delays in receiving hospital treatment—whether because women waited longer to call for help or were not taken to hospital as quickly as men—were associated with a higher risk of dying.

Women were nearly twice as likely as men to die in the hospital, 12% vs. 6%. Women's risk of dying remained higher even after the researchers accounted for factors such as age, treatments received, and heart disease risk factors.

The study also found that women were slightly less likely than men to undergo treatment to open clogged arteries, which tend to be most effective in the first hour after a heart attack strikes.

After being admitted to the hospital, there were no major differences between women and men in the average time it took them to receive clot-busting drugs or balloon angioplasty to open blocked arteries.

33

The study was presented at the annual meeting of the American College of Cardiology in San Diego.

Heart Attack Symptoms May Differ In Women

One reason why women may delay seeking treatment is a lack of "classic" signs of heart attack, such as intense chest pain. Instead, they may have shortness of breath, nausea or vomiting, or pain in the back, neck or jaw, and their symptoms may develop slowly over hours or days or even come and go, according to the researchers.

For more information on heart attack in women, visit the website of the U.S. Office on Women's Health, *www.womenshealth. gov.* Search "heart attack signs."

Cardiac Rehab Saves Lives—But Women Don't Get It

Jillian Colbert, MD, cardiology fellow in training, University of Calgary, and James A. Stone, MD, PhD, cardiologist, Cardiac Wellness Institute of Calgary, both in Alberta, Canada. Their study was presented at the 2013 annual meeting of the American College of Cardiology.

There's a proven way for men and women to slash their risk of dying from heart disease, yet few women take advantage of the opportunity—often because their doctors don't tell them about it. Called cardiac rehabilitation, it's a simple program that's widely available and hugely helpful, yet vastly underused. A new study shines a spotlight on the dark facts.

Study participants included nearly 26,000 patients with coronary artery disease (CAD), a buildup of waxy plaque in the arteries that deliver blood and oxygen to the heart. CAD affects about 20% of people age 65 and older and is the leading cause of death for both women and men. Cardiac rehab typically is a 12-week outpatient program appropriate for

people who have been diagnosed with CAD, have suffered a heart attack or have some other heart problem. It is an individualized program that includes supervised exercise sessions, nutrition counseling, stress-management training, smoking-cessation assistance and encouragement to make permanent lifestyle changes. For the study, researchers reviewed medical records spanning up to 15 years to see who attended cardiac rehab and how much it helped boost patients' survival.

Findings: The good news was that women with CAD who attended rehab were 66% less likely to die than women who did not attend. Rehab also benefited men with CAD, but not to as great a degree. However, only 31% of the women in the study were ever even referred to a cardiac rehab program by their doctors, compared with 42% of men. Physicians don't deserve all the blame, though—because among the patients who did get a rehab referral, only 50% of women (versus 60% of men) bothered to go.

Though the study didn't look at why so few women were referred to cardiac rehab, it could be that many doctors as well as patients still mistakenly think of heart disease as "mostly a man's problem"…or that some doctors refer only their healthier female heart patients to rehab, assuming that sicker ones are too ill to be helped.

As for why women who were referred declined to go? Researchers speculate that women may feel that they have too many family obligations and other responsibilities to make time for rehab…and that women tend to put their own health needs on the back burner. That's ironic, though—because if women with CAD don't take care of themselves, they won't be around to take care of their families.

Though this new research was conducted in Canada, smaller studies have shown that the same problem occurs in the US.

Self-defense: Male or female, if you have CAD or some other cardiovascular problem (for instance, a history of heart attack, bypass, angioplasty, stenting, angina, valve surgery or heart transplant), don't wait for your doctor to bring up the subject of cardiac rehab—come right out and ask whether it's appropriate for you. If the doctor says you don't need it, request a detailed explanation…and consider getting a second opinion, too. And if you are referred for cardiac rehab, go! Programs are offered at many hospitals and medical centers and typically are covered by Medicare and other health insurance.

How Heart Patients Can Lower Risk for Early Death by 55%!

When cardiac patients talked with nurses and doctors about their treatment and other concerns…did relaxation exercises…and/or participated in music therapy during their hospitalization or rehabilitation, they were 55% less likely to die or have another cardiovascular event after two years, in a recent study.

How heart patients can get this type of support: Ask health-care providers more questions about their treatment…and seek out

activities, such as music or exercise programs, group psychotherapy and meditation.

Zoi Aggelopoulou, PhD, RN, head of continuing education, NIMTS Veterans Hospital of Athens, Greece.

Hospitalized for Heart Attack? Make Sure They Check You for Diabetes

Suzanne V. Arnold, MD, MHA, assistant professor at Saint Luke's Mid America Heart Institute and the University of Missouri at Kansas City. Her study was presented at the 2014 annual meeting of the American Heart Association.

It's well-known among health-conscious people that heart disease and diabetes are linked, so it seems a shame to be hearing news from the American Heart Association that 10% of Americans who've had a heart attack probably have undiagnosed diabetes. What's worse, though, is news that doctors are missing opportunities to detect and treat diabetes in people even when they are hospitalized for a heart attack.

Are so many doctors this clueless?

Although it might be a great challenge for health-care professionals to identify everyone with diabetes before complications, such as heart attack, occur, a basic precaution can at least help those who do land in the hospital because of heart attack. So if you've had a heart attack or have cardiovascular disease—or you want to be prepared to give yourself the best odds if you ever have a heart attack in the future—here's what you need to insist that your medical-care team does for you, especially if you land in the hospital…

A Simple Overlooked Test

It comes down to getting a simple blood test. Doctors who order a hemoglobin A1c test when a patient is being treated for heart attack are making the right move to ensure that diabetes won't be missed and the heart attack can be treated correctly, said Suzanne

V. Arnold, MD, MHA, an assistant professor at the University of Missouri in Kansas City. She led a study on undiagnosed diabetes in heart attack patients that was reported at this year's American Heart Association meeting. The hemoglobin A1c test shows average blood sugar levels for the preceding three months and is widely used to diagnose both type 1 and type 2 diabetes and monitor how well blood sugar is being controlled after diagnosis.

In her study, Dr. Arnold and her team took 2,854 patients who were hospitalized for heart attacks but had never received a diabetes diagnosis and arranged for them to have the hemoglobin A1c test. Both the hospitalized patients and the doctors treating them were kept in the dark ("blinded" in scientific speak) about the test results, and doctors were left to their business-as-usual patient care. Diabetes was considered "recognized" by the researchers if a patient either received diabetes education while hospitalized and/or diabetes medication when sent home.

The study results were a real eye-opener. Sure, Dr. Arnold's team discovered that 10% of these patients had diabetes and didn't know it, but the far bigger issue that patients and their families need to know about was that doctors failed to recognize diabetes in 69% of these previously undiagnosed patients.

That's a major fail—especially when all it took for the treating doctors themselves to discover diabetes was to order the same simple, inexpensive A1c test that Dr. Arnold's team had already ordered for their study.

Six months down the road, the researchers checked in on the patients they themselves knew had diabetes. They found that 71% of the patients whose diabetes had also been discovered by a doctor during their hospital stays were getting diabetes care. As for the patients whose diabetes had not been discovered by doctors treating them in the hospital, only 7% were getting diabetes care, meaning that the likelihood was strong that no one, except Dr. Arnold's team, had yet checked these folks for diabetes. This left them at high risk for more cardiovascular complications, including additional heart attacks.

Knowledge That Can Also Guide Heart Attack Treatment

Knowing that a heart attack patient has type 2 diabetes is important in the moment because it determines treatment decisions, explained Dr. Arnold. For example, patients with multivessel coronary artery disease and diabetes may do better with bypass surgery (rather than stents) and particular blood pressure medications, such as ACE inhibitors.

Dr. Arnold's advice for people who have heart attacks and survive...but don't know whether they have diabetes...is that they insist on having a hemoglobin A1C test during their hospitalization. She does not advocate routine hemoglobin A1C screening for everyone, though, calling it "impractical," although it's certainly something you can bring up with your doctor if you know you have heart disease. And although you may be in-the-know about diabetes and heart disease prevention, this seems like a good place to include a refresher for you or a loved one. You can assess your risks and the warning signs of diabetes with these checklists from the American Diabetes Association:

Your chances of diabetes increase if you...

- **Have a family history of type 2 diabetes**
- **Don't get much exercise and are otherwise physically inactive**
- **Are overweight**
- **Have high blood pressure**
- **Have low HDL cholesterol and high triglycerides**
- **Don't watch your diet and feast on high-calorie, fatty, sugary and low-fiber foods**
- **Smoke**
- **For women, had diabetes during pregnancy**

These are warning signs of diabetes...

- **Unquenchable thirst**
- **Excessive urination**
- **Increased appetite, despite eating**
- **Unexpected weight loss**

- **Tingling, pain and/or numbness in your hands and/or feet**
- **Blurred vision**
- **Cuts and bruises that take a long time to heal**
- **Extreme fatigue**

It's not very challenging for health-conscious people to avoid type 2 diabetes and heart disease, but keeping this bit of information on a simple blood test in mind can protect you or a loved one even more.

Tomatoes Keep Blood Vessels Strong

Getting a daily dose of the antioxidant *lycopene* improved the inner linings of blood vessels (endothelia) in people with heart disease, a new study has found. Healthy endothelia help curb the progression of heart disease. The study participants received a lycopene extract (7 mg daily). You can, of course, get lycopene from food—enjoy tomatoes (your body will absorb more of the antioxidant if they're cooked)…watermelon…and apricots.

Joseph Cheriyan, MD, associate lecturer in medicine, University of Cambridge, UK. The research appeared in *PLOS ONE*.

Heart-Device Danger

Jeffrey L. Williams, MD, medical director of electrophysiology at The Good Samaritan Hospital, with a private practice at Lebanon Cardiology Associates, both in Lebanon, Pennsylvania. He is author of *What Is a Pacemaker?*

Too many people are getting heart defibrillators.

Unsettling fact: A large study concluded that more than 20% of people who have an implanted cardioverter defibrillator (ICD) don't meet the expert guidelines for who should have the device.

An ICD is a pacemaker-like device that delivers a brief shock when it detects ventricular fibrillation, a life-threatening arrhythmia that can cause cardiac arrest and sudden death. The device is recommended for patients with ventricular defibrillation…those who have already suffered from cardiac arrest…and those with an ejection fraction (a measure of the heart's pumping ability) below 35% that doesn't improve with other treatments.

Researchers at Duke University examined nationwide data involving nearly 112,000 patients. Those who received ICDs who did not meet the guidelines were more likely to suffer infections and complications. They spent more time in the hospital and were more likely to die in the hospital.

Why don't more doctors follow the guidelines? Some simply don't keep up with the latest recommendations. There also is concern that because Medicare pays $50,000 for the procedure, some hospitals might simply be cashing in. The Department of Justice opened an investigation of ICD overuse in 2010 that is still ongoing.

The guidelines specify a 40-day waiting period after a heart attack before implanting an ICD. If your doctor recommends an ICD sooner than this or if you don't meet the guidelines above, ask him/her why you need the device. In the study, electrophysiologists (who have the most experience with ICDs) were more likely to follow the guidelines than other doctors.

Lifesaving Vest

A lifesaving vest that delivers electrical shocks to keep the heart beating is more comfortable—and possibly more reliable—than older wearable defibrillators worn by heart patients. The vest, still in development, can be worn under clothes and washed at home.

Johns Hopkins University.

Better Pump for Heart Failure

The FDA recently approved a new pump, which is implanted in the patient's chest near the heart, to treat heart failure. In clinical trials of the device, called the HeartWare Ventricular Assist System, 91% of 140 advanced heart-failure patients were alive six months after the new pump was implanted—these survival rates are comparable to those for patients using the currently available left ventricular assist device (LVAD). This older device, however, must be placed in the abdomen, which is not suitable for some heart-failure patients.

Edward K. Kasper, MD, director of clinical cardiology, The Johns Hopkins Hospital, Baltimore.

What Doctors Don't Tell Women About Sex After a Heart Attack

Emily M. Abramsohn, MPH, public health researcher, University of Chicago. Her study was published in Journal of the *American Heart Association*.

If you suffer a heart attack, your doctor is likely to give you all sorts of guidelines about what is and is not safe when it comes to diet, exercise, work, travel and more.

And if you're a man, there's a good chance that your doctor also will tell you whether it's safe to have sex again.

But if you're a woman? Don't count on your doctor to initiate that important discussion about physical intimacy—because with female heart attack patients, a new study shows, physicians are strangely mum on the topic of sex. That's a crying shame, because their silence is leading to lots of unnecessary confusion and fear in the bedroom for women—and for their partners.

Phone Sex Interview

For this study, researchers turned to a registry of heart attack survivors to investigate how women tended to fare sexually in the aftermath of their heart attacks. They sent letters to invite participation, and then they started dialing. The respondents were women between the ages of 43 and 75. Generally they rated their health as good to very good. All were in monogamous relationships, either marriage or a long-term same-sex partnership.

The women were asked a number of questions, including "Has your doctor ever talked to you about sex after having a heart attack?"—and the answer to that query raised red flags. *Here's why...*

• **The majority of women surveyed did not recall any discussion with their doctors about resuming sex.** That's sad—because previous research showed that patients who are not counseled about sex are much less likely to be sexually active one year after their heart attacks than patients who are counseled.

The few women who did recall such a conversation said that they had initiated the discussion themselves—and that the instructions they got were befuddling. For instance, one woman said, "I asked the doctor point-blank when could I have sex again,

---

Watch for Depression

Heart attacks are more likely to cause depression in women than in men. Survivors of both genders report more sadness, worry and stress in life. But the gap between feelings before and after the heart attack is greater in women. And significantly more women who had heart attacks (35%) were diagnosed with depression than men who had heart attacks (24%).

Bottom line: Both men and women—but especially women—need extra social support after a heart attack.

Results of 353,492 interviews by Gallup-Healthways Well-Being Index, reported in *USA Today*.

and he said, 'When you can climb two flights of stairs without getting out of breath.' Well, I could…hardly climb two flights of stairs before I had a heart attack." In other cases, the instructions given were so vague as to be meaningless. Another survey respondent recalled, "The day before I left the hospital I said, 'You didn't tell me when I could have relations.' So then he says, 'Well, that's going to be up to you, how you feel.' But that's not giving me an answer."

It was odd and frustrating to the patients that doctors did not discuss sex, particularly since they provided detailed guidelines for many other activities. As one woman said, "They tell you not to run the vacuum cleaner, not to do this or that for so many months after. Why not say, 'As far as your sexual activity, hold off for four weeks'?"

• **Although hospital discharge instructions can be overwhelming,** the women generally felt that the discussion about sex should start at the time of discharge and then be continued during follow-up care. One woman suggested that doctors should ask about sex at every follow-up appointment, especially at the one-month visit: "It sets a precedent. Just knowing that [sex] is an open topic would go a long way in encouraging women to discuss it."

• **When those important conversations don't take place, fear can take over.** In fact, fear was the driving factor behind women's loss of sexuality following a heart attack. For instance, one respondent reported, "My heart beat real fast and it scared me"…another said, "Fear is not conducive to a healthy romp." The women's partners were fearful, too. One

woman recalled, "At first he was afraid because he thought I would have another heart attack. I told him I'd rather die with a smile on my face…I had to convince my husband that I wasn't going to die in bed."

Guidelines Go Ignored

Both the American Heart Association (AHA) and the American College of Cardiology recommend that physicians counsel their patients—notice that's "patients," not "male patients"—about resuming sex after a heart attack. Yet based on the results of this survey, it seems that doctors just aren't following the guidelines. And that's really too bad, because such conversations would most likely put women (and their partners) at ease.

Reason: The AHA says that sex is generally safe after a heart attack provided that a patient is in stable condition and has no complications…and that heart attacks rarely occur during sex because sexual activity is usually relatively short in duration.

One caveat, dear readers: Research shows that when a heart attack does occur during sex, it is usually during extramarital sex, not sex with one's spouse.

What you can do: First, for more background info, read AHA's article "Sex and Heart Disease." Then, to find out whether sex is safe for you, prepare a list of questions for your doctor and insist on frank, detailed answers that take your individual situation into account—and don't leave the doctor's office until all your questions have been answered to your satisfaction.

Chapter 2

BEST WAYS TO BEAT THE BIG C: BREAKTHROUGHS IN BREAST CANCER AND MORE

Do You Really Need a Mammogram?

While American doctors follow guidelines that screening should be offered at least every two years to women who are 50 to 74 years old, and although we definitely know that risk of breast cancer increases with age, do you really need a mammogram when you hit 70? A Dutch study says no. In fact, it found that breast cancer screening for women age 70 and older may actually cause more harm than good, leading to unnecessary treatment that puts elderly women at even higher risk than they already are for anemia, gastrointestinal problems, fatigue, infection, memory loss, effects of bone loss (osteoporosis) and heart disease. This all boils down to quality of life in your later years.

And statistics bear this out.

If 1,000 women started biennial mammography screening when they were 50 years old and continued for 10 years, one to three breast cancer deaths would be prevented over the next 15 years. If 1,000 60-year-old women had biennial screenings for 10 years, three or four deaths would be prevented over the next 20 years. For women in their mid-70s,

however, their average remaining life expectancy—about 13 more years—is shorter than the 17-year lag time in which a death attributed to breast cancer could be prevented. Suddenly the number of women being helped by screening starts going down, not up.

But maybe you are 72 and expect to live until 102. Fair enough. In that case, breast cancer screening and next steps if breast cancer is detected should be a personal, individualized decision between you and your health-care provider, according to Russell Harris, MD, MPH, professor of medicine at University of North Carolina School of Medicine.

Approaching Breast Cancer Detection from Another Angle

Dr. Harris said he is not suggesting that all breast cancer screening guidelines should completely go out the window and leave women and their doctors high and dry. His wish—and what he expects to happen, based on discussions with his colleagues in the public health field—is that for older women, at least, there will be new, more individualized guidelines that will be conveyed to

Russell Harris, MD, MPH, professor of medicine and adjunct professor of epidemiology, University of North Carolina School of Medicine and Gillings School of Global Public Health, Chapel Hill, North Carolina.

gynecologists and primary-care physicians over the next few years. *The same broad leeway being proposed for elderly women should be extended to all women, of every age—and these downsides of breast cancer screening are the rationale...*

●**Cumulative radiation exposure.** Although the amount of radiation received per mammogram is minimal, every time you get a mammogram or are otherwise exposed to radiation in the medical setting, it has a cumulative effect on your body.

●**Possible unneeded treatment.** Some breast cancers are so slow-growing that they would not have caused any harm if they had gone undetected.

●**Side effects of treatment.** As we all know—cancer therapy itself is wrought with side effects. Surgery, radiation, chemotherapy and hormone therapy all come with risks that become riskier with age. Radiation to the breast can damage the heart and lead to lung cancer, and hormone therapy raises a woman's risk for serious blood clots and stroke. For some women, the treatment can be just as devastating as the disease it's meant to conquer.

Why It's a Personal Decision

Each woman—young, old and in between—needs to evaluate the pros and cons of her own screening in relation to her personal health, family history and life situation. The physician's role is to help women make informed, individualized decisions about breast cancer screening—not to automatically pressure them into decisions based on screening statistics.

Part of being informed means recognizing that screening isn't the only way to protect yourself. There are other approaches to prevention that we've de-emphasized at our peril. It's time to stop putting all our eggs in the screening basket. Screening is not our only hope to reduce the scourge of breast cancer. Maintaining a healthy weight, remaining physically active, not smoking, being moderate in our drinking habits and proactively working with a gynecologist and

High Cholesterol...Big Danger for Breast Cancer

●**High cholesterol increases risk.** A recent British study found that women diagnosed with high cholesterol, defined by counts higher than 200 mg/dL, were 64% more likely to develop breast cancer than women without high cholesterol. Researchers reviewed the medical records of 664,159 female patients between 2000 and 2013. The researchers decided to do the study after a mouse study last year linked aggressive breast cancer to a chemical created by the body's processing of cholesterol. Further research is needed to confirm the findings. In the meantime, there is strong evidence that exercising regularly and maintaining a healthy weight can help lower the risk of developing breast cancer after menopause. The British study also suggests that taking statins (prescription drugs to reduce high cholesterol) could help prevent breast cancer, but a clinical trial of the use of statins for breast cancer would need to be conducted before statins could be prescribed for that.

Rahul Potluri, MD, honorary clinical lecturer in cardiology, Aston Medical School, Aston University, Birmingham, England. He is lead author of the *ACALM* study presented at the Frontiers in CardioVascular Biology 2014 Conference in Barcelona.

●**High cholesterol increases severity.** The molecule 27HC, a derivative of cholesterol, mimics estrogen, a hormone that increases breast cancer risk and reduces the effectiveness of anti-estrogen treatments for breast cancer such as aromatase inhibitors and tamoxifen. Women with breast cancer and high cholesterol should talk to their doctors about lowering cholesterol with statins and/or dietary changes.

Donald McDonnell, PhD, chairman of the department of pharmacology and cancer biology at Duke University School of Medicine, Durham, North Carolina. He is lead author of a study published in *Science*.

primary-care physician to know and address personal risk factors are important ways for women to protect themselves against cancer, stay all-around healthy and have a great quality of life.

Better Breast Cancer Detection

Mammograms using digital radiography (DR) are slightly more effective than computer radiography mammograms (CR) for detecting breast cancer.

Recent finding: DR detected 4.9 cancers per 1,000 mammograms, while CR detected 3.4.

Study of 816,000 mammograms carried out on 688,000 women, ages 50 to 74, by researchers at several cancer care centers in Ontario, Canada, published in *Radiology*.

New Device May Make Mammograms More Comfortable

Lusi Tumyan, MD, chief of breast imaging, City of Hope Cancer Center, Duarte, CA.

Woutjan Branderhorst, PhD, researcher, Academic Medical Center, Amsterdam, and clinical application scientist, SigmaScreening, Amsterdam, the Netherlands.

Radiological Society of North America 2014 annual meeting, Chicago.

Dutch researchers have developed a device that may reduce the discomfort many women feel during a mammogram while preserving the quality of the image.

Breast compression is necessary in mammography for imaging purposes, but it can be painful. The new device displays the average pressure during compression, so the pressure can be adjusted and standardized, which reduces pain, according to the researchers.

Background

Currently, mammographers can only estimate the pressure applied to the breasts, according to study researcher Woutjan Branderhorst, PhD, from the Academic Medical Center in Amsterdam and a scientist at SigmaScreening, the company developing the device.

Those who perform mammograms have a difficult task, Dr. Branderhorst explained. They must "adjust the applied compression force to breast size, composition, skin tautness and pain tolerance," he said.

Currently, he said, the technologist doing the mammogram can only use visual and tactile clues to estimate the pressure on the breast. This results in large variations, Dr. Branderhorst said.

"Especially for small breasts, this can lead to extremely high pressure," he added.

Study on New Device

In their study, Dr. Branderhorst and his team performed mammograms on more than 400 women undergoing routine mammograms. The researchers theorized that a protocol based on pressure, not force, would make the tests more comfortable.

Using the new device, they did four compressions on each woman. Three were standardized to a specific force; one was standardized to a specific target pressure.

The mammogram targeted for pressure was rated as less painful, on average, by the women. The pressure-targeted mammogram didn't reduce image quality, Dr. Branderhorst noted.

"The device used in our study measures and displays the pressure in real time, which provides an objective guide for the technologists and enables standardization of the pressure," Dr. Branderhorst said.

This makes the procedure less uncomfortable because high, painful pressures are avoided, he said.

Dr. Branderhorst presented the results of the study at the annual meeting of the Radiological Society of North America in Chicago.

Pink Ribbon, an organization that supports breast cancer research and awareness, and SigmaScreening, a spin-off company of the Academic Medical Center, provided funding for the study.

Expert Commentary

Lusi Tumyan, MD, chief of breast imaging at the City of Hope Cancer Center in Duarte, California, reviewed the findings. "It looks promising and it looks interesting, but it is too early to tell," she said.

Currently, she said, mammographers use visual clues to determine how much pressure to apply. "If a patient is uncomfortable we don't press as much."

If the research bears out, she said, the device might also help standardize the mammograms from year to year.

However, Dr. Tumyan said, since the number of women in this study was small, more studies would be needed.

Good News

Existing mammography machines could be upgraded with the device, Dr. Branderhorst said, and the device could be integrated into new machines. The extra costs would be minimal, he predicted.

To learn more about what to expect during a mammogram, visit the Web site of the National Cancer Institute, *cancer.org*, and search "mammogram."

Tomatoes vs. Breast Cancer

In a new study, postmenopausal women at increased risk for breast cancer ate about 25 mg of lycopene (the amount in one cup of tomato juice) every day. After 10 weeks, they had increased blood levels of the protein adiponectin, which has been linked to reduced breast cancer risk. Besides tomatoes, other good sources of lycopene include apricots, watermelon and papaya. Cooked tomatoes have even more lycopene than raw, so also enjoy tomato soup or red pasta sauce.

Adana Llanos, PhD, MPH, assistant professor of epidemiology, Rutgers, The State University of New Jersey, New Brunswick.

Vitamin D Deficiency Linked to Increased Breast Cancer Death Risk

Study titled "Meta-analysis of vitamin D sufficiency for improving survival of patients with breast cancer," published in *Anticancer Research*.

Vitamin D is often in the news because most Americans get too little of it... and because deficiencies are associated with increased risk for cardiovascular disease, diabetes, Alzheimer's disease, osteoporosis and many other serious health problems. And now here we go again—because too-low levels of that same vitamin are linked to nearly double the risk of dying from breast cancer, a new study shows.

Here's what you (or the woman you love) should know...

Bras Do Not Cause Cancer

Bras do not raise risk for breast cancer. Some media reports have suggested that wearing a bra may inhibit lymph circulation and drainage, boosting breast cancer risk.

But: A recent study found that there is no connection between wearing a bra and breast cancer risk.

Study of more than 1,000 women by researchers at Fred Hutchinson Research Center, Seattle, published in *Cancer Epidemiology, Biomarkers & Prevention*.

Pooling Results to Settle the Score

Many studies have looked at the association between vitamin D levels and the risk of developing breast cancer, but there has been little exploration of the link between vitamin D and the odds of surviving breast cancer. To address that oversight, researchers looked for studies that investigated a link between breast cancer survival and levels of a vitamin D precursor called 25-hydroxyvitamin D, or 25(OH)D for short. The blood test for 25(OH)D is considered the most accurate way to measure how much vitamin D is in a person's body. Five studies met the researchers' criteria, but their results varied. *However, when the researchers pooled the data from these studies and did a statistical analysis, they found that...*

●**Breast cancer patients with higher levels of 25(OH)D** at the time of their diagnoses had a substantially lower risk of dying from their disease during the study periods, which averaged about 10 years.

●**Women with the highest levels, around 30 nanograms per milliliter (ng/mL),** had a 44% lower risk of dying from breast cancer than women with the lowest levels, around 17 ng/mL.

●**There was a strong dose-related response,** meaning that higher vitamin D levels were consistently associated with reduced mortality risk.

What this Means for You

It's important to point out that this study does not prove that 25(OH)D actually helps protect against death from breast cancer. It could be the other way around—the more deadly forms of breast cancer might cause vitamin D to become depleted, making 25(OH)D a marker for disease severity. However, the researchers consider this unlikely because no other studies suggest that cancer reduces 25(OH)D levels. Furthermore, the evidence in support of vitamin D's protective mechanism is bolstered by the fact that cancer death rates are lower in areas of the US (and the world) with ample sunlight, the most abundant catalyst for naturally sufficient vitamin D levels.

Just how might higher 25(OH)D improve survival for cancer patients? Perhaps by the same mechanism through which it is thought to help prevent cancer in the first place. Lab studies have shown that vitamin D by-products interfere with cancer during three critical phases of development—by helping to maintain cell differentiation (well-differentiated cancer cells look more like normal cells and tend to grow and spread more slowly than poorly differentiated cells)...promoting apoptosis (normal programmed cell death)... and inhibiting angiogenesis (formation of blood vessels) that would feed tumors. It's also possible that restoring 25(OH)D to normal levels may increase the function of E-cadherin, a protein that helps cells stick together to form organized tissue and suppress tumor growth.

Don't DIY with D: The average blood level of 25(OH)D for breast cancer patients in the US is 17 ng/mL—which is too low. The researchers stated that blood levels "in all patients with breast cancer should be restored to the normal range [of] 30 to 80 ng/mL." However, it's important for cancer patients—and everyone else who wants to protect his or her health by optimizing vitamin D levels—to not take a do-it-yourself approach. As we've been warning you for several years, too much vitamin D can be dangerous, increasing the risk for blood vessel calcification, heart rhythm abnormalities and kidney damage.

Prudent: Ask a nutrition-oriented doctor to check your 25(OH)D level and, if necessary, to prescribe an appropriate dosage for supplementation.

Unhealthy Insulin Levels May Boost Breast Cancer Risk

Marc Gunter, PhD, associate professor, cancer epidemiology and prevention, Imperial College London School of Public Health, London, England.

Allison DiPasquale, MD, fellow, and Courtney Vito, MD, associate clinical professor, breast and surgical oncology, City of Hope Cancer Center, Duarte, California.

Cancer Research.

After menopause, unhealthy insulin levels may predict breast cancer risk even more than excess weight, new research suggests.

The new findings suggest "that it is metabolic health, and not overweight per se, that is associated with increased risk of breast cancer in postmenopausal women," said study co-author Marc Gunter, PhD. He is an associate professor of cancer epidemiology and prevention at Imperial College London School of Public Health in England.

While high insulin levels often occur in overweight or obese women, some very heavy women have normal levels of the hormone, experts say. And some normal-weight females have metabolically unhealthy insulin levels.

The study was published in a January 2015 issue of the journal *Cancer Research*.

Study Details

To assess insulin's role in breast cancer risk, Dr. Gunter studied more than 3,300 women without diabetes, 497 of whom developed breast cancer over eight years. He analyzed information on their weight, fasting insulin levels and insulin resistance, in which the body does not respond properly to insulin. Insulin helps the body use digested food for energy. A body's inability to produce insulin or use it properly leads to diabetes.

Overweight for the study was defined as a body mass index (BMI) of 25 or more. BMI is a calculation of body fat based on height and weight.

"The women who are overweight but who do not have metabolic abnormalities [as assessed by insulin resistance] are not at increased risk of breast cancer compared to [normal-weight] women," Dr. Gunter said.

"On the other hand, normal-weight women with metabolic abnormalities were at approximately the same elevated risk of breast cancer as overweight women with metabolic abnormalities," he added.

Dr. Gunter said this seemingly strong link between insulin and breast cancer is not a reason for women to ignore excess pounds. Being overweight or obese does increase the chances of developing insulin problems, he said.

In his study, high fasting insulin levels doubled the risk of breast cancer, both for overweight and normal-weight women.

In addition, women who were overweight and insulin-resistant had an 84% greater risk of breast cancer than overweight women who weren't insulin-resistant, he found.

Other research has found that up to 10% of women at a healthy weight may have insulin problems, he said.

Dr. Gunter said more research is needed to explain the findings. Insulin can cause cells, including cancer cells, to grow, so that could be a factor, he said. Other hormones related to insulin can also be higher in overweight women, and they could contribute to breast cancer risk, he said.

Expert Comment

The overall findings are not surprising, said Courtney Vito, MD, associate clinical professor of surgical oncology at City of Hope Cancer Center in Duarte, California.

"Fat is not inert," she said. "It is a metabolically active organ and we've known this from many other studies." There is much that experts still don't know about fat, she said.

The study is interesting, Dr. Vito said, although she agreed that more research is needed before the results can be considered conclusive. She played no role in the study.

Dr. Gunter's earlier research also found that higher insulin levels boost breast cancer risk in postmenopausal women. What may surprise some is the information about higher cancer risk in slender women with insulin problems, said Allison DiPasquale, MD, a fellow at City of Hope, who wasn't involved in the study.

Future studies, Dr. DiPasquale said, should look more closely at four subgroups: overweight women with and without insulin problems and normal-weight women with and without insulin problems.

Meanwhile, all three experts agreed the take-home point for women is to eat a healthy diet and to exercise regularly, so weight and insulin levels are more likely to stay normal. Also, women need to ask their doctors to screen them for insulin resistance, no matter what their weight or other risk factors.

The American Diabetes Association has more about insulin resistance at *http://www. diabetesforecast.org/2011/jun/understanding-insulin-resistance.html.*

Women Testing Negative for the Breast Cancer Gene Still May Be at Risk

It was originally thought that women who come from families with BRCA mutations but who test negative for any BRCA mutations had the same risk for breast cancer as the general population.

Recent finding: Women from such families with negative BRCA2 mutation had four times the risk for breast cancer as the general population.

Gareth Evans, MD, honorary professor of medical genetics and a cancer epidemiologist at The University of Manchester in England and lead author of a study of 800 families, published in *Cancer Epidemiology, Biomarkers & Prevention.*

Is It Breast Cancer or Not?

Melissa A. Lazar, MD, assistant professor of surgery at Thomas Jefferson University Hospital and a surgeon who specializes in the treatment of benign and malignant breast disease at the Jefferson Breast Care Center, both in Philadelphia.

It's scary to know that something suspicious appeared on what you thought was a routine mammogram. If your doctor recommends a biopsy, you obviously want to hear that everything's normal after all. But what if it's not? The medical language that's used in these reports can make things sound worse than they really are.

Here are common breast findings and what they really mean...

Lobular or Ductal Hyperplasia

The lobules in the breasts are milk-producing glands. The ducts are passages that milk travels through to get to the nipples. Many women will eventually develop lobular or ductal hyperplasia. It means that there is an overgrowth of cells in one of these areas.

Is it a worrisome finding? Probably not, as long as the cells don't appear atypical (see below). When researchers at the Mayo Clinic looked at almost 9,000 women who had had benign breast biopsies, about one-third had these proliferating cells.

Hyperplasia is not cancer. It typically does not increase a woman's risk of getting breast cancer. I advise women not to worry about it.

Atypical Hyperplasia

This is a little different from the situation described above. Atypical hyperplasia (also known as proliferative changes with atypia) is not a cancer. However, women who have been diagnosed with this condition do have to take precautions.

As the name suggests, "atypical" cells don't quite resemble normal cells. Atypical hyperplasia increases a woman's lifetime cancer risk, even in the unaffected breast, making the risk four to five times higher than that of the general population. *My advice…*

•If the cells were discovered during a core needle biopsy (a sampling of tissue taken from the suspicious area), I usually advise women to have an excisional biopsy. It will remove the entire area that contains the abnormal cells.

Editor's note: You might want to obtain a second opinion on the biopsy results given the findings of a recent study (see "Beware: Breast Biopsy Results May Not be Accurate" next page).

•Premenopausal women with atypical hyperplasia are advised to take the drug tamoxifen for five years. It will reduce their risk for breast cancer by about two-thirds. Postmenopausal women will get a similar benefit when they take *raloxifene* (Evista) or *exemestane* (Aromasin). Discuss possible side effects of the drugs, such as blood clots and risk for stroke, with your doctor.

•Screening guidelines from the National Comprehensive Cancer Network include annual mammograms and a clinical breast exam (a manual exam by a doctor) every six to 12 months.

Lobular Carcinoma In Situ (LCIS)

Don't let the word "carcinoma" throw you. Some doctors prefer the term lobular neoplasia because LCIS isn't a cancer—it is a risk factor.

The term "in situ" means that abnormal cells within the breast lobules haven't broken through the lobule wall and migrated into adjoining tissues or into the bloodstream.

Yet there is a risk. Women with LCIS are more likely to eventually develop breast cancer. The risk increases by 1% every year. A woman diagnosed with LCIS in her 40s is about 20% to 25% more likely to get breast cancer within 15 years than a woman who never had it.

Some women feel that any increase in breast cancer risk is unacceptable. They might ask their doctors if they should have a preventive (prophylactic) mastectomy. It's a difficult decision, particularly because the mastectomy would have to be bilateral (removing both breasts). Women with LCIS are just as likely to develop cancer in one breast as the other.

My advice: I don't recommend mastectomy for most women with LCIS, with the possible exception of those with a strong family history of breast cancer or other risk factors.

Better: Watchful waiting. Your doctor can monitor you closely. If a cancer does eventually develop, it can be treated quickly.

Get an annual mammogram…a clinical breast exam twice a year…and possibly take tamoxifen, raloxifene or exemestane. Women with LCIS who take one of these drugs can reduce their breast cancer risk by about 50%.

Ductal Carcinoma In Situ (DCIS)

Unlike LCIS, DCIS is a cancer. About 60,000 women in the US each year are found to have DCIS. The abnormal cells are confined inside the milk ducts and thus are not considered invasive. But if you're diagnosed with DCIS, you have to get treated. Treatment options include a lumpectomy followed by radiation to kill any cancer cells that were left behind…or, in some cases, a mastectomy (with or without breast reconstruction). Your surgeon might recommend a mastectomy if the DCIS is extensive or multicentric (more than one tumor, often in different areas of the breast). Once the carcinoma is removed, you will need to be followed closely. There always is the risk for a recurrence, which is 5% to 10% following lumpectomy with radiation and 1% to 2% following a mastectomy.

If the DCIS is estrogen receptor-positive, taking tamoxifen for five years is recommended to reduce your risk for recurrence and a new breast cancer.

Beware: Breast Biopsy Results May Not Be Accurate

Study led by researchers at University of Washington School of Medicine and Fred Hutchinson Cancer Research Center, both in Seattle, published in *The Journal of the American Medical Association*.

Breast biopsy findings may not be reliable when it comes to subtle abnormalities, according to a new study.

Researchers asked 115 pathologists to examine biopsy slides, then compared their diagnoses with those from a panel of leading experts who had seen the same slides. The panel of experts was made up of internationally recognized pathologists with highly regarded experience in research and continuing medical education on diagnostic breast pathology.

The outside pathologists were very good at diagnosing invasive breast cancer and agreed with the expert panel in about 96% of cases. For benign findings, they agreed with the experts in 87% of cases. When it came to diagnosing DCIS, they agreed with the experts about 84% of the time.

But with atypical ductal hyperplasia, the pathologists were in line with the experts only 48% of the time. They diagnosed atypia in 17% of readings where the experts had not and missed it in 35% of readings.

Too Few Breast Cancer Patients Getting Radiation After Mastectomy

Quyen Chu, MD, professor of surgery, Louisiana State University Health Sciences Center, Shreveport. American College of Surgeons, news release.

Many American women with locally advanced breast cancer do not receive recommended radiation therapy after mastectomy, a new study finds.

Recommendation for Radiation

Experts at the U.S. National Cancer Institute currently recommend that breast cancer patients who undergo mastectomy receive radiation therapy if their cancer has spread to four or more nearby lymph nodes.

New Study Findings

However, in the new study, which tracked nearly 57,000 such breast cancer cases in the United States between 1998 and 2011, researchers found only 65% of patients received follow-up radiation therapy.

The researchers "were quite startled by the finding," said lead author Quyen Chu, MD, professor of surgery at Louisiana State University Health Sciences Center in Shreveport.

Factors such as race/ethnicity, income and education level, health insurance, where patients lived or where they were treated, or the presence of other health problems did not influence whether these patients received radiation therapy, the team found.

One factor, however, showed a strong association with receiving radiation therapy: chemotherapy. Women who had received chemotherapy had more than five times the odds of getting radiation treatment compared to those who had not, the study found.

About 82% of the patients in the study received chemotherapy. Dr. Chu theorized that women who decided to skip chemotherapy might also be less willing to undergo radiation therapy.

Still, the exact reasons why more than a third of patients forgo post-op radiation remains unclear.

"From this study, we could not tease out whether patients refuse treatment or there is a lack of awareness among women and physicians about the need for radiation therapy after mastectomy for locally advanced breast cancer," Dr. Chu said.

The study was published in the *Journal of the American College of Surgeons*.

Important

If women with locally advanced breast cancer plan to have a mastectomy but are not offered follow-up radiation therapy, they should ask their doctor why, he recommended.

The U.S. National Library of Medicine has more about mastectomy at *nlm.nih.gov*. Search "mastectomy."

When It's Too Much Radiation...

Many breast cancer patients get radiation for longer than they need. Three to five weeks of post-lumpectomy radiation is now recommended for women over age 50 who have not had chemotherapy or lymph node involvement.

However: About two-thirds of women in this group are receiving the less intense conventional treatment, which lasts five to seven weeks. The two schedules involve about the same total amount of radiation, have similar side effects and are equally effective—but the shorter treatment is more convenient for patients and less expensive (average difference: $2,894).

Justin Bekelman, MD, assistant professor of radiation oncology at Perelman School of Medicine, University of Pennsylvania, Philadelphia, and lead author of a study of 15,643 lumpectomy patients, published in *JAMA*.

Gel Offers Better Breast Cancer Treatment

Women with the most common form of noninvasive breast cancer who rubbed a tamoxifen gel into their breast tissue daily for six to 10 weeks had similar antitumor effects as those who took oral tamoxifen daily.

Possible reason: The drug was present in equal amounts in the breast tissue of both groups.

Bonus: Blood levels in the gel group were much lower than in those taking oral tamoxifen, which could result in fewer side effects, such as blood clots.

Seema A. Khan, MD, professor of surgery, Northwestern University Feinberg School of Medicine, Chicago.

Heart Danger from Herceptin

The breast cancer drug Herceptin may cause heart problems, but these problems typically reverse once treatment is over. Herceptin caused a reduction in the heart's pumping force in 5% of patients who took the drug for one year. Congestive cardiac failure occurred in less than 1% of patients. Women should have a cardiac assessment before starting Herceptin and cardiac monitoring while taking it.

Brian Leyland-Jones, MBBS, PhD, vice president of molecular and experimental medicine, Avera Cancer Institute, Sioux Falls, South Dakota.

Breast Cancer Rehab: Vital Therapies Survivors Need But Don't Get

Julie K. Silver, MD, associate professor, department of physical medicine and rehabilitation, Harvard Medical School, Boston. She also is the founder of Oncology Rehab Partners, creator of the STAR Program Certification and author of *After Cancer Treatment: Heal Faster, Better, Stronger. JulieSilverMD.com*

For many breast cancer patients, the challenges don't end on the last day of treatment. They continue to suffer from the aftereffects of the disease and its treatments—pain, fatigue, physical limitations, foggy thinking, fear. In fact, according to a recent study in the journal *Cancer*, almost two-thirds of breast cancer patients report cancer complications that linger for many years.

It doesn't have to be that way…but sadly, it often is. "After treatment is over, many patients are sent away by their oncologists, having been told only to exercise and come back for a checkup every three to six months. That's not good enough!" said Julie K. Silver, MD, an associate professor of physical medicine and rehabilitation at Harvard Medical School, author of *After Cancer Treatment: Heal Faster, Better, Stronger* and a breast cancer survivor herself.

What could help breast cancer survivors recover more fully? Cancer rehab, a program of individualized, targeted, multidisciplinary therapies. "Cancer rehab is far more than standard follow-up care. It's a way of dealing with and minimizing the long-term impairments that breast cancer and its treatment can cause," said Dr. Silver.

You might think that breast cancer patients would be getting rehab services as a matter of course, but that's not the case. Dr. Silver cited one recent study showing that, while 90% of breast cancer survivors need rehabilitative care, fewer than 30% are getting it. The reason is that many patients—and many doctors—are unaware of this vital resource.

Lingering Problems

Breast cancer survivors typically suffer some if not all of the following long-term difficulties…

• **Pain in the chest wall where muscles and other tissue were cut for a mastectomy or lumpectomy.**

• **Frozen shoulder (adhesive capsulitis),** a condition characterized by stiffness and pain in the shoulder joint.

• **Lymphedema**—swelling, discomfort and/or loss of function in the arm closest to the affected breast, which result from lymph node removal and scarring that allow fluid to build up.

• **Neuropathy,** a nerve problem that causes pain and numbness, typically in the hands and/or feet.

• **"Chemo brain,"** the well-documented phenomenon of feeling less mentally sharp than before chemotherapy.

• **Generalized weakness,** which makes it difficult to lift things or carry out other normal tasks.

• **Excessive fatigue that interferes with the ability to exercise,** work, socialize or enjoy life.

• **Fear, anxiety or depression** brought on by the battle with breast cancer and continuing concerns about a possible recurrence.

Dr. Silver said that many patients recovering from breast cancer (and other cancers) come to her after enduring years of discomfort…and they blame themselves, saying, "I should have asked my doctor for a rehab referral."

But, she said, "I tell those patients that they shouldn't have to ask—rehab should be a routine part of treatment for all cancer patients, regardless of what type of cancer they had."

Good news: Starting in 2015, it will be routine—because the American College of Surgeons' Commission on Cancer (CoC) has mandated that all hospitals provide aftercare plans for cancer patients. If an institution fails to have such a plan in place, it will not be accredited by the CoC.

If you are currently being treated for breast cancer or are a breast cancer survivor experiencing lingering complications, there is absolutely no reason to wait until 2015 to demand a rehab plan. Most cancer rehab services are already covered by insurance and Medicare.

What Rehab Can Do for You

The exact services provided in rehab depend on the type of cancer and on each individual patient's needs. *Breast cancer rehab typically includes care from any or all of the following types of specialists…*

• **Physiatrist,** a physician who specializes in nerve, muscle and bone problems that affect how you move. After breast cancer, a physiatrist's care might center on reducing the effects of neuropathy and easing ongoing pain. For example, physiatrists can order specialized tests and prescribe medications or physical therapy to help.

•**Physical therapist (PT),** who can develop an individualized exercise program that accommodates current limitations while focusing on restoring stamina and strength… increasing range of motion in the affected arm and shoulder…and addressing problems with balance that can result from chemotherapy's effects on the nervous system. In addition, a PT can provide hands-on therapies that minimize lymphedema.

•**Occupational therapist (OT),** who can help overcome challenges in performing tasks of daily living. For instance, in the case of shoulder problems or lymphedema, an OT can help a breast cancer survivor master difficulties related to getting dressed, grooming and carrying packages. For a patient experiencing chemo brain, an OT can suggest strategies for improving concentration, memory and organizational skills.

•**Speech-language pathologist,** who can help breast cancer patients recover speech or language skills that have been altered by cancer treatments. Speech therapists also may treat cognitive problems, including chemo brain.

•**Psychologist,** who provides counseling to ease fear, anxiety and a sense of isolation or loss—so survivors can get back to enjoying their lives to the fullest.

Gold STAR: After recovering from cancer herself, Dr. Silver developed the STAR Program (Survivorship Training and Rehabilitation) Certification for hospitals and cancer centers, which involves a protocol for best practices in cancer rehab. More than 100 hospitals and cancer centers nationwide have signed up for STAR Program certification so far, and it is offered at several hundred sites. For information and/or a referral to a STAR Program in your area, visit the Web site of Oncology Rehab Partners, an organization founded by Dr. Silver and dedicated to advancing survivorship care.

Keep It Dark

Resistance to certain chemotherapy drugs is a growing problem among some cancer patients.

Possible reason: Lab studies have found that exposure to even dim light at night can trigger resistance to *tamoxifen* (widely used for breast cancer) and another common chemotherapy drug (*doxorubicin*) by suppressing production of the hormone melatonin, which is needed for the drugs to work properly.

If you take tamoxifen or doxorubicin: Keep your bedroom completely dark at night, or wear a sleep mask.

Steven M. Hill, PhD, codirector, Circadian Cancer Biology Group, Tulane University School of Medicine, New Orleans.

Prevent Breast Cancer Recurrence

Breast cancer survivors have a one in six chance of developing cancer in the other breast.

New animal study: A moderate dose of radiation delivered to the unaffected breast reduces the cancer risk by threefold.

PLoS ONE.

Advanced Breast Cancer Has Nearly Tripled in Young Women

Over the past 30 years in the US, the rate of metastatic breast cancer in women under age 40 has increased from about 250 cases in 1976 to about 850 cases in 2009. Researchers are now trying to determine why.

Study of 936,497 women who had breast cancer from 1976 to 2009 by researchers at Seattle Children's Hospital, published in *The Journal of the American Medical Association.*

PBJ Is OK!

Young girls who eat peanut butter reduce their risk of developing benign breast disease. Eating peanut butter or nuts three days a week between the ages of nine and 15 lowered the risk for breast disease by 39% 15 years later. Benign breast disease—noncancerous changes in the breast tissue—affects about one-fourth of all women and is considered a risk factor for later development of breast cancer.

Graham Colditz, MD, DrPh, associate director for cancer prevention and control, Alvin J. Siteman Cancer Center and professor of medicine, Washington University School of Medicine, both in St. Louis, and leader of a study of 9,039 schoolgirls, published in *Breast Cancer Research and Treatment*.

4 New (and Delicious) Cancer-Fighting Foods

Alice G. Bender, MS, RDN, associate director for nutrition programs at the American Institute for Cancer Research (AICR), a nonprofit organization that analyzes research and educates the public on the links between diet, physical exercise, weight loss and the prevention of cancer. *AICR.org*

Researchers are continually investigating foods that may help prevent cancer. But which ones have the strongest evidence?

The American Institute for Cancer Research (AICR), a nonprofit group that keeps tabs on cancer and diet research, recently identified the following foods as being among those having the strongest scientific evidence for fighting cancer.*

Pumpkin

Under the hard rind, orange pumpkin flesh is rich in carotenoids such as beta-carotene,

*The studies cited in this article are only a small portion of the research supporting these cancer-fighting foods. The AICR and its international panel of experts review a much larger spectrum of research.

alpha-carotene, lutein and zeaxanthin. A high intake of foods containing carotenoids has been linked to a lower incidence of many cancers, including those of the esophagus, mouth and larynx. Scientists have recently uncovered another protective compound in pumpkins—*cucurmosin*, a protein that has been shown to slow the growth of pancreatic cancer cells.

Smart idea: Eat pumpkin (plain, canned pumpkin is a convenient option) and the seeds.

What to do: Eat a handful of pumpkin seeds (store-bought are fine) daily as a snack. To prepare your own, rinse fresh seeds in water, air-dry, add a touch of oil and bake at 350°F for 10 to 20 minutes.

Grapefruit

Grapefruit is a rich source of dietary fiber and vitamin C. The pink and red varieties also contain carotenoids (such as beta-carotene and lycopene) that decrease the DNA damage that can lead to cancer.

Scientific evidence: Strong research shows that foods like grapefruit help reduce risk for colorectal cancer. Other evidence suggests that it reduces risk for such malignancies as those of the esophagus, mouth, lung and stomach.

Helpful: Put red or pink grapefruit slices in a green salad with avocado. The tart grapefruit and creamy avocado are delicious together—and the fat in the avocado boosts the absorption of lycopene.

Caution: Grapefruit contains *furanocoumarins*, compounds that block a liver enzyme that breaks down some medications. (More than 85 medications interact with grapefruit, including cholesterol-lowering statins.) If you're thinking about eating more grapefruit and currently take one or more medications, talk to your doctor first.

Apples

An apple a day is good for you—but two may be even better!

Hazardous Hair Dyes

Exposure to toluidines and other potential carcinogens in dye and perm products could explain the higher risk for bladder cancer in hairdressers. Always wear gloves when using these products.

British Medical Journal.

Scientific evidence: In a study published in the *European Journal of Cancer Prevention*, people who ate an apple a day had a 35% lower risk for colorectal cancer—and those who ate two or more apples had a 50% lower risk.

Apples are protective because they contain several anticancer nutrients (many of them found in the peel), including fiber, vitamin C and flavonoids such as quercetin and kaempferol—plant compounds that have stopped the growth of cancer in cellular and animal studies. Research does not specify any particular type of apple as being more protective, so enjoy your favorite variety.

A quick and easy apple dessert: Core an apple, stuff it with raisins and cinnamon, top the stuffing with one tablespoon of apple cider or water, cover the apple with waxed paper and microwave for two minutes.

Mushrooms (Used in a Surprising Way)

When it comes to preventing cancer with diet, it's not only what you eat—it's also what you don't eat.

Scientific evidence: The evidence is convincing that eating too much red meat is linked to colorectal cancer. The AICR recommends eating no more than 18 ounces a week of cooked red meat (such as beef, pork and lamb).

A cancer-fighting meal extender: An easy, delicious way to lower your intake of red meat is to replace some of it in recipes with mushrooms. They're a perfect meat extender, with a savory, meaty taste and texture.

What to do: In a recipe that uses ground meat, replace one-third to one-half of the meat with chopped or diced mushrooms.

In a recent study, people who substituted one cup of white button mushrooms a day for one cup of lean ground beef consumed 123 fewer daily calories and lost an average of seven pounds after one year.

If you're heavier than you should be, losing weight means decreasing cancer risk—the AICR estimates that 122,000 yearly cases of cancer could be prevented if Americans weren't overweight or obese.

Cancer Risk You Can Prevent

Prediabetes is linked to a 15% higher risk for cancer overall. Prediabetes, which is increasingly common, is indicated by a blood sugar level between 100 mg/dL and 125 mg/dL. Prediabetes is associated with a 100% higher risk for liver cancer...60% for endometrial cancer...55%, stomach/colorectal cancer...19%, pancreatic cancer...and 19%, breast cancer (see page 45 for more). It does not increase risk for bladder, kidney, lung, ovarian or prostate cancer.

Self-defense: Cut blood sugar levels with diet and exercise.

Joel Zonszein, MD, professor of clinical medicine at Albert Einstein College of Medicine and director of the Clinical Diabetes Center at Montifiore Medical Center, the Bronx, New York.

Diabetes Medications That Lower Cancer Risk

In a recent finding, women with type 2 diabetes taking insulin sensitizers, including the diabetes medication *metformin* (Glucophage), or thiazolidinediones, such as *pioglitazone* (Actos), had 21% lower risk for cancer than women taking insulin secretagogues. Insulin secretagogues include sulfonylureas, such as *glimepiride* (Amaryl), and meglitinides, such as *nateglinide* (Starlix).

Sangeeta Kashyap, MD, endocrinologist and associate professor of medicine at the Cleveland Clinic's Endocrinology & Metabolism Institute. She is lead author of a study published in *Diabetes, Obesity and Metabolism*.

Ob-Gyns: Use Ultrasound to Assess Pelvic Symptoms

Beryl Benacerraf, MD, clinical professor in obstetrics, gynecology and reproductive biology and radiology at Harvard Medical School and Brigham and Women's Hospital, Boston.
Steven Goldstein, MD, professor of obstetrics and gynecology at New York University School of Medicine.
American Journal of Obstetrics & Gynecology, news release.

Ultrasound should be the first type of imaging used to assess pelvic symptoms in women, a group of U.S. experts says.

Background

Currently, many women with pelvic pain, masses or flank pain first undergo CT scans, and sometimes MRIs, noted lead author Beryl Benacerraf, MD, who is also a clinical professor in obstetrics, gynecology and reproductive biology and radiology at Harvard Medical School and Brigham and Women's Hospital in Boston.

CT and MRI Versus Ultrasound

However, CT scans and MRIs of the pelvis often result in unclear findings that require further clarification using ultrasound, she said.

Moreover, the growing use of CT raises safety concerns, added article co-author Steven Goldstein, MD, professor of obstetrics and gynecology at NYU School of Medicine.

"The use of CT scans has tripled since 1993," Dr. Goldstein said, noting that radiation associated with CT may pose a cancer risk.

It's estimated that 29,000 future cancers could be related to CT done in the United States in 2007 alone, Dr. Goldstein added. And nearly half of those predicted cancers were attributed to CT of the pelvis and abdomen, he said.

"For example, patients with suspected kidney stones frequently have a CT scan first, despite the associated radiation burden. In a recent study, most of the patients evaluated first by ultrasound did not ultimately need a CT scan, sparing radiation exposure," Dr. Goldstein noted.

Ultrasound imaging uses sound waves rather than radiation.

Conclusion

Ultrasound is safer and more cost-effective than other types of imaging for diagnosing pelvic symptoms, the team of obstetricians and gynecologists concluded in an article published in the *American Journal of Obstetrics & Gynecology*.

They support an American Institute of Ultrasound in Medicine initiative called Ultrasound First, which urges doctors to use ultrasound when evidence shows that it is equally, if not more, effective compared to other imaging methods for the area on the patient's body that requires examination.

"This recommendation applies particularly to obstetric and gynecologic patients. A skillfully performed and well-interpreted ultrasound usually eliminates the need to perform additional more costly and complex cross-sectional imaging techniques," said Dr. Benacerraf.

The U.S. National Institute of Child Health and Human Development has more information about pelvic pain at *www.nichd.nih.gov/health/topics/pelvicpain*.

Cervical Cancer Is More Common

Cervical cancer is much more common than previously reported. Earlier estimates included women who had had hysterectomies. When they were excluded from the statistics, the actual rate of cervical cancer rose to 18.6 cases per 100,000 women. The US Preventive Services Task Force recommends that women ages 21 to 65 have a Pap smear every three years...and women ages 30 to 65 be tested for HPV every five years.

Anne F. Rositch, PhD, MSPH, assistant professor in the department of epidemiology and public health at University of Maryland School of Medicine, Baltimore.

Use of the Pill Tied to Higher Risk for Rare Brain Cancer

David Gaist, MD, PhD, professor, department of neurology, Odense University Hospital, Odense, Denmark.
Evan Myers, MD, MPH, professor of obstetrics and gynecology, division of clinical and epidemiological research, department of obstetrics & gynecology, Duke University Medical Center, Durham, North Carolina.
British Journal of Clinical Pharmacology, online.

The risk for developing a rare form of brain cancer known as glioma appears to go up with long-term use of hormonal contraceptives such as the Pill, new Danish research suggests.

Women under 50 with a glioma "were 90% more likely to have been using hormonal contraceptives for five years or more, compared with women from the general population with no history of brain tumor," said study leader David Gaist, MD, PhD.

How Large a Concern Is Glioma?

However, the Danish study couldn't prove cause-and-effect, and Dr. Gaist stressed that the findings "need to be put in context" for women because "glioma is very rare."

Only five out of every 100,000 Danish women between the ages of 15 and 49 develop the condition each year, according to Dr. Gaist, a professor of neurology at Odense University Hospital. He said that figure in-

cludes women who take contraceptives such as the birth control pill.

So, "an overall risk-benefit evaluation favors continued use of hormonal contraceptives," Dr. Gaist said.

The findings were published online in the *British Journal of Clinical Pharmacology*.

Study Details

In the study, Dr. Gaist's team looked at government data on all Danish women between the ages of 15 and 49 who had developed a glioma between 2000 and 2009.

In all, investigators identified 317 glioma cases, among whom nearly 60% had used a contraceptive at some point. They then compared them to more than 2,100 glioma-free women of similar ages, about half of whom had used contraceptives.

Use of the Pill or other hormonal contraceptive did appear to bump up the risk for glioma, the researchers reported, and the risk seemed to rise with the duration of use.

For example, women who had used any type of hormonal birth control for less than one year had a 40% greater risk for glioma compared with non-users. And those who had used the drug for five years or more saw their risk nearly double compared to non-users, the findings showed.

In addition, Dr. Gaist's team found that glioma risk seemed to go up most sharply for women who had used contraceptives containing the hormone progestogen, rather than estrogen.

Expert Comment

Evan Myers, MD, MPH, is a professor of obstetrics and gynecology at Duke University Medical Center in Durham, North Carolina. He described the Danish study as "really well-done."

However, he stressed that the study couldn't prove a cause-and-effect relationship between hormonal contraception use and risk for glioma. Dr. Myers also suggested that future research focus on a number of indirect factors—such as the progesterone found in some types of IUDs (intrauterine devices)—that might also play a critical role in driving up glioma risk.

And in the end, "even if hormonal contraception does increase the relative risk of glioma, the absolute risk—the actual increase in the chances of having a glioma diagnosed—is quite small," Dr. Myers stressed.

According to his own statistical breakdown, Dr. Myers said that between 2000 and 2011, glioma affected less than two out of every 100,000 American women between the ages of 15 and 29.

"To put that in perspective," he said, "that's about one-tenth the risk of death from trauma in women aged 15 to 44, and a little over twice the risk of dying from a complication of pregnancy."

Dr. Myers said his number crunching suggests an even lower risk profile when looking specifically at women who are taking the Pill or another form of hormonal contraception.

"Without going through the math, it's about 8.5 [cases of glioma] per million" for that subset of women, Dr. Myers said.

The American Brain Tumor Association has more on gliomas at *http://www.abta.org/ brain-tumor-information/types-of-tumors/ glioma.html.*

Study Finds Most Uterine Cancers Are Preventable

Regular physical activity—at least 30 minutes a day—and maintaining a healthy weight can prevent nearly 60% of cancers of the lining of the uterus, a recent study reports. Dietary choices also matter—drinking one cup of coffee a day, regular or decaf, can reduce risk by 7%…but eating lots of sugary foods and processed grains can raise cancer risk.

Study published by American Institute for Cancer Research and World Cancer Research Fund International.

Advisers Endorse HPV Test for Cervical Cancer Checks

Society of Gynecologic Oncology, news release. American College of Obstetricians and Gynecologists.

An HPV test recently approved by U.S. health officials is an effective way to check for cervical cancer, according to two leading women's health organizations.

The groups said the HPV test is an effective, one-test alternative to the current recommendation of screening with either a Pap test alone or a combination of the HPV test and a Pap test.

The American Cancer Society estimates 12,900 new cases of invasive cervical cancer diagnoses in 2015, and about 4,100 women will die from the disease.

According to the cancer society, cervical cancer was once a leading cause of cancer death for American women. But in the last three decades the death rate has dropped more than 50%. The Pap test is the big reason cited for the decline.

Not all experts are in agreement with the single-test decision. The largest ob-gyn group in the United States, the American College of Obstetricians & Gynecologists (ACOG) is still recommending that women aged 30 to 65 be screened using either the Pap test alone, or "co-tested" with a combination of both the HPV test and a Pap test.

The new, so-called interim guidance report was issued by two other groups—the Society of Gynecologic Oncology and the American Society for Colposcopy and Cervical Pathology. It followed U.S. Food and Drug Administration approval in 2014 of the Cobas HPV test as a primary test for cervical cancer screening.

The HPV test detects DNA from 14 types of HPV—a sexually transmitted virus that includes types 16 and 18, which cause 70% of cervical cancers.

The two medical groups said the interim guidance report will help health care providers determine how best to include primary HPV testing in the care of their female patients until a number of medical societies update their guidelines for cervical cancer screening.

"Our review of the data indicates that primary HPV testing misses less pre-cancer and cancer than cytology [a Pap test] alone. The guidance panel felt that primary HPV screening can be considered as an option for women being screened for cervical cancer," interim guidance report lead author Dr. Warner Huh said in a news release from the Society of Gynecologic Oncology. Dr. Huh is director of the University of Alabama's Division of Gynecologic Oncology

The FDA approved the Cobas HPV test in April 2014 as a first step in cervical cancer screening for women aged 25 and older. Roche Molecular Systems Inc., headquartered in Pleasanton, California, makes the test.

The recent interim report recommends that primary HPV testing should be considered starting at age 25. For women younger than 25, current guidelines recommending a Pap test alone beginning at age 21 should be followed.

The new recommendations also state that women with a negative result for a primary HPV test should not be tested again for three years, which is the same interval recommended for a normal Pap test result. An HPV test that is positive for HPV 16 and 18 should be followed with colposcopy, a procedure in which the cervix is examined under illumination and magnification.

"The introduction of cervical cytology screening [the Pap test] was truly one of the great breakthroughs in medicine, and has saved countless lives," Dr. Herschel Lawson, chief medical officer at the American Society for Colposcopy and Cervical Pathology, said in the news release.

"We are lucky that we have so many tools available now to improve cervical cancer prevention efforts and afford patients options depending on their individual situations.

We'll continue to work to find the best way to combine screening tools with other prevention efforts like HPV vaccines, for the early detection and treatment of cervical cancer," he said.

"The most important message for providers and the community is that women should be screened for cervical cancer. Screening saves lives," Dr. Lawson added.

However, experts at ACOG said Thursday that it's too early to move to an HPV test-only screening model. They are standing by their recommendation for a combination of the HPV test and the Pap smear.

The reason? HPV infection is common among younger women, and often resolves on its own, so a positive test result might lead to too many invasive follow-up tests. While it's possible that the HPV test "can" replace the Pap smear altogether, there's not enough evidence at this time to say that it "should," ACOG said.

HPV is thought to cause the majority of cervical cancers. Certain strains, such as HPV 16 and 18, are most strongly tied to these tumors. The virus also causes genital warts in both men and women and certain head and neck cancers.

The interim guidance report was published online in the journals Gynecologic Oncology, the *Journal of Lower Genital Tract Disease and Obstetrics and Gynecology*.

The U.S. National Cancer Institute has more about cervical cancer screening at *http://www.cancer.gov/cancertopics/pdq/screening/cervical/Patient/page3*.

Poor Oral Health Is Linked to Higher Rates of Human Papillomavirus (HPV)

People with swollen gums, mouth sores, missing teeth and other indicators of poor oral health are more likely to be infected during oral sex with the virus, which can cause cancers of the cervix, mouth and throat.

Study of 3,489 people by researchers at The University of Texas Health Science Center at Houston, published in *Cancer Prevention Research.*

Mouthwash and Dentures Linked to Increased Risk of Oral Cancer

Study titled, "Oral health, dental care and mouthwash associated with upper aerodigestive tract cancer risk in Europe: The ARCAGE study," published in *Oral Oncology.*

You wouldn't dream of leaving the house in the morning or going to bed at night without brushing your teeth. And ideally, you give your pearly whites a good daily flossing, too. But if you're also accustomed to swishing some mouthwash—to sweeten your breath, whiten your teeth, fight infection or make your mouth "feel really clean"—it's important that you take two specific precautions.

Another alert: If you're a denture wearer, you also need to be on guard. *Here's why…*

Researchers Sink Their Teeth Into the Data

For a recent study, researchers from nine European countries interviewed nearly 2,000 men and women who had been recently diagnosed with oral cancer—malignancies of the mouth, larynx (voice box), pharynx (throat) or esophagus. For comparison's sake, they also interviewed a similar number of age-matched but cancer-free people who served as controls.

All of the participants were asked about various lifestyle and dietary habits…their oral hygiene habits…and their medical and dental history. When the researchers analyzed this data (and adjusted for smoking and alcohol consumption, two known risk factors for oral cancers), they came to some predictable conclusions—for instance, that failing to brush teeth twice daily or to visit the dentist at least annually was associated with significantly increased risk for oral cancer. *But they also found two surprising risk factors…*

• **Wearing dentures.** Even partial dentures were associated with increased risk. And people who wore complete upper and lower dentures had nearly double the risk of people who did not wear dentures. Oral cancer risk was especially high among those who started wearing dentures before they were 55 years old.

• **Frequent use of mouthwash.** Compared with people who did not use mouthwash, those who rinsed their mouths with mouthwash three or more times each day had about triple the risk for oral cancer. However, there was no increased risk found among people who used mouthwash less frequently than three times a day.

Noteworthy: Unfortunately, this study did not distinguish between mouthwash that contained alcohol and mouthwash without alcohol. Some previous, smaller studies suggested that both alcohol-containing and alcohol-free mouthwash may increase oral cancer risk, but other studies found increased risk only with mouthwashes that contain alcohol…and as pointed out previously, alcohol is a known carcinogen.

Double jeopardy: For people who both wore dentures and used mouthwash three or more times daily, the risk for oral cancer was multiplied more than seven times!

For optimal oral health…

• **Clean your teeth well every day.**

• **Visit your dentist two or more times each year.**

• **If you are a fan of mouthwash,** there's probably no need to stop using it altogether—but it may be wise to stick with brands that are alcohol-free and limit your swishing to no more than once or twice a day.

• **What if you have dentures?** You can't change that—but you can be extra vigilant about watching for possible signs of oral cancer, such as a slightly raised white or red patch in the mouth…an unexplained lump in the neck…discomfort on one side of the throat…subtle changes in voice…unexplained and persistent ear pain…or difficulty or mild pain with swallowing. Remember, as with many diseases, the earlier oral cancer is caught and treated, the better the outcome generally is.

Blood Pressure Medicines Can Cause Lip Cancer

Some common blood pressure drugs, including the diuretic *hydrochlorothiazide*, the calcium channel blocker *nifedipine* and the ACE inhibitor *lisinopril*, increase sun sensitivity and can make users more likely to develop lip cancer. But lip cancer is rare, curable and rarely spreads—in most cases, the drugs' benefits outweigh the risk.

Study comparing 712 patients with lip cancer who were taking blood pressure drugs with 22,904 people who did not have lip cancer by researchers at Kaiser Permanente Northern California Division of Research, published in *Archives of Internal Medicine*.

Ovarian Drug Shrinks Tumors

New ovarian cancer drug shrinks tumors for eight months, on average. Lynparza (*olaparib*) is for women who have received at least three rounds of chemotherapy for advanced ovarian cancer associated with abnormal inherited BRCA genes. Trials are ongoing.

Edward J. Pavlik, PhD, director of the ovarian screening research program, Markey Cancer Center, Lexington, Kentucky.

Irregular Periods Can Mean a High Cancer Risk

Women with irregular periods may have double the risk for ovarian cancer, compared with women who have regular monthly periods.

Best: If you have irregular periods or if you have a condition called polycystic ovarian syndrome, ask your doctor if you should be screened for ovarian cancer.

Study of more than 14,000 women led by Barbara A. Cohn, PhD, MPH, director of Child Health and Development Studies at the Public Health Institute in Oakland, California, presented at the annual meeting of the American Association for Cancer Research, San Diego.

Vitamin B-12 and Cancer

A new study found that people with elevated vitamin B-12 levels (above 800 pg/mL) had an increased risk for such cancers as leukemia and malignancies of the lung or bladder. None of the study participants were taking B-12 supplements.

Theory: Elevated B-12 levels may result from some not-yet-identified cancer-related process. If your blood work consistently indicates higher-than-normal levels of vitamin

B-12: Discuss your cancer risk with your doctor.

Johan Arendt, researcher, Aarhus University Hospital, Denmark.

Better Screening for Lung Cancer

New risk-calculating software that was used when reading the CT scans of nearly 2,700 current or former smokers predicted with more than 90% accuracy which nodules were benign or malignant.

Implication: After an initial CT scan, doctors can now better determine what type of follow-up is needed—a second CT scan, biopsy or surgery.

If you need a CT scan to screen for lung cancer: Your doctor can use the risk-calculating spreadsheet at Brocku.ca/Lung-Cancer-Risk-Calculator.

Stephen Lam, MD, professor of medicine, The University of British Columbia, Vancouver, Canada.

Better Way to Detect Pancreatic Cancer

Pancreatic cancer has an overall five-year survival rate of 6%, partly because it causes few symptoms in the early stages.

New study: Genetic biomarkers for pancreatic cancer were found in 90% of adults in the early stages of the disease but not in those who did not have it. Until the new test becomes available in a few years, be sure your doctor knows if you're at increased risk for pancreatic cancer due to family history, obesity and/or smoking.

Nita Ahuja, MD, associate professor of surgery, The Johns Hopkins University School of Medicine, Baltimore.

New Urine Test Predicts Bladder Cancer Recurrence

A urine test that measures genetic biomarkers was 80% successful in predicting when bladder cancer would return in a recent study of 90 cancer survivors. Current tests, which include biopsy and cystoscopy, are 15% to 35% successful in predicting cancer recurrence. The new urine test may become available in the next year or two. To participate in a clinical trial for this urine test, go to *ClinicalTrials.gov*.

Gangning Liang, PhD, associate professor of urology, USC Norris Comprehensive Cancer Center, Los Angeles.

Do Statins Help or Harm Thyroid Cancer Risk?

Study titled "Statin use and thyroid cancer: a population-based case-control study" from the department of otolaryngology, Taipei Medical University, Taiwan, published in *Clinical Endocrinology*.

Do statin drugs lower your risk for certain kinds of cancer? Some doctors think they do. But when a group of Taiwanese researchers recently looked at statin use and a particular kind of common cancer—something never examined before—their findings were especially alarming for women.

The Thyroid Cancer Connection

Researchers from Taipei Medical University reviewed Taiwan's health insurance database to find 500 people in whom thyroid cancer had been diagnosed between 2008 and 2011. They compared each person with five people of the same age and gender who didn't have thyroid cancer. Then, the researchers looked through the medical insurance records of all of these people to see who was ever given a prescription for a statin and how often they took it. They also examined whether high cholesterol itself might be associated with development of thyroid cancer.

The results. The odds of getting thyroid cancer were 40% higher in women who were "regular" statin users—defined as people who were on statins for at least 60 days within six months of getting the cancer diagnosis. Men who regularly used statins and people who used them less often than regularly had no increased risk of thyroid cancer. The researchers could not explain why women were affected and men not.

Cause for Concern?

The role of statins in the development of colorectal, breast and prostate cancers and leukemia has already been studied, with some studies showing that statins decrease the risk of certain cancers and others suggesting that statins have no effect on cancer risk. Although more studies need to be done to better clarify whether statin use puts a person at higher risk for thyroid cancer, the new study's findings are yet another reason to consider alternatives when a doctor suggests you take a statin—especially if you are a woman.

Thyroid Cancer: An Epidemic of Disease... Or Overdiagnosis?

Juan Pablo Brito, MBBS, assistant professor and Health Care Delivery Scholar, division of endocrinology, diabetes, metabolism and nutrition, and coinvestigator of the Knowledge and Evaluation Research Unit, Mayo Clinic, Rochester, Minnesota. Dr. Brito's recent study on thyroid cancer was published in *BMJ*.

Put the word cancer after anything—brain cancer...pancreatic cancer...lung cancer—and it raises everyone's level of alert, especially when a particular cancer appears to be on the rise. But the alert that centers around thyroid cancer isn't really about an epidemic of the disease itself.

Coffee: More Good News

An analysis of more than 3,000 adults found that drinking one to three cups of caffeinated coffee daily reduced liver cancer risk by at least 40%.

Theory: Coffee has been shown to reduce the risk for diabetes, which has been linked to liver cancer.

Carlo La Vecchia, MD, head of epidemiology, Istituto di Ricerche Farmacologiche Mario Negri, Milan, Italy.

Instead, what has many experts worried is a possible epidemic of overdiagnosis and overtreatment.

Why are they so concerned? Because most people diagnosed with thyroid cancer will never even develop symptoms, much less have their lives threatened by the disease. Yet they are being treated with surgery, radiation and/or medication—treatments that carry serious risks of their own. There's also considerable expense, inconvenience and anxiety associated with the diagnosis and treatment...all of which could be completely unnecessary in a significant number of cases.

Will you or a loved one wind up being pushed down that path? You could be, given that thyroid cancer is now the most commonly diagnosed endocrine cancer in the US. *Here's what you should know before that happens...*

Looking at the Numbers

The thyroid cancer diagnosis rate in this country has nearly tripled since 1975, going from 4.9 cases per 100,000 people to about 14.3 per 100,000 people. But despite the massive increase in the rate of people diagnosed with the disease, the rate of people dying from thyroid cancer hasn't changed at all over the same time period.

You might assume that the explanation is that thyroid cancer treatment has improved so much over the past 30-plus years that essentially all of the additional cases have been successfully treated. But in fact, the treatment for thyroid cancer is pretty much the same as it has been. So the more likely explanation is a dramatic rise in diagnosis—or, as many experts now caution, in overdiagnosis. *Here's why...*

The numbers, the risks: More than 60,000 people will be diagnosed with thyroid cancer in the US this year, with women outnumbering men three to one. Almost all of these patients will have surgery to remove their thyroid glands, which carries a risk for nerve damage that can lead to permanent hoarseness or weak voice...and requires them to take medication for the rest of their lives to replace the hormones their thyroid glands previously produced. In addition, many of these patients will be given radioactive iodine to conquer any remaining thyroid cancer cells—a treatment that can cause dry eyes and altered taste and more than quintuple the risk of developing leukemia.

Those risks would be worth it if the treatments saved lives. But most of these patients would not have died of thyroid cancer anyway!

Evidence: Studies involving autopsies have shown that thyroid cancer is detected in as many as one in three people who died from any other cause, yet in the US, thyroid cancer accounts for only about one in every 200,000 deaths overall! This means that the number of people who die with thyroid cancer—but not because of it—is staggering.

Not All Thyroid Cancers Are Created Equal

As cancers go, thyroid cancer is one of the least deadly, claiming fewer than 1,900 lives in the US each year. *There are four different types of thyroid cancer...*

•**Papillary cancer accounts for 85% of cases and has an excellent prognosis,** with 98% of patients alive 20 years after diagnosis.

•**Follicular cancer accounts** for 11% of cases and has a 10-year survival rate of more than 95% in patients younger than age 40 at diagnosis.

•**Medullary cancer accounts for 3% of cases.** It has a 10-year survival rate of 75% for those under age 40 at diagnosis, and 50% rate for older patients.

•**Anaplastic cancer accounts for just 1% of cases.** It is the most aggressive type, with a one-year survival rate of 20%.

What's Really Driving the Increase?

Papillary cancer (the least dangerous type) that is driving the increase in thyroid cancer diagnosis.

Rates of the other forms of cancer have barely changed. *There are several likely reasons why more papillary cancers are being found...*

•**More doctors are screening for the disease,** looking for cancer in people with no symptoms. During a routine exam, the doctor might examine the patient's neck, feeling for thyroid nodules (solid or fluid-filled lumps within the thyroid gland), which are common. When the doctor's fingers find a nodule, he then schedules an ultrasound to get a better look at it, and then perhaps a biopsy is taken with a needle. Thyroid cancer is found in about 10% of people with nodules.

•**Thyroid nodules and cancers also are detected incidentally,** during an imaging test for another condition—and these imaging tests are being done more and more often. For example, a CT exam of the chest or an ultrasound of the carotid artery can easily pick up a tiny two-millimeter nodule in the neck. Such incidental findings explain, at least partially, why nearly 40% of thyroid cancers now being found are smaller than one centimeter across (technically called microcarcinomas)...whereas back in 1989, just 25% of known papillary cancers were smaller than one centimeter.

The diagnostic cascade also explains some of the increased incidence.

Example: A patient tells her doctor that she's feeling sluggish and gaining weight. The doctor's endocrine antenna goes up, and he suspects that an underactive thyroid

New Colon Cancer Test

•**The FDA has approved Cologuard, a noninvasive screening test for colorectal cancer for adults over age 50.** The new test screens stool samples for red blood cells and DNA mutations that may indicate the presence of cancer or precancerous growths. In a recent study of more than 10,000 adults, Cologuard detected more cancers and more advanced adenomas than the fecal occult blood test that is widely used in annual physicals. Routine colonoscopies are still recommended.

N. Jewel Samadder, MD, assistant professor of gastroenterology and hepatology, University of Utah School of Medicine, Salt Lake City.

•**New colorectal-cancer test is covered by Medicare.** The Cologuard test studies a patient's stool sample to see if there is DNA that suggests precancerous polyps or colorectal cancer. People who don't have symptoms of colon cancer can have the Cologuard test once every three years at no cost. It is covered under Medicare Part B for people who are 50 to 85 years old…show no signs or symptoms of colorectal disease… and are at average risk for colorectal cancer, which means no personal or family history of cancer, inflammatory bowel disease, adenomatous polyps or certain other conditions.

Medicare.gov.

with a family history of thyroid cancer…those who had previous head or neck exposure to radiation from, for instance, medical radiation therapy or heavy industrial exposure (not just dental X-rays)…or those in whom the lymph nodes or ultrasound of the neck seem particularly suspicious. For patients who meet one of these exceptions and for those with larger nodules, a biopsy is recommended.

If the biopsy reveals cancer, the patient is sent for surgery. For some, what's recommended is a total thyroidectomy (removal of the entire thyroid gland)…or, for some patients with the low-risk papillary cancer, what's suggested according to the guidelines is a partial thyroidectomy (removal of just the part of the thyroid with the nodule).

Despite these guidelines, however, many patients who are candidates for partial thyroidectomy instead opt for the complete thyroidectomy. Perhaps they feel nervous when they hear the word cancer and think, Take out the whole darn thing! And then they risk the treatment complications described previously. These patients would be better able to make informed choices if they understood the extremely low likelihood of ever developing symptoms or dying from thyroid cancer.

No one is suggesting that we simply ignore papillary cancer. *But to cut back on overdiagnosis and overtreatment, we need…*

•**Risk assessment.** Doctors need better tools to identify which papillary cancers carry higher risks so they can send the right patients—rather than all of them—to the operating room. The signs that should raise the level of alert, especially in a patient with a family history of thyroid cancer, include a visible, palpable mass…radiation exposure during childhood…difficulty swallowing…a change in the voice…and certain features found during an ultrasound.

•**Large studies.** Clinical trials showing what happens when people with small, low-risk papillary cancers choose to skip surgery and instead adopt an active surveillance ("watchful waiting") approach, similar to what's often done with prostate cancer, are needed in the US. In one study from Japan,

gland is causing those vague symptoms. If a lump is felt in the thyroid or seen on an ultrasound, the doctor might order a biopsy, and then the results might show papillary cancer—even though the patient's thyroid may have had absolutely nothing to do with the fatigue and weight gain.

Scared Patients Ignoring Guidelines?

The American Thyroid Association recommends against biopsies for thyroid nodules smaller than a centimeter, except for people patients with papillary microcarcinoma did not have surgery, but instead were followed with annual or biannual ultrasounds and measurements of blood markers for thyroid disease. Over the next 10 years, the tumors actually shrank in some patients. One-third of the participants ended up having thyroidectomies, mainly because their tumors had grown—but none of these patients had a recurrence of cancer after surgery and there were no deaths.

• **Renaming.** Many experts think that it would be appropriate to call small, low-risk papillary tumors something other than cancer—to reduce the anxiety that comes with a cancer diagnosis and the subsequent overtreatment. A name such as papillary lesions of indolent course (PLIC) might enable less emotionally charged conversations about the benefits and harms of the various treatment options. There's precedent for this. Such renaming has already occurred with other "cancers," he pointed out—for instance, what is now known as cervical intraepithelial neoplasia used to be lumped together with full-blown cervical cancer.

Self-defense: If you have a thyroid nodule or a small, low-risk papillary cancer, you do not need to rush into treatment. Thoroughly discuss the pros and cons with your doctor—show him this article, if you need to, to get his full attention on the matter—and consider getting a second opinion from a thyroid cancer specialist.

Danger After a Colonoscopy

Karen Larson, editor of *Bottom Line/Personal*. BottomLinePersonal.com

What's the best part of a colonoscopy? When it's over, of course. But for one of my colleagues, the end of a colonoscopy was just the start of a medical misadventure—she fainted two days after the procedure and wound up in the emergency room due to dehydration.

That's not uncommon, says Leo Galland, MD, founder and director of the Foundation for Integrated Medicine in New York City. The incident points to a troubling gap in colonoscopy communication—patients are told how to prepare for this procedure but often not what they should do afterward. *Dr. Galland's advice...*

• **Drink eight to 16 ounces of fruit juice right after the procedure.** Ask if the health facility will have juice. If not, bring your own. Any beverage will help with dehydration, but fruit juice also wards off hypoglycemia—low blood sugar. Drink another 48 ounces of fluid during the day and 64 ounces the day after.

• **Eat a light snack as soon as you feel able.** Bring a sandwich or an energy bar with you to the health facility, too. Avoid foods with high fat content—fats are difficult to digest.

• **Take a probiotic supplement.** Take one just before your first meal following the procedure and twice a day for the next 10 days at the start of a meal. Consuming probiotics can reduce bowel irritation and promote good overall digestive health. Try a few different ones well before your colonoscopy to find one that seems to aid your digestion.

Women Who Smoke Are At Greater Risk for Colon Cancer Than Men Who Smoke

In a recent finding, women who smoked or who had ever smoked had nearly 20% higher risk for colon cancer than women who never smoked. Men who smoked had an 8% higher risk for colon cancer than men who never smoked.

Study of data on more than 600,000 people ages 19 to 67 over 14 years by researchers in the department of community medicine, University of Tromsø, Norway, published in *Cancer Epidemiology, Biomarkers & Prevention.*

Colon Cancer Alert

Using current screening guidelines, about one in 10 colon malignancies was missed among people with a family history of advanced colon polyps (precursors of colon cancer), in a recent study.

If you have a first-degree relative (a parent, sibling or child) who had advanced polyps diagnosed at any age: Talk to your doctor about getting screened more often than the current recommendation (once every five years beginning at age 40).

N. Jewel Samadder, MD, assistant professor of medicine, Huntsman Cancer Institute, University of Utah, Salt Lake City.

Alcohol: The Drink That's Linked to Deadly Melanoma Skin Cancer

Study titled "Alcohol drinking and cutaneous melanoma risk—A systematic review and dose-risk meta-analysis," to be published in *British Journal of Dermatology.*

You know that cavorting in the sun without adequate protection from clothing and sunscreen is a big mistake when it comes to preventing melanoma...and you know that this kind of skin cancer can kill. But did you know that what you drink affects your melanoma risk, too? When it comes to alcohol, it's true—in fact, your skin cancer risk rises with as little as one serving of alcohol a day, according to new research. *Here's the startling connection...*

Imbibers Beware

It's well-established that the leading cause of melanoma is intermittent, intense, sunburn-causing exposure to the sun's ultraviolet rays. Even sunburns from childhood can come back to haunt you decades later, increasing your skin cancer risk. But other factors (a fair complexion, the presence of moles, advancing age, etc.) enter into the risk equation, too...and researchers decided to see whether alcohol also played a role. To that end, they conducted a meta-analysis, pulling together 16 previous studies that investigated a possible relationship between alcohol consumption and melanoma. The data they examined represented a total of 6,251 cases of this type of skin cancer.

Because the various studies used different measures to describe levels of alcohol consumption, the researchers looked at the grams of ethanol consumed each day, designating one drink as 12.5 grams of ethanol. (For comparison's sake, in the US, one drink is generally defined as 14 grams of ethanol—the equivalent of a 12-ounce beer, a five-ounce glass of wine or a 1.5-ounce shot of 80-proof liquor.) For the new study, light drinking was defined as no more than 12.5 grams of ethanol per day...moderate-to-heavy consumption was defined as anything in excess of 12.5 grams per day. Although there was limited data on heavy drinking, this level of consumption was defined as more than 50 grams of ethanol (four drinks) per day.

What the researchers discovered: Compared with people who never or seldom drank, people who did drink were 20% more likely to get melanoma. As alcohol intake

Fiber-Based Laxatives Are Best

People who regularly use fiber-based laxatives have a 56% lower colorectal cancer risk than people who don't use laxatives. But regular users of nonfiber laxatives have a 49% higher risk. Fiber-based laxatives, which boost the water content and bulk of stool, include Citrucel, Fiberall and Fibercon. Nonfiber or stimulant laxatives, which force the colon to contract, include Correctol, Ex-lax and Dulcolax.

Jessica S. Citronberg, MPH, predoctoral fellow at Fred Hutchinson Cancer Research Center, Seattle, and leader of a study published in *The American Journal of Gastroenterology.*

went up, so did the danger—light drinking was associated with a 10% increase in melanoma risk…moderate-to-heavy drinking was associated with an 18% increase in risk…and heavy drinking was associated with a 55% increase in risk.

What explains the link? You may assume that people who are imbibing at the beach, barbecue or ball game don't want to interrupt their fun, so they don't bother to refresh their sunscreen…or else they're so buzzed that they're oblivious to how sunburned they're getting. And no doubt that plays a part—in fact, other research suggests that nearly one-fifth of sunburns in American adults are attributable to alcohol consumption.

But drunk-induced sunburns don't tell the whole story, the new study's authors suggested.

Their theory: Alcohol intake may reduce the strength of the immune system, allowing the sun's UV rays to do greater harm to cells. That's because soon after ethanol is consumed, it's converted to a substance that makes skin even more sun-sensitive and vulnerable to oxidative stress, which in turn damages DNA and increases cancer risk.

Self-defense for your skin: If you plan to drink alcohol when you're outdoors, you'd be wise to slather on the sunscreen beforehand and wear plenty of protective clothing…set a timer on your watch or phone to remind you to refresh your sunscreen every few hours…and limit alcohol consumption to no more than one drink per day. Need even more motivation? Remember that alcohol is linked to numerous other malignancies, including cancers of the mouth, esophagus, stomach, colon, liver, breast and prostate—so in that regard, what's good for your skin is good for the rest of your body, too.

5 Sunburns = More Risk

If you had five or more blistering sunburns before age 20, watch out. This increases lifetime risk for melanoma by 80%, according

The "20-Mole Test"

If you have a total of 20 or more moles on both your arms, your risk for melanoma is more than six times higher than the risk for people with fewer moles, according to a recent study of more than 2,000 dermatology patients.

Why: Having a lot of arm moles indicates that you may have many on your entire body, raising the risk for DNA changes that can lead to the deadly skin cancer. Only moles were counted—not freckles or age spots.

Giuseppe Argenziano, MD, associate professor of dermatology, Second University of Naples, Caserta, Italy.

to a new study of nearly 109,000 Caucasian women.

Why: Sudden, massive amounts of sun exposure may damage pigment cells in the skin.

If you had many bad sunburns in your youth: Be particularly vigilant about further sun exposure and annual skin exams, which should be performed by a board-certified dermatologist.

Abrar Qureshi, MD, MPH, professor of dermatology, Warren Alpert Medical School, Brown University, Providence.

Don't Ignore That Itch

Pain or itching can be signs of skin cancer, warns Gil Yosipovitch, MD. People often are told to be on the lookout for visual changes to their skin, but it is important not to overlook changes in how skin feels.

Recent findings: More than one-third of skin cancer lesions itch—these can be a sign of basal cell carcinoma. About 30% are painful, and these can indicate squamous cell carcinoma.

Gil Yosipovitch, MD, chair of dermatology at Temple University School of Medicine and director of Temple Itch Center, both in Philadelphia, and leader of a study published in *JAMA Dermatology*.

Advanced Melanoma Treatment Cuts Risk of Death

New immunotherapy for advanced melanoma is now available.

Recent finding: Patients who took *Opdivo* (nivolumab) were 58% less likely to die within one year than patients who used a standard chemotherapy drug. Opdivo, which uses the body's immune system to fight cancer, also has fewer side effects. It was approved by the FDA in March 2015.

Georgina Long, MD, PhD, associate professor of melanoma biology and translational research at Melanoma Institute Australia at University of Sydney. She is coauthor of a study published in *The New England Journal of Medicine.*

Got Cancer? Don't Make All Those Decisions on Your Own

Mitch Golant, PhD, senior consultant for strategic initiatives at the Cancer Support Community and a clinical psychologist in Los Angeles. He helped develop the Open to Options counseling program. Dr. Golant is also coauthor of *The Total Cancer Wellness Guide: Reclaiming Your Life After Diagnosis.*

"You have cancer" are three of the most frightening words a person can hear.

A hidden challenge: While cancer patients are still reeling from the emotions of a potentially life-threatening diagnosis, they are asked to make some of the most important decisions of their lives. Even with the support of loved ones, all the treatment decisions that must be made can feel overwhelming.

Good news: There's now a unique approach that can help cancer patients feel less alone.

Where to Start

Most cancer-treatment decisions are made within a few weeks of the initial diagnosis.

Beware of Nail Salon Dryers

Dryers with lights, especially those used for gel manicures, emit ultraviolet (UV) rays. Multiple exposures can result in premature age spots, wrinkles and a slightly increased risk for skin cancer on the hands and fingers.

Self-defense: Apply sunscreen before using the dryer. Or wear special manicure gloves (available online).

Chris G. Adigun, MD, clinical assistant professor and attending nail clinic physician at New York University Langone Medical Center, New York City.

Patients who aren't thinking clearly are expected to understand what's happening and make difficult decisions.

A resource worth trying: A free, evidence-based counseling program, called Open to Options, is available nationwide. Developed by the Cancer Support Community (CSC), a nonprofit group based in Washington, DC, the program matches cancer patients with paid professional counselors (psychologists, social workers and marriage and family therapists) throughout the country. They are specially trained to help patients better communicate with their doctors by formulating questions about their treatment options during that difficult period between diagnosis and treatment.

What research shows: Studies of nearly 200 patients have found that those who worked with Open to Options counselors were more informed during meetings with their doctors and were less likely to have second thoughts after treatment decisions were made.

How It Works

To find professional counselors in their areas, newly diagnosed cancer patients can use the CSC website, *CancerSupportCommunity. org*, or call the Cancer Support Helpline at 888-793-9355. They can meet with counselors face-to-face or communicate by phone or e-mail.

Counselors in this program do not answer medical questions or give medical advice. Rather, the counselors are trained to help patients decide what issues are most important to them and should be discussed with their doctors.

After the counselor and patient meet, the counselor creates a one-page summary agenda that the patient will share with his/her doctor. (The agenda can be faxed or e-mailed to the doctor before the patient's appointment.)

What the Program Covers

When working with a counselor, a patient creates a list of all her questions: "Will I suffer from the mental fog ('chemo brain') that sometimes goes along with chemotherapy?" "How long will I be treated?" "How can I minimize side effects?" "When can I return to work?" "Will my concentration or ability to travel be affected?"

When a patient speaks with a counselor, he'll be guided through a series of steps to answer questions such as...

•**What's your situation?** You already know you have cancer, and your doctor probably has a good sense of how he will recommend treating it. But your personal situation and values will also influence your decisions.

Example 1: Your doctor might be inclined to treat your cancer with a particular form of chemotherapy, one that sometimes causes hand neuropathy as a side effect. If you mention that you're an artist and can't make a living without the use of your hands, he might choose another treatment instead.

Example 2: Your doctor tells you about a new effective oral chemotherapy that costs $20,000 a month. Your insurance covers only 80%. What are the possibilities for payment, financial assistance and therapy?

•**What are your options?** These will depend on your health history and the type of cancer. The counselor will help you formulate some of the most important questions.

Example: You may want to continue working for the next several years. Will you do better with surgery, chemotherapy or radiation? Are the survival rates similar with each treatment? How long will it take to recover from each? What will the side effects be?

Important: Don't forget to ask the doctor whether a clinical trial (a study of a new treatment) is appropriate. Many people avoid clinical trials because they assume that they might be assigned to a "control" group that receives no treatment. However, in a typical clinical trial, participants are assigned to different groups—one is given the current standard care, and the other is given the new treatment being studied. Placebos are never given in place of treatment.

•**What are your goals?** This goes beyond "surviving" or "being healthy." Other factors are equally important—or even more important for some people.

Example: You might want to treat your cancer aggressively but not before you've attended your daughter's wedding. Your objective might be simply to wait a bit before starting treatment. You'll ask your doctor what the ramifications might be.

•**Who is in your support network?** Think about everyone who might be involved in your care—health professionals, your spouse, friends, helpful neighbors, etc.

•**Will you have someone to help you on the days of your scheduled treatments?** Maybe your spouse is available only on certain afternoons. Let your doctor know this—most cancer centers or hospitals have social-work departments that can help you solve logistical problems.

•**What comes next?** You'll probably have many questions as your treatment progresses. Write them down as you go. If you're not sure how to formulate your questions—or you're not even sure what you should know—ask your counselor for help. Even though most patients use the Open to Options program immediately following their diagnoses, they can rely on it anytime a treatment decision must be made. If they like, patients can also work with a specific counselor each time they ask for help.

Important: Even though you may feel inclined to act immediately if you've just gotten a cancer diagnosis, research shows that patients have better treatment outcomes and less anxiety when they are well-informed and partner with their doctors in determining the best treatments for them. This may take a bit longer, but the benefits far outweigh the risks.

Does Chemo Make Patients Smell Bad?

Joanne Mortimer, MD, vice chair and professor, medical oncology and therapeutics research, and director, Women's Cancer Programs, City of Hope (a comprehensive cancer center), Duarte, California.

Lise N. Alschuler, ND, board-certified naturopathic oncologist in practice at Naturopathic Specialists, LLC in Scottsdale, Arizona. A breast cancer survivor, she is coauthor of *The Definitive Guide to Thriving After Cancer: A Five-Step Integrative Plan to Reduce the Risk of Recurrence and Build Lifelong Health* and cocreator of *FiveToThrivePlan.com*, a website about integrative cancer care. *DrLise.net*

Outrageous! A mom with breast cancer was banned from her daughter's school because her chemotherapy made her smell bad. Patients battling cancer have enough to worry about without having nasty people complain that they stink.

Little research has been done on the phenomenon of chemo-induced body odor. In one study of 518 cancer patients receiving chemotherapy, 41% reported scent changes. And the online chat rooms for cancer patients are full of plaintive comments like, "I smell bad! Has this happened to anyone else?" Patients complain that their skin, sweat, urine, clothes and bed linens reek from the chemo. Some describe the smell as metallic or chemical...others liken it to mothballs or bad cologne...still others call it ickily sweet or overwhelmingly foul. Yet there are also those who say the odor problem is "all in the patients' heads."

Here's help from Joanne Mortimer, MD, vice chair and professor of medical oncology at City of Hope, a comprehensive cancer center in Duarte, California...and Lise N. Alschuler, ND, a Scottsdale, Arizona–based naturopathic oncologist.

Question: Is "chemo smell" an actual odor that chemo patients develop...or does chemotherapy alter patients' perception of smell, so that their own bodies smell bad to themselves but smell fine to others?

Answer: It's probably a bit of both. Chemo drugs definitely can cause changes in sensory perception by directly altering or damaging the olfactory receptor cells responsible for our sense of smell, Dr. Mortimer said.

For some patients, odor perception becomes distorted (a phenomenon called dysomia) or hyper-acute...others may perceive odors when no actual odor exists (phantosomia). In some cases, the changes are "hedonic," meaning that a scent formerly considered pleasant is now perceived as unpleasant. In addition, patients may experience a psychological response, brought on by the anxiety associated with their cancer and its treatment, that makes them imagine they are perceiving odors associated with a hospital setting.

There also are several possible reasons why a cancer patient's scent actually does change. For one thing, cancer itself can have a musty, sharp odor, quite apart from any medications used to treat it. *In addition, chemo can alter scent in the following ways...*

Lung Cancer Can Lie Dormant

Lung cancer can lie dormant for more than 20 years and then become aggressive. In a small study of smokers, former smokers and people who never smoked, researchers found that the initial genetic errors that cause cancer can go undetected for many years, and the cancer can become active when triggered by new mutations.

Study by researchers at Cancer Research UK, published in *Science*.

•**As chemotherapy drugs get metabolized in the body,** some metabolites are eliminated through the skin, where they gain odor themselves or trigger the release of other odiferous toxins in the skin, Dr. Alschuler said. For instance, when ferrous iron reacts with human skin cells, it produces compounds that have a metallic smell.

•**Skin contains fatty acids and inflammatory cytokines that,** under normal circumstances, help protect it against infectious bacteria and other pathogens. However, when chemo suppresses the immune system, the skin's normal immune response is altered…and rather than guarding the skin, the cytokines and fatty acids instead contribute to rashes and inflammation. As a result, chemo patients may harbor more or different bacteria than usual on their skin, in turn producing a different odor, Dr. Alschuler said.

•**Chemotherapy can cause dry mouth,** mouth sores and vomiting, all of which can lead to bad breath.

•**Urine might smell foul because,** as the body is breaking down chemotherapy agents and metabolizing them into new compounds, some of those compounds that are eliminated in urine have their own odor.

•**When patients receive chemo,** their blood cell counts drop, which may make them prone to fungal infections—and these infections smell, Dr. Mortimer added.

Quench the Stench

Patients on chemo can combat treatment-related odors by taking the following steps…

•**To help your body eliminate odor-causing toxins,** exercise regularly (with your doctor's OK)—and do so intensely enough to work up a good sweat. Perspiration is one way the body removes toxins.

Important: Drink plenty of water before and during workouts to facilitate ample sweating (and of course, be sure to bathe afterward). If you don't have the energy to exercise hard, another way to encourage sweating (again, with your doctor's OK) is to take a sauna or steam bath, Dr. Alschuler said.

Aspirin May Reduce Cancer Cell Growth

In recent research, aspirin and other non-steroidal anti-inflammatory drugs (NSAIDs) were found to help prevent the growth of cancer cells when taken at least once a week for six months.

Study led by researchers at University of California, San Francisco, published in *PLoS Genetics*.

•**Eat plenty of fruits and vegetables.** These provide detoxification support for the liver, where the metabolism of chemo drugs primarily occurs. Dr. Alschuler particularly recommended beets, parsnips, dark leafy greens, avocados and chicory—in addition to being good detoxifiers, these foods have antimutagenic (mutation-fighting) effects.

•**To further aid the elimination of the chemo drugs' toxins, keep your digestive system running well.** That means drink enough fluids to keep your urine nearly clear (which also reduces the smell)…and get enough fiber to maintain bowel regularity.

•**Be diligent about hygiene.** Bathe two or three times a day if you like, using scented soap. Slather on a body lotion that smells good to you (but note that Dr. Alschuler advised choosing one that's free of parabens and phthalates, which have been linked to cancer). Brush your teeth often or chew sugarless gum to freshen your breath. Launder garments after each wearing. Change bed linens and especially pillowcases frequently. Even if you are the only one who perceives an odor, these steps can help you feel your freshest and reduce the distress associated with chemo smell.

•**Talk to your doctor.** Research shows that cancer patients often do not report concerns about smell perception or changed body odor to their doctors—perhaps because they are embarrassed or think it's a trivial complaint. By speaking up, you give your doctor a chance to assess any odor problem and make additional suggestions that could improve the situation or at least put your mind more at ease.

•**Consider taking zinc supplements,** which can help normalize the perception of odors as well as tastes.

Important: Excessive zinc (above 40 mg per day) may reduce immune function and interfere with certain medications. Get your doctor's OK before taking any type of supplements, as they may affect the potency of your chemotherapy.

•**Try to be patient.** Once chemo ends, the smell problem generally fades away within six to nine months.

Hyperthermia Therapy Makes Cancer Treatments Work Better

Jennifer Yu, MD, PhD, radiation oncologist and cancer researcher in stem cell biology and regenerative medicine, Cleveland Clinic, Cleveland. She also is the director of the Cleveland Clinic Center for Hyperthermia.

A treatment for cancer used in ancient Egypt is proving to be effective in 21st-century America. That's right—the first known mention of therapeutic hyperthermia, which involves using hot water to heat a tumor and the surrounding area, appeared in a 5,000-year-old papyrus! Today, doctors at some cancer centers are using noninvasive mild-heat hyperthermia to boost the effectiveness of other cancer therapies, especially radiation, without increasing the dosage and subsequent risk for unwanted side effects.

How it works: Mild-heat hyperthermia combats cancer several ways. *For instance, it…*

•**Disables certain enzymes,** impairing the cancer cells' ability to repair the DNA damage caused by radiation.

•**Improves blood flow to the area where the tumor is,** bringing more oxygen to the tissues, which in turn increases the effectiveness of radiation.

•**Damages proteins and structures within cancer cells,** causing tumors to shrink—while doing minimal damage to normal tissues.

•**Kills cancer stem cells that often are resistant to radiation.**

•**May enhance the effects of certain anticancer drugs.**

•**Supports the immune system,** increasing the body's ability to fight off the cancer.

What happens during treatment: Hyperthermia is added to a course of radiation. For instance, suppose a patient is scheduled to undergo five radiation sessions per week for four weeks. If he/she is receiving hyperthermia, he also would get two sessions of the mild-temperature hyperthermia therapy, administered immediately before the radiation (the other three days per week, radiation would be administered alone).

Typically hyperthermia is applied with hot-water bags that are carefully positioned and precisely heated with an external microwave unit and temperature monitors. Temperatures are maintained at slightly above "fever range," or around 110°F. The patient lies in a darkened room for an hour during the hyperthermia treatment. It feels like a heating pad. Many patients take a nap during the treatment. Once the hyperthermia session is over, the patient immediately moves on to the radiation.

Risks and side effects are minor. In about 10% of cases, small blisters develop. This is most common on the skin near a cancer surgery site because blood flow in scarred areas is reduced, so heat is not carried away by the circulating blood as efficiently as it normally would be. This is usually a minor discomfort, though. Spilling coffee on yourself would probably hurt more, and these blisters usually heal on their own. They're not so severe that treatment has to be stopped.

Types of cancer treated: Mild-heat hyperthermia is most often used to treat cancers that occur near the surface of the body, such as breast cancer, melanoma, and head and neck cancers. It also is increasingly being used for other types of cancer as well, including cancers of the cervix, prostate, rectum, pancreas, brain, bladder and liver.

Though hyperthermia can help patients who are facing their first bouts with cancer, research suggests that it is especially beneficial for people with recurring cancer where radiation didn't help as much as doctors had hoped initially. For instance, according to one study from Duke University Medical Center that looked at patients with recurrent breast cancer, hyperthermia combined with radiation successfully eradicated tumors in 65% of cases, versus just 42% for radiation alone. For patients whose cancer has metastasized, whole-body hyperthermia may be done using warm-water immersion.

Where to get treatment: Most insurance companies cover hyperthermia therapy. However, the treatment requires a large team of specialized practitioners—at the Cleveland Clinic, for example, it includes a physician, medical physicist, and nurses and therapists specially trained in hyperthermia and repeat radiation. Unfortunately, this safe and effective treatment isn't widely available. Many places do not have the personnel or infrastructure to run these types of facilities, and few young physicians are trained in how to deliver hyperthermia. If you are interested in having a consultation with a doctor who provides this treatment, enlist your oncologist's aid in finding a practitioner.

Though cancer is a very complex disease, it's heartening to know that something as simple as hot water could help you treat it.

Lymphoma Breakthrough

In a recent study, cancer patients with chemotherapy-resistant, large B-cell lymphoma who were treated with *azacitidine* (Vidaza)—a DNA methyltransferase (DNMT)

inhibitor—responded to chemo after taking the drug and then went into remission.

Possible reason: DNMT inhibitors genetically reprogram cancer cells, which seems to help chemo drugs work better. Larger studies are under way to see if DNMT is effective for other cancers.

Leandro Cerchietti, MD, assistant professor of medicine, Weill Cornell Medical College, New York City.

5 Supplements That Help Prevent Cancer Recurrence

Lise N. Alschuler, ND, board-certified naturopathic oncologist, Naturopathic Specialists (*Listenandcare. com*), Scottsdale, Arizona. A breast cancer survivor, she is coauthor of *The Definitive Guide to Thriving After Cancer: A Five-Step Integrative Plan to Reduce the Risk of Recurrence and Build Lifelong Health.* DrLise.net

It's a top question on the minds of many cancer survivors: What will help keep the cancer from coming back? Unfortunately, conventional medicine often doesn't have much of an answer beyond, "Take care of yourself, and try not to worry." Naturopathic medicine, however, does have some specific recommendations for cancer survivors—and dietary supplements play a key role.

The reason: Dietary supplements are able to fit into the "nooks and crannies" of our biochemical pathways, creating specific changes that influence our bodies on a cellular level.

The five supplements listed below comprise a "foundational supplement plan" for just about every cancer survivor—and for just about every person who wants to reduce the odds of ever getting cancer in the first place. *Each of the five supplements helps reduce cancer risk through five key pathways...*

- **Boosting immune system function.**
- **Reducing inflammation.**
- **Improving insulin sensitivity.**

- **Supporting digestion and detoxification.**
- **Reducing stress-induced hormone imbalances.**

Although dietary supplements are available over-the-counter, before you start taking them, it is essential to check with a naturopathic doctor (ideally one with additional board certification in naturopathic oncology) or an integrative medical doctor with specific expertise in integrative cancer care. These providers have training in nutritional biochemistry as it relates to cancer. They can confirm that the following supplements are appropriate for you and determine the dosages and the specific brands that will best suit your needs.

For my own post-cancer patients, I typically prescribe all five of the following supplements, to be taken daily starting as soon as conventional treatment is completed. Some patients may be advised to start taking some of these supplements during their conventional treatment, but that should be done only under the guidance of an integrative health-care physician.

The top five cancer fighters include…

- **Omega-3 fatty acids.** These essential fatty acids—found in supplements of fish oil, flaxseed oil and algae-based oil—positively influence all five of the key pathways mentioned above. However, they are especially important for reducing chronic inflammation, which is one of the precursors of cancer. Think of inflammation as a burning ember in your body that can change your tissues in ways that favor the growth of abnormal cells. Omega-3s quench that fire.

Though omega-3s are helpful for survivors of all types of cancer, studies show particular benefits for patients who have battled colon, prostate, breast or lung cancer. A typical daily dosage is 1,000 mg to 3,000 mg of omega-3 oil.

Caveat: Omega-3s can increase bleeding, so it's vital to get your doctor's OK before taking omega-3s if you are on blood-thinning medication or are anticipating any surgery.

- **Probiotics.** Beneficial bacteria in the intestinal tract help metabolize nutrients, bind waste products for removal in stool and regulate immunity. When beneficial bacteria are depleted, the digestive tract is overrun with harmful bacteria and a condition called dysbiosis develops. This negatively impacts all five of the body's key pathways, contributing to an increased risk for cancer recurrence. Studies have shown that supplementing with beneficial intestinal bacteria called probiotics can reduce the risk for infection after surgery and improve the immune system's response.

You can get some probiotics from eating yogurt and fermented foods such as fresh sauerkraut, miso, tempeh and kefir. However, to fully support my patients' beneficial digestive bacteria, I typically prescribe a supplement that combines several types of probiotics at a dosage of at least one billion colony-forming units (CFU) daily.

Caution: Probiotics are not appropriate for people whose white blood cell count is below normal—some evidence suggests that probiotics can increase the risk for blood infection in those individuals.

- **Polyphenols.** Healthful, colorful fruits and vegetables get their rainbow hues from the naturally occurring plant compounds called polyphenols (also referred to as flavonoids). Three polyphenols are particularly important in the fight against cancer…

- **Green tea catechins,** which may lower the risk for cancers of the digestive tract, breast, bladder, lung, blood and prostate.

- **Curcumin,** the bright yellow flavonoid found in turmeric root, which appears to inhibit cancer formation ina variety of ways, helping protect against the majority of cancer types.

- **Resveratrol,** which gives color to red grapes and some berries, has shown promise against breast, colorectal and liver cancers by activating tumor suppressor genes and increasing the rate of apoptosis (normal programmed cell death).

Your doctor may prescribe a combination supplement that contains all three of these polyphenols, or you may take each one separately. Many high-quality brands also include other polyphenols. But watch out for what I call "window-dressing" supplements that list 20 to 30 different polyphenols—because the amount of each one will be so small that you might as well just eat a salad.

•**Antioxidants.** Look at metal that's been exposed to rain and sunlight—it starts to rust because it's being oxidized. That's essentially what happens to our bodies from exposure to "free radicals," or oxidative toxins. Antioxidants guard against this by binding to oxidative toxins so they can be eliminated…and they also stimulate cell repair and normal apoptosis. Cancer treatment can deplete your antioxidant capacity because cancer drugs themselves exert their cancer-killing effects via oxidation. *A plant-based diet provides antioxidants, but cancer survivors should get additional support by taking…*

•**Glutathione,** the body's "master antioxidant," which is critical for the elimination of environmental toxins. A typical dosage is 250 mg to 500 mg daily.

•**Coenzyme Q10 (CoQ10),** which is associated with decreased risk for breast and thyroid cancer, as well as melanoma, studies show. A typical daily dosage is 30 mg to 100 mg.

•**Vitamin D.** Numerous studies have shown the cancer-preventing potential of this vitamin, which promotes proper cell maturation and regulates inflammation, among other activities. "Without adequate levels of vitamin D, it's hard for our bodies to maintain good blood sugar control or reduce inflammation," said Dr. Alschuler.

Although it's often called the sunshine vitamin, many people in the northern hemisphere cannot get enough vitamin D just from being outdoors, especially during cooler seasons. Ask your doctor to measure your blood level of vitamin D—that information will help determine the right dosage for you.

Caution: If you take the heart medication digoxin, be especially sure to talk with your doctor before taking vitamin D because the combination could lead to abnormal heart rhythms.

Important: Dietary supplements are called "supplements" for a reason—they are meant to supplement the diet, not to replace healthy eating. Over time, they provide targeted molecular support that gently but radically alters the terrain in your body, creating an environment that impedes cancer recurrence…so you can get back to the business of living your life.

Better Skin Lesion Treatment

Precancerous skin lesions are better treated with photodynamic therapy (PDT) than with cryotherapy, reports Daniel Eisen, MD. In cryotherapy, lesions are frozen with liquid nitrogen. With PDT, the entire treatment area is "painted" with medication and then a special light is directed on it to activate the drug that kills the precancerous cells. Patients may require up to three sessions. Studies show that PDT is 14% more likely to completely clear the area in three months.

Daniel Eisen, MD, clinical professor of dermatology at University of California Davis Health System, Sacramento.

Feel Your Best After Cancer…How to Get the Care You Need…

Sheetal Kircher, MD, oncologist and clinical director of the Cancer Survivorship Institute at the Robert H. Lurie Comprehensive Cancer Center of Northwestern University in Chicago.

You beat cancer. Now what? For the 14 million cancer survivors in the US, this is no small question.

Once you've given that sigh of relief for having survived a possibly life-threatening illness, you're immediately confronted with a new set of concerns: How should you protect yourself against the dangerous aftereffects of cancer treatments? What about nagging emotional issues, including depression? And what can be done to keep cancer from coming back?

Latest development: Cancer survivors have traditionally lacked coordinated follow-up care by their physicians after completing their treatments. But there's now a new option for getting specialized aftercare. Hospitals and cancer centers across the US are offering survivorship-care programs that give patients state-of-the-art methods for keeping tabs on their health and reclaiming their emotional equilibrium after battling cancer.*

Getting On with Your Life

At a cancer-survivorship program, a team of medical doctors, physical therapists, psychologists, nutritionists and other health professionals focus exclusively on the individual needs of each cancer patient. This includes monitoring for complications that can result from cancer treatment. *Among the most important to watch for...*

•**Heart damage.** Chemotherapy and radiation can harm any organ, notably the heart. It doesn't necessarily happen right away—a potent class of drugs called anthracyclines, commonly used to treat some lymphomas, breast cancer and certain rare types of cancer like sarcoma, can cause cardiomyopathy (weakening of the heart) decades after treatment is completed.

Radiation that reaches the heart, as often occurs, for example, with lung cancer, can cause damage, too. Similarly, a study appearing in the *Journal of Clinical Oncology* attributed up to 25% of the deaths of former Hodgkin's disease patients to heart disease caused in some part by radiation.

Best self-defense: Depending on the treatment you received, your doctor may

*To find a cancer-survivorship program near you, go to the National Cancer Institute (NCI) website, *CancerCenters.Cancer.gov.* Cancer-survivor programs are often used in conjunction with care from one's primary care doctor and are covered by most health insurers.

recommend one or more tests, such as MRI, ultrasound and/or electrocardiogram, to closely monitor your heart health.

•**Infection.** Chemo, radiation and stem cell transplants used to treat cancer suppress the immune system, increasing risk for infection.

Best self-defense: Vaccines must be used carefully in cancer survivors. For example, "live" vaccines (such as Zostavax for shingles) should not be used in cancer patients with weakened immunity—they are at increased risk of contracting the infectious disease from the live organism in the vaccine. Cancer patients should talk to their doctors about the vaccines they need.

•**Fatigue.** Up to 82% of cancer survivors are affected by persistent fatigue, brought on by chemo and/or radiation or as a result of stress or chronic pain.

Best self-defense: It's common for individuals who have received chemo and/or radiation to suffer mild to moderate fatigue for up to a year. However, other conditions not directly related to the cancer itself—for example, an underactive thyroid, anemia, arthritis or insomnia—or even the use of pain medication may be partially to blame.

If these possibilities are ruled out, the best defense is often a carefully designed exercise program. A physical therapist on staff at a cancer-survivorship program will be knowledgeable about the issues that cancer survivors confront.

For best results: Pace yourself! Start with just 20 minutes of brisk walking and/or resistance training one to three days a week...and gradually increase to 20 to 60 minutes up to five days a week.

•**Pain.** More than one-third of cancer survivors experience chronic pain—often due to chemotherapy, radiation or surgery.

Best self-defense: Don't rely on just one pain-fighting strategy. A combination of approaches, such as physical therapy, exercise, oral painkillers, lidocaine (injections, creams or patches) and massage, may be recommended.

•**Depression.** This is also common after cancer treatment.

Best self-defense: Don't shrug off worrisome symptoms, such as trouble sleeping, an inability to focus, lingering feelings of sadness and anger or an overwhelming sense of isolation or fear. These are all red flags that depression may have taken hold.

The psychologists, social workers and other mental health professionals at survivorship programs are trained to identify and treat cancer-related complications, such as fatigue and pain, that may contribute to depression. In addition, therapy and/or medication may be needed to treat the depression.

•**Additional postcancer issues.** Cancer-survivorship programs also treat sexual dysfunction...cognitive decline...and sleep problems.

Risks for Recurrence

Up to 70% of cancer survivors report having significant fear of a cancer recurrence.

If you have survived cancer, the best way to catch a recurrence early—when the malignancy would be most treatable—is to stay on top of follow-up visits to your doctors.

How often? Follow-up visits are generally recommended every three to four months for the first few years following treatment and once or twice annually after that. However, the exact schedule depends on such factors as the type of cancer you had, the treatments you received and your age.

Which tests? It's crucial to have an after-cancer screening plan that may include specific tests (such as blood tests and MRI and/or CT scans) that are sometimes used to help detect cancer recurrences.

Best resource: Guidelines from the National Comprehensive Cancer Network. Go to *NCCN.org/default.aspx*. Under "NCCN Guidelines," click on "NCCN Guidelines for Patients."

Chapter 3

STROKE: RISKS, SYMPTOMS, AND SECRETS TO RECOVERY

Never Have a Stroke

For women, stroke prevention is even more important than it is for men. There are steps you can take now to reduce your risk.

Reasons: Between the ages of 45 and 54, women are more than twice as likely as men to have a stroke, according to a study from the University of California. Even when treated with state-of-the-art medication, women of all ages are at greater risk than men for suffering serious disability after a stroke. And regardless of age, female stroke patients are more likely to die than male stroke patients are. *What you need to know…*

Stroke Prevention Strategies

A stroke is a "brain attack" that occurs when a blood vessel that carries oxygen and nutrients to the brain gets blocked by a clot (an ischemic stroke) or leaks or bursts (a hemorrhagic stroke). Either way, cells in the affected area of the brain are starved of oxygen. This can impair a person's ability to function, often irreparably.

Risk factors for stroke build up over years, even decades. *To slash your stroke risk…*

1. Know your numbers. Get a checkup that includes tests for the risk factors below.

Discuss with your doctor how your results compare with these ideal measurements…

- **Blood pressure**—less than 130/80.
- **Total cholesterol**—less than 200.
- **LDL (bad) cholesterol**—no more than 100 for most women.
- **HDL (good) cholesterol**—greater than 50.
- **Triglycerides (blood fats)**—less than 150.
- **Fasting blood glucose (sugar)**—less than 100.
- **Body mass index (a ratio of height to weight)**—18.5 to 24.9, with higher numbers indicating excessive weight. Calculate your body mass index at *www.nhlbi.nih.gov* (search "BMI calculator").
- **Waist circumference**—35 inches or less.

2. Determine your risk level based on new American Heart Association (AHA) guidelines. This will help you and your doctor develop a personalized prevention program.

Lori Mosca, MD, PhD, MPH, director of the New York–Presbyterian Hospital Preventive Cardiology Program in New York City, *Hearthealthtimes.com.* She is professor of medicine at Columbia University Medical Center and author of *Heart to Heart: A Personal Plan for Creating a Heart-Healthy Family.*

•**You're at high risk if you've already had a stroke...**or have diabetes or coronary heart disease.

•**You're at risk if you smoke...**have high blood pressure...or have a condition called metabolic syndrome, characterized by symptoms such as a thick waist, higher-than-normal blood glucose, high triglycerides and low HDL cholesterol.

•**Your risk factor level is optimal if you eat a heart-healthy diet...**exercise regularly...and have none of the risk factors listed above.

For more risk-assessment tools, visit *www. hearthealthtimes.com*, the website for the New York–Presbyterian Hospital Preventive Cardiology Program.

3. Exercise every day at moderate intensity. Being active helps lower blood pressure and keeps your weight in check.

Concern: Being overweight by as little as 10 pounds boosts stroke risk. To lose weight, you should log 60 to 90 minutes of exercise daily. Consistency is important because it keeps blood vessels healthy and metabolism functioning optimally.

4. Eat to beat stroke. Build your diet mostly on fruits, vegetables and whole grains. Eat fish twice a week, preferably fatty kinds, such as herring. Limit sodium to less than 2,300 mg a day by reducing salt added to foods and avoiding high-sodium prepared foods (check nutrition labels). Avoid trans fats, such as partially hydrogenated vegetable oils and shortening. Keep saturated fat low—less than 7% of total calories if possible—by limiting meats and nonskim dairy foods. Consume no more than 300 mg daily of dietary cholesterol. Limit alcohol to one drink daily. Avoid fried foods. Opt for baked, boiled, broiled, steamed or sautéed foods.

5. Make informed decisions about medications that affect hormones. Taking estrogen for menopausal symptoms or a selective estrogen receptor modulator (SERM), such as tamoxifen, for breast cancer treatment may raise stroke risk. The longer you take such medications, the greater your risk.

6. Consider aspirin. For women age 65 and over, taking aspirin daily (typically 75 mg to 162 mg) may prevent the blood clots that cause the most common type of stroke and may protect against heart disease. Aspirin therapy also may make sense for women under age 65 who are at high risk for stroke.

Do not take aspirin without first discussing it with your doctor. Aspirin therapy can increase your risk for stroke if you have uncontrolled high blood pressure. It also can cause gastrointestinal bleeding. That's why women under age 65 who are not at high risk for stroke generally are advised against taking daily aspirin—the risks may outweigh the benefits.

7. Stop smoking. Smoking increases blood pressure and blood clotting, both of which can set the stage for stroke. Women who smoke and take oral contraceptives are at even greater risk for stroke. Studies show that the more individual, group or telephone smoking-cessation counseling you get, the better your chances of quitting.

Helpful: Use medication, such as nicotine replacement, to reduce cravings.

8. Don't ignore troubling symptoms, such as heart palpitations. A common risk factor for stroke is atrial fibrillation (AF)—an irregular, rapid heart rhythm that causes abnormal blood flow and increases the likelihood of a clot. AF increases a woman's stroke risk fivefold. Other AF symptoms include light-headedness, weakness, confusion and/or difficulty breathing. If you have symptoms of AF, see your doctor—blood-thinning drugs, such as aspirin or *warfarin* (Coumadin), can lower your risk for clots and stroke.

9. Talk to your doctor about other medications that reduce risk factors. If efforts to improve your lifestyle habits aren't enough to reduce your risk, talk to your doctor about adding drug therapy. For instance, thiazide diuretics and other prescription drugs can help control blood pressure...niacin or fibrate medication can increase HDL (good) cholesterol.

One Word That Can Save a Life—FAST

Stroke is a medical emergency that requires immediate care. Brain cells starved of oxygen die and do not regenerate. To remember the sudden symptoms of stroke, think of the word "FAST"…

●**Face.** Sudden numbness or weakness of the face, especially on one side…severe headache…dizziness…vision trouble.

●**Arm and leg.** Sudden numbness or weakness of the arm and/or leg, especially on one side…trouble walking…loss of coordination.

●**Speech.** Sudden confusion and trouble speaking or understanding speech.

●**Time.** Time is critical—if you think you or someone else is having a stroke, call 911.

Many Women Unaware of Female-Specific Stroke Symptoms

Ohio State University Wexner Medical Center, news release.

Stroke is the third leading cause of death in women, but many are unaware of warning signs and symptoms that are unique to females, a recent study says.

Of 1,000 women surveyed, only one in 10 was aware that hiccups that occur with unusual chest pain is an early warning sign of stroke in women, said researchers from Ohio State University Wexner Medical Center, in Columbus.

Although men and women share some risk factors for stroke—such as smoking, being sedentary and having high blood pressure—others are specific to women, the researchers explained.

But only 11 percent of women polled knew that pregnancy, lupus, migraine headaches, birth-control pills and hormone replacement therapy increase their stroke risk, the study found.

"I think we have a ways to go when it comes to educating women about stroke and their unique risk factors," Diana Greene-Chandos, MD, a neurologist and director of neuroscience critical care, said in a medical center news release.

"Things like pregnancy, hormone replacement therapy and even something as trivial as a case of the hiccups can all play an important role when it comes to strokes in women, and we need to be more aware of it," she added.

Other stroke symptoms the researchers say are unique to women include…

●**Dizziness not associated with vertigo,**

●**Headaches,**

●**Numbness over the entire body that is more severe on one side.**

"Women may have more headaches with their strokes. They actually can have hiccups with a little bit of chest pain with their stroke symptoms, sometimes sending them down the pathway of looking for either heart disease or indigestion," said Dr. Greene-Chandos.

"Pregnancy also increases their risk of stroke, particularly in the final months and the immediate period after delivering the child," she said.

Signs of stroke in both men and women can include sudden confusion; trouble speaking or understanding; sudden trouble seeing; sudden difficulty walking; or loss of balance and coordination.

Identifying symptoms of a stroke early on and seeking immediate medical attention is critical because clot-busting drugs are only an option within three hours of the onset of a stroke, the researchers cautioned.

"Women do not think they are going to have a stroke. They think of it as a man's disease," said Dr. Greene-Chandos. "You have to know when you are having a stroke, you have to recognize that it's a stroke and you have to get to the emergency room and receive the medication."

Nearly half of those surveyed also said they didn't know that following a stroke, many women experience nerve damage, problems swallowing and depression, which can prevent them from getting needed rehabilitation.

Each year more than 137,000 Americans die from stroke, about 60 percent of them women, according to the American Heart Association and American Stroke Association.

The National Stroke Association (*Stroke. org*) provides more information on stroke symptoms unique to women.

Better Stroke Prevention

Fewer than one in three stroke survivors are able to consistently control their blood pressure. But those who can keep blood pressure below 140/90 mmHg most of the time reduced their risk for a second stroke by 54%, according to a recent study of 3,680 stroke survivors.

Best practices: Check blood pressure twice a day at home and share logs of your readings with your doctor. Also, lower your salt intake…eat a healthful diet…exercise regularly…and be sure to take all prescribed medication.

Amytis Towfighi, MD, assistant professor of neurology, Keck School of Medicine, University of Southern California, Los Angeles.

Women, Reduce Stroke Risk with Potassium

Sylvia Wassertheil-Smoller, PhD, Dorothy and William Manealoff Foundation and Molly Rosen Chair in Social Medicine Emerita, department of epidemiology and population health, Albert Einstein College of Medicine in Brooklyn. Her study was published in *Stroke*.

Bananas are rich in it, dried fruits such as raisins, prunes and apricots are, too. Potatoes, white beans and tomato sauce are great sources as well. You may have guessed the nutrient I'm talking about—po-

tassium. And what does getting enough potassium do besides help your muscles move and regulate your blood pressure and heartbeat? It's crucial to heart health, especially for postmenopausal women. And a recent study showed that postmenopausal women who consumed more potassium were less likely to have strokes.

In this study, women who consumed the most potassium (at least 3,194 milligrams [mg] per day) were 12% less likely to suffer any type of stroke than women who consumed the least potassium (less than 1,926 mg per day). And they were 16% less likely to suffer an ischemic stroke, the most common type, caused when a blood clot blocks oxygen and nutrients to the brain. For women who kept their blood pressure and weight in check and knew to bulk up on potassium, protection against ischemic stroke was more than doubled (a 27% to 30% lower risk) compared with women who consumed a minimum of dietary potassium. That is a huge risk reduction.

Incidentally, even the high-range number for potassium intake mentioned above—around 3,200 mg per day—may be considered on the low side. The World Health Organization recommends 3,510 mg…while the US Department of Agriculture (USDA) recommends 4,700 mg a day. But the sad fact is that most postmenopausal women are nowhere near that goal. In the latest study, the average daily intake of potassium among the 90,000-plus participants was only 2,611 mg—that's barely more than half the daily amount that the USDA says we need!

Are You Getting Enough?

The irony is that potassium is found in nearly all food groups, especially fruits, vegetables, dairy products and fish and seafood. You can make every meal—breakfast, lunch and dinner—potassium-rich. *See for yourself…*

•**Breakfast or Snack Time.** A banana provides 422 mg of potassium. A cup of cantaloupe, 430 mg. Eight ounces of yogurt gives you up to 579 mg. Toss in a cup of strawberries and you get 255 mg more. Prune juice packs 707 mg in a cup (a cup of stewed prunes, 796 mg). And a cup of orange juice will provide 496 mg. Dried apricots or peaches are sweet and tasty sources of potassium, too, delivering between 378 mg and 398 mg per quarter cup.

●**Lunch and Dinner.** A small baked potato, including the skin, has 738 mg of potassium, a medium sweet potato with skin, 542 mg. Tomato products are great sources of potassium...one-half cup of tomato sauce provides 405 mg. All types of beans, especially white beans (595 mg per half-cup) are excellent sources, too. And a cup of cooked spinach packs 840 mg. Fish and seafood are also great. For example, three ounces of yellowfin tuna provides 484 mg of potassium.

That's just a small sampling, but you can see how having a deliciously varied diet of healthful foods can provide all the potassium you need for heart health and stroke risk reduction. For more information on the potassium content of foods, check out this cheat sheet of low-calorie, high-potassium foods from the University of Massachusetts School of Medicine.

Do You Need a Supplement?

The benefits of potassium come from dietary intake. Supplements do not seem to have the same beneficial effect, said Sylvia Wassertheil-Smoller, PhD, who participated in the study on potassium and stroke risk in postmenopausal women. Dr. Wassertheil-Smoller is chair of social medicine at Albert Einstein College of Medicine in Brooklyn, New York. She and other experts agree that having too much potassium in the blood can be dangerous to the heart. So do check with your doctor before taking a potassium supplement. If a potassium supplement is recommended to you, your doctor should monitor your blood potassium levels to make sure they do not go higher than what is healthy and normal.

Tasty Foods That Help Prevent Stroke...

●**Red peppers fight stroke.** Eating red peppers and other vitamin C–rich fruits and veggies may reduce your risk for intracerebral hemorrhagic stroke (a blood vessel rupture in the brain). And what's so great about red peppers? At 190 mg per cup, they contain three times more vitamin C than an orange. Other good sources of vitamin C—broccoli and strawberries. Researchers believe that this vitamin may reduce stroke risk by regulating blood pressure and strengthening collagen, which promotes healthy blood vessels.

Stéphane Vannier, MD, neurologist, Pontchaillou University Hospital, Rennes, France, from research being presented at the annual meeting of the American Academy of Neurology.

●**Apples really help you live longer.** A British study found that eating one apple a day could prevent 8,500 deaths a year from heart attacks and strokes in people over age 50 in the UK. Apples act like statins to reduce LDL "bad" cholesterol, a risk factor for heart attacks and stroke.

Study by researchers at University of Oxford, England, published in the *BMJ*.

●**Eat this protein to reduce stroke risk.** Certain types of protein may protect against stroke, a recent study has found. In a review of the diets of nearly 255,000 people, those who ate the most protein (at least 20 g per day) were 20% less likely to have a stroke than those who ate less.

Possible explanation: Protein helps lower blood pressure.

However: Those who ate fish benefited the most. Plant protein sources (such as beans) were less protective, and red meat has been linked to increased risk for stroke.

Xinfeng Liu, MD, PhD, professor of neurology, Nanjing University School of Medicine, China.

Could a Jolt to the Neck Cause a Stroke?

Rebecca Gottesman, MD, associate professor of neurology and epidemiology at The Johns Hopkins University School of Medicine and director of clinical research at Johns Hopkins Bayview Neurology, both in Baltimore.

Most strokes occur due to years of high blood pressure...or when the gradual buildup of fatty substances (plaque) in the arteries cuts off blood flow to the brain.

An unusual and little-recognized trigger: Some people get strokes from simply moving the neck in an extreme way or holding it in an odd position. This sort of neck movement might occur during a car accident, for example—but it might also be caused by normal activities such as riding a roller coaster, craning your neck to paint a ceiling or leaning back to have your hair shampooed at a hair salon (the so-called "beauty parlor syndrome").

The culprit in such strokes is a vertebral artery dissection (VAD), a tear in the innermost or middle layer of the three-layered vertebral artery wall, which can disrupt blood flow to the brain. Sometimes, the damage is minor and the artery repairs itself without difficulty. In other cases, however, the arterial injury leads to a stroke.

Recent development: The American Heart Association (AHA) recently issued a warning that neck manipulation (used, for example, during certain chiropractic or physical therapy treatments) has been linked to stroke due to such arterial injuries. While no direct cause-and-effect relationship has been found, the AHA now advises health-care practitioners to inform their patients of the association before performing neck manipulation.

When an Artery Shreds

The right and left vertebral arteries run up the back of the neck and into the skull, carrying blood to the brain. A stroke-inducing arterial tear can result from virtually any sudden and/or extreme movement that turns or stretches the neck excessively. But in many cases, people with VAD can recall nothing more unusual than a sneeze or vigorous sexual activity in the preceding days, and sometimes there is nothing to blame it on.

Why the cause can be elusive: Some people are apparently more vulnerable to VAD than others. It is more common in those with known connective tissue disorders such as Marfan's syndrome or fibromuscular dysplasia. Also, some studies have found that artery walls in people who have suffered dissections look subtly abnormal under the microscope, suggesting a congenital abnormality.

But practically speaking, there is no way to predict who will get a VAD or what will cause it. There are warning signs, though. And if you've already suffered a VAD, there are steps you can take to help prevent another one.

Red Flags for VAD

Each year, approximately 4,500 Americans suffer VAD. The condition is a leading cause of stroke in adults under age 45. VAD also can occur, though less commonly, in older adults. Of course, the best course is to spot a VAD early-—before it can cause a stroke.

Recent finding: An analysis of 75 studies involving nearly 2,000 people diagnosed with VAD found that dizziness or vertigo was the most common symptom, reported

---

20-Second Stroke-Risk Test

Balance on one leg for at least 20 seconds. Difficulty balancing may mean that tiny strokes or bleeds have already occurred, increasing your risk for more serious strokes.

Recent finding: Among those who had two or more tiny strokes, about one-third had trouble balancing.

Yasuharu Tabara, PhD, associate professor, Center for Genomic Medicine, Kyoto University Graduate School of Medicine, Japan, and lead author of a study published in *Stroke*.

by 58% of sufferers, with headache (51%) and neck pain (46%) close behind.

The trouble is that dizziness, headache and neck pain are extremely common and can be caused by many different conditions. And you can't run to the doctor to check out every headache or dizzy spell.

When to be concerned: If you have a headache that is more severe than usual…suffer extreme dizziness…have neck pain that is unusual for you…or if any of these symptoms occur at the same time or last longer than a day. Call or visit your doctor without delay.

When to be very concerned: If you develop symptoms such as double vision, difficulty walking, speaking or swallowing, and/or weakness on one side of your face or body, particularly if they occur with dizziness, neck pain or headache. These could be signs that a stroke or transient ischemic attack (TIA), a temporary blockage of brain circulation, is occurring.

A sudden and severe "thunderclap" headache (the kind that people describe as "the worst headache of my life") may indicate that a brain hemorrhage is imminent or has happened.

Prompt emergency care in these situations could mean the difference between complete recovery and disability or death.

Preventing an Arterial Tear

If you have ever had an episode of VAD, you are at increased risk for another. This doesn't mean that you should stop all exercise or keep your neck in a brace, but you may want to pass on activities that could easily lead to a neck injury, such as mountain biking and skydiving.

Also, if you've had a VAD, avoid any situations where your neck is stretched out for prolonged periods—for example, try to avoid hyperextending your neck at an extreme angle backward while getting your hair shampooed or styled. Don't give up yoga, but skip postures that stress your neck. If you receive chiropractic care, it's safest for manipulations to be performed below neck level.

Diagnosing and Treating an Arterial Tear

If your doctor suspects that you've suffered a vertebral artery dissection (VAD), he/she will probably order a CT scan or MRI. Treatment for a VAD usually includes a drug to keep clots from forming, most commonly *warfarin* (Coumadin). If you have a VAD, it's common to take the drug for three to six months. If symptoms persist, your doctor may recommend that a stent or coil be surgically placed in the damaged artery.

Precautions: While VAD is less likely to cause a stroke once you begin taking an anticoagulant, anticlotting drugs themselves carry the risk of bleeding. Your doctor should advise you what activities to avoid during this time—this usually includes anything that could cause head injury. Patients on oral anticoagulants also should have their blood levels checked regularly and need to maintain a regular diet in order to keep their blood thin enough while they are taking this medication.

Having Shingles Can Increase Risk for Stroke Later in Life

People who had shingles after age 40 had a 10% higher risk for heart attack and a 15% higher risk for mini-stroke, or transient ischemic attack. People who had shingles prior to age 40 were at much greater risk—they had a 50% higher risk for heart attack…were 2.4 times more likely to have a mini-stroke… and had a 74% higher risk for stroke.

If you have had shingles: Get a cardiovascular checkup, and be screened for risk factors, such as high cholesterol and high blood pressure.

Judith Breuer, MD, professor of virology at University College London, and lead author of a study published in *Neurology*.

Protect Yourself from Having Your Stroke Missed in the ER

David E. Newman-Toker, MD PhD, associate professor, department of neurology, The Johns Hopkins University School of Medicine, Baltimore. His study appeared in the journal *Diagnosis*.

You may know all about the "classic" signs of a stroke—sudden one-sided weakness…a loss of balance, speech or coordination…paralysis. But not all strokes come with those clear signs that raise a red flag. More generalized symptoms that could be caused by lots of things—such as headache and dizziness or temporary numbness—can also be symptoms of a stroke. Doctors in the emergency room (ER) are responsible for deciding whether such symptoms are benign, related to some other ailment or whether the person in front of them is having a stroke or transient ischemic attack (a TIA, or prestroke).

Too often, doctors get it wrong. According to new research from The Johns Hopkins School of Medicine in Baltimore, tens of thousands of strokes and TIAs are probably missed and diagnosed as something else each year in hospital ERs. Those mistakes put people at great risk for future strokes. What's more, certain population groups, such as women and minorities, are more at risk than others for being misdiagnosed when they come to the ER and actually are having a stroke.

Calculating Missed Strokes

To get to the bottom of how often strokes are missed and misdiagnosed in ERs—and which patients are involved—the researchers searched a database that included ER, hospital-admission and hospital-discharge records from nine states dating back to 2009. The team identified 187,188 patients who landed in the hospital with a diagnosis of stroke. Then they looked back through the records of those patients to see which ones had visited the hospital's ER within the past 30 days with symptoms that might have been those of a stroke or a TIA but were diagnosed as something else.

Of these 187,188 patients, it was discovered that 23,809—or 13%—were possibly having a stroke during their earlier ER visit, but the examination they got in the ER—or the ER physician's suspicion that a stroke was happening—wasn't strong enough to make a stroke diagnosis stick. I'm sure you have been in a position where a doctor needs more time and trial and error to find out what's wrong with you…but you want a doctor to be especially thorough and on the ball now if you have a life-threatening condition! And the study found out that a more thorough approach is exactly what's needed in the ER.

Are You At Risk for a Missed Stroke?

Your stroke symptoms might be confused for something else. For example, the Johns Hopkins study revealed that women are 33% more likely to be misdiagnosed than are men. Why? Mainly because generalized symptoms, such as headache and dizziness, are naturally more common in women, and therefore are less likely to be considered possible signs of stroke.

More shocking, though…if you are black, Asian or Hispanic, your stroke symptoms might be overlooked because you didn't receive as thorough an examination as what a white person with the same symptoms might've gotten. In these two ethnic groups, the risk of misdiagnosis in the ER ranged from 18% to 30%! So if you are black, Asian or Hispanic, it is especially important that you be proactive about knowing what kind of care you and family members are entitled to and making sure you receive it.

Young people have strokes, too. Although less likely to have a stroke than older people, those 18 to 45 years old were seven-fold more likely than the elderly (people age 80 and older) to be misdiagnosed when stroke was probably the true cause of their symptoms.

These Stressors Can Cause a Stroke...

•**Keep the noise down.** Ongoing and lengthy exposure to everyday noises, such as cell phone rings or traffic, increases heart rate and decreases heart rate variability—two risk factors for cardiac problems and stroke.

Self-defense: Take deep breaths to ease your body's response to noise. Block out loud noises with earplugs, sound-blocking headphones and/or white noise.

Seth Goldbarg, MD, electrophysiologist, New York Hospital, New York City, writing in *Prevention.*

•**Insomnia increases stroke risk.** According to a recent study, people who have insomnia have a 54% higher risk for stroke than people who do not have insomnia—even after known risk factors such as diabetes, hypertension and obesity are taken into account. Adults ages 18 to 34 with insomnia had eight times higher risk for stroke. If you have insomnia, talk to your doctor about steps to take.

Demetrius Lopes, MD, surgical director of Rush University Comprehensive Stroke Center, Chicago.

•**Get your emotions in order.** People with the most stress, depression, anger and/or hostility were up to twice as likely to suffer a stroke or transient ischemic attack (TIA), also known as a "ministroke," as those with the lowest levels of those traits, according to a new 11-year study.

Why: Chronic psychological problems are just as significant as traditional stroke risk factors, such as smoking and high blood pressure.

Susan Everson-Rose, PhD, MPH, associate professor of medicine, University of Minnesota, Minneapolis.

Another alarming finding from the study was that across all ethnic and age groups on average, if you use an ER of a nonteaching hospital—that is, a hospital that is not connected to a medical college—you face rather high odds of having a stroke missed: 45%. And, worse, if you are in a low-volume ER—meaning one that doesn't see very many patients compared with other hospitals—the odds of being misdiagnosed increase to 57%! The take-home message here is that, if at all possible, use a busy university hospital when you need to get to an ER.

Nipping a Stroke in the Bud

Early recognition and treatment of a stroke improves outcomes and reduces the risk of future strokes by as much as 80%. Diagnosing a stroke correctly, quickly and early is, therefore, crucial.

The researchers are not recommending that every patient who comes through the ER with a headache or dizziness have a CT scan or MRI to definitively rule out a stroke—that has been proven to be a highly inefficient way to identify patients at risk for stroke, in addition to driving up health-care costs. In fact, CT scans done only a few hours after stroke symptoms begin are commonly normal, with the damage caused by stroke showing up days later. Even MRI scans miss strokes in the first 24 hours up to 20% of the time. Instead, the research team is recommending that ER doctors use proven methods to identify strokes at the patient's bedside—get a thorough history of symptoms that have occurred over time and do a physical exam that doesn't depend on race or age and specifically focus on symptoms (such as carefully inspecting specific eye movements if dizziness is the main symptom). And, given the high rate of misdiagnosis in black, Asian and Hispanic people, the researchers recommend that doctors be vigilant, regardless of a patient's race, ethnicity, gender or age, so that everyone has a strong chance of a correct diagnosis. You are entitled to nothing less.

What You Must Know About Unruptured Brain Aneurysm Removal

Seppo Juvela, MD, PhD, neurosurgeon, department of neurosurgery, University of Helsinki, Finland. His study was published in *Stroke*.

What if you had some reason for needing a brain scan? Maybe you got shook up in a car accident or maybe you have ringing and pressure in one of your ears that affects your hearing. So you get the scan, and the doctor comes back with good and bad news...

It turns out that you don't have a brain injury or an acoustic neuroma (a tumor in the ear that affects hearing) or whatever you had the brain scan for, but you do have an unruptured intracranial aneurysm (UIA)—a bulging blood vessel smack in the middle of your brain! An estimated 6 million people in the United States have a UIA, and one of those UIAs bursts every 18 minutes. If you have a UIA and it bursts, causing a hemorrhagic stroke, there's a 40% chance you won't survive more than 30 days. So surgery to remove it before it bursts sounds pretty attractive. Yet, when small UIAs (one-quarter inch or smaller) are found on brain scans, docs usually leave them alone, believing that their risk of bursting is small. In fact, the unruptured aneurysm lodged in your brain might not ever burst—but not necessarily because of its size. A Finnish study found that certain telltale characteristics determine whether or not a UIA should be removed. And this is a key point that American doctors have not been in the know about. For them, size is what matters most, even though small aneurysms have been known to burst, too.

Top Reason to Have That UIA Removed

So which people with UIAs are really most at risk for a hemorrhagic stroke? Being a cigarette smoker topped the list. Compared with ex-smokers and nonsmokers, smokers had three times the risk. Since most of us don't know if we are walking around with UIAs, the findings of this study make smoking even more of a game of Russian roulette. If warnings about lung cancer, heart disease and premature aging aren't incentive enough to quit, the risk of brain damage or death from hemorrhagic stroke should be.

It also turns out that women, smokers or not, are more vulnerable than men when it comes to a bursting UIA. Age at diagnosis is also a big factor—men and women who were younger than 50 when the UIA was diagnosed were more than three times as likely to suffer a hemorrhagic stroke as people who were older than 50. If nothing else, these findings are clear—if you are a smoker or younger than 50 and told you have a UIA, you ought to have it removed no matter what the size, according to the researchers. If you are a non-smoker and older than 40, especially if you are a man, you probably can safely take that watch-and-wait approach, they said.

Getting Rid of UIAs

Microsurgical clipping and endovascular coiling are two common ways that UIA are surgically taken care of. In microsurgical clipping, a hole is drilled through the skull to get

---

MRI Predicts Stroke

An MRI of the carotid artery is better than ultrasound (the test most often used for this purpose) for predicting whether a person will have a stroke or heart attack. In fact, a recent study shows that MRI scans are 7% more accurate in predicting stroke over a five-year period than ultrasound or traditional risk factors alone, such as family history.

Reason: MRI can help determine the thickness of the artery wall and identify deposits of calcium or fat within plaque—all are linked to increased risk for stroke.

David Bluemke, MD, director of radiology and imaging sciences, National Institutes of Health Clinical Center, Bethesda, Maryland.

to the aneurysm. Then a small metal clip is permanently placed at the base of the aneurysm to stop blood flow into it. Endovascular coiling, on the other hand, doesn't involve open brain surgery. Instead, a microcatheter is snaked through an artery in the groin to the site of the aneurysm in the brain. An x-ray technology called fluoroscopy is used to guide the microcatheter into place and make it release one or more tiny platinum coils attached to it into the aneurysm. The coils cause the blood in the aneurysm to clot, cutting off blood flow into the bulge.

The most serious complication of these procedures is rupture of the aneurysm. Incidence is not that common, occurring 2% to 3% of the time. And, naturally, recovery for microvascular clipping is longer than it is for endovascular coiling because microvascular clipping involves open brain surgery.

After clipping, most patients spend a night in the intensive care unit and then a few days in a private hospital room. Although patients will be able to be up and about after they leave the hospital, they do have to take it easy for the next four to six weeks to fully recover.

After endovascular coiling, patients also spend a night in the intensive care unit but get to go home the next day. Within a few days, they are fully back to all of their normal activities. One drawback to endovascular coiling, though, is that the UIA can come back. So patients having this procedure are required to visit their doctors for imaging tests on occasion to make sure all is well.

In any case, no matter what your health status, sex or age, there's no guarantee that a brain aneurysm won't burst, and it's ultimately up to you to decide whether to have surgery. The Finnish researchers came to their conclusions after they examined 118 people given a diagnosis of UIA before 1979 and followed them until they had hemorrhagic strokes or died of old age or other causes. The Finns were in a unique position to study what happens to people when UIAs, large or small, are just left alone. Up until 1979, instead of removing at least large UIAs, Finnish doctors just left them alone.

Their study found that women, especially women who smoke and have large UIAs (more than one-quarter of an inch in size) are most at risk for a hemorrhagic stroke. In fact, the risk of hemorrhagic stroke in women with large UIAs was 73%. If the woman also smoked, her risk increased to 100%. Meanwhile, men who smoked and had an aneurysm of this size had half the risk of their female counterparts...50%. Risk was virtually nil for men who didn't smoke regardless of the size of their aneurysms...and nonsmoking women had a 31% risk.

Importantly for those people who learn that they have a UIA, this information can help them and their doctors make crucial decisions about whether to go through a risky procedure to remove it. If you do not have any of the risky characteristics, your safest option may be to do nothing at all—be sure to have a thorough discussion about this with your doctor.

Faster Stroke Test

A helmet called Strokefinder uses microwaves to examine brain tissue. It can accurately tell within 10 minutes if a stroke is caused by bleeding or clots even before patients arrive at the hospital. Testing is under way.

Chalmers University of Technology.

An Epilepsy Drug May Be the Answer to Stroke Survival

Mark S. Shapiro, PhD, professor, and Sonya M. Bierbower, PhD, postdoctoral fellow, department of physiology, University of Texas Health Science Center, San Antonio. Their study was published in *The Journal of Neuroscience*.

Fast action is needed to survive a stroke. Once brain cells die due to lack of oxygen during an ischemic stroke (a stroke caused by a blood clot), there's no saving them, and reactive oxygen species released by the dying cells injure nearby brain tissue. A quick dose of the clot buster tPA can come to the rescue, but it has to be given within the first four hours after a stroke, and its use is limited because its blood-thinning effects are so powerful. It is not an option for patients who have high blood pressure, a history of bleeding or weak blood vessels. But a drug used to treat another serious health condition that works in an entirely different way may allow many more people to survive strokes with minimal disability.

Turning an Available Drug Into a New Lifesaver

The drug is *retigabine* (also called *ezogabine*, brand name Potiga), an antiseizure drug for certain forms of epilepsy. Researchers from the University of Texas studied its effects in mice that, for the sake of human health, were experimentally given either catastrophic strokes or less severe transient ischemic attacks (ministrokes). Mice given a single dose of retigabine after their strokes were compared with nontreated mice and mice that were not given strokes (controls). The treated mice were divided into groups and each given the drug at a different time, ranging from immediately to six hours after the stroke. Twenty-four hours after the strokes occurred, the mice that had had mini-strokes were tested for balance and coordination by having them walk on a balance beam and on a tiny ladder. (All of the mice had mastered these tasks before their strokes.) Since the mice that had had major strokes were not able to complete these tasks due to the severity of stroke injuries, they were not tested for motor function.

The results: The ministroke mice that didn't receive retigabine slipped and fell several times, but the mice that did receive retigabine were able to traverse the balance beam and ladder just as well as control mice.

All the mice were then euthanized over a period of one to five days after their strokes so that the area of the infarct (the dead brain tissue resulting from the strokes) could be examined. All of the mice that had been given retigabine, whether for a mini-stroke or a major one, had much smaller infarcts than the mice that hadn't been given the medication. Although the greatest benefits were found when the drug was used within three hours post-stroke, retigabine was effective when given up to six hours after the stroke. And even though the infarct size can continue to increase for days after a stroke because dying cells release destructive molecules, mice given retigabine showed no increase in infarct size, suggesting that the drug stops stroke damage in its tracks.

Soothes Brain Cells

Retigabine treats epilepsy by reducing the electrical activity of nerve cells that are out of control because of excessive electrical firing during an epileptic seizure. The researchers theorized that retigabine may reduce damage to the brain in stroke patients by decreasing the excitability of the dying nerve cells and preventing the cells from firing when they really should be preserving their strength.

The researchers are not entirely sure that the drug will have the same effect in people as it did in mice, but retigabine has been on the market and used in humans since 2011 for treating epilepsy. Although the drug isn't currently FDA-approved to treat ischemic strokes, doctors can use the drug off-label for conditions other than epilepsy and may consider doing so if evidence mounts about retigabine's lifesaving potential. Like all drugs, it can cause side effects, which can include mild and temporary imbalance, drowsiness or confusion, vision loss, and pain or difficulty urinating. Whereas the drug is used on a daily basis in patients with epilepsy, it would be used, like tPA, as a one-time emergency medication in stroke patients and so any side effects would not persist longer than a day or two. However, the research suggests that the prevention of brain damage would be permanent. Thus the benefits will need to be weighed against risks as research about the drug for stroke patients continues.

In the meantime, researchers are planning clinical trials of the drug for stroke patients that will likely compare its effectiveness and safety to tPA. If you know that you are at high risk for stroke, you may want to speak with your doctor about participating in a clinical trial of retigabine and also discuss what emergency-care plan is in place for you should you have a stroke.

Bed Position Helps Stroke Recovery

Doctors must evaluate the type of stroke and initial progress of the patient to decide what bed position in the first 24 to 48 hours is best for recovery. Sitting upright can harm some patients by decreasing blood flow to the brain. For those patients, lying flat can improve blood flow. But if a stroke increases brain swelling, sitting upright can improve blood drainage and make damage from the swelling less likely. Ask your doctor which position is best for you.

Murray Flaster, MD, PhD, neurologist and stroke specialist at Loyola University Medical Center, Maywood, Illinois. He reported on stroke-care issues in *MedLink Neurology*.

Delay Surgery After Stroke

In more than 480,000 surgeries, patients who underwent elective, noncardiac procedures following an ischemic stroke had the lowest risk for complications if their surgeries took place more than nine months after their strokes, a recent analysis found. Patients who received surgery within the first three months after their strokes were at highest risk of suffering another stroke or even death. Risk gradually decreased after three months, possibly due to stabilization of blood flow to the brain.

Mads Jorgensen, MB, research assistant, The Cardiovascular Research Center, Gentofte Hospital, Denmark.

Better Surgery Prep for Heart Patients

Among adults with severe heart disease who underwent noncardiac surgery, those given beta-blocker drugs beforehand were 40% less likely to have a stroke or heart attack or die during the 30 days following surgery than those who did not take these drugs.

Possible reason: Beta-blockers lower blood pressure and slow heart rate, which can help ease stress on the heart during and after surgery.

If you have heart disease and need noncardiac surgery: Ask your doctor if you should take a beta-blocker.

Charlotte Andersson, MD, PhD, cardiology researcher, Gentofte Hospital, Hellerup, Denmark.

Watch Out for Warfarin

A new study of atrial fibrillation (AF) patients found that within the first 30 days of beginning the anticlotting drug, they had a 71% higher risk for stroke than those who didn't take the medication. Risk peaked on the third day after starting warfarin.

Possible reason: Warfarin stops two anticoagulant proteins, which can temporarily increase blood stickiness in some people.

If you have AF and are prescribed warfarin: Ask your doctor to closely monitor your blood levels of the drug for the first month, or discuss the use of a "bridge" medication, such as heparin.

Laurent Azoulay, PhD, project leader, Lady Davis Institute for Medical Research, Jewish General Hospital, Montreal, Quebec, Canada.

Two-Pill Treatment Cuts Stroke Risk by One-Third After a TIA

S. Claiborne Johnston, MD, PhD, director, Clinical and Translational Science Institute, University of California, San Francisco. His study was published in *The New England Journal of Medicine.*

If you recently suffered a transient ischemic attack (TIA), also known as a ministroke or warning stroke, your strokelike symptoms might have lasted only a few minutes, and you may have emerged without permanent damage. But you're not home free—because 10% to 20% of TIA patients go on to have a full-blown stroke within 90 days.

Breakthrough: Now there's a way to reduce that risk by one-third. It involves adding a second type of pill to the standard pill that TIA patients take. But to work best, the dual treatment should begin right away after a TIA. That's why you need to know about it—so you'll be prepared in case you or a loved one ever suffers a TIA.

Dynamic Drug Duo

The vast majority of strokes are ischemic strokes, the type caused by a blood clot. That's why it's standard for TIA patients to start taking a daily aspirin, because aspirin is known to help prevent clots. Aspirin's benefits in this regard, though, are rather modest. So researchers set out to determine whether adding the anticoagulant drug *clopidogrel* (Plavix) would help. Like aspirin, clopidogrel works by preventing platelets (a type of blood cell) from collecting and forming clots. Clopidogrel is not risk-free—it can cause significant bleeding—but researchers wanted to see whether its benefits outweighed its risks for TIA patients.

The new study included 5,170 people who had had a TIA or a similar kind of ministroke called an acute minor ischemic stroke within the previous 24 hours. All patients received aspirin right away. The first dose ranged from 75 milligrams (mg) to 300 mg, depending on their doctors' decisions, then the dose was dropped to 75 mg from day two onward.

Patients were randomly divided into two groups. In one group, patients received daily aspirin plus a placebo through day 90. In the other group, patients received clopidogrel at a dose of 300 mg on day one and 75 mg on days two through 90, plus daily aspirin for 21 days. In this dual-therapy group, aspirin was discontinued after 21 days to minimize the risk for bleeding.

Here's what happened over the course of the 90 days…

●**Stroke occurred in 12% of patients in the aspirin-only group,** but in only 8% of the patients in the clopidogrel-plus-aspirin group—meaning that the likelihood of suffering a stroke was one-third lower in the clopidogrel-plus-aspirin group.

●**Fatal or disabling stroke occurred in 7% of aspirin-only users…**but in only 5% of clopidogrel-plus-aspirin users.

●**Hemorrhagic stroke** (the type caused by bleeding rather than a clot) occurred at an identical rate of 0.3% in both groups… and other severe bleeding events (such as bleeding that required surgery or transfusion) occurred at an identical rate of 0.2% in both groups. This was important—because it meant that adding the 90-day clopidogrel therapy to the 21-day aspirin therapy did not increase patients' risk for hemorrhagic stroke or other severe bleeding problems. The rate of mild bleeding events (such as bruising or oozing from puncture sites) was slightly higher among the clopidogrel-plus-aspirin users.

Timing Matters Big Time

Because this study was conducted in China, some experts would like to see the results confirmed before the two-pill therapy becomes the standard of care in the US. It's also worth noting that, because the study follow-up period lasted 90 days, it's not known whether any participants went on to have strokes later—but remember, the riskiest period for stroke occurs right after a TIA. That's why the researchers said that starting treatment with clopidogrel-plus-aspirin as soon as possible after TIA symptoms appear is likely to produce the greatest benefit. Note that doctors generally recommend that TIA patients stay on antiplatelet therapy indefinitely.

What to watch for: The most typical warning signs of a TIA are exactly the same as those of a stroke—sudden numbness or weakness of the face, arm or leg, especially on one side of the body…sudden confusion or trouble speaking or understanding speech…sudden loss of balance or coordination or difficulty with walking…sudden problems with vision in one or both eyes…and/or a sudden, severe headache with no known cause.

As soon as symptoms appear: Seek emergency medical help without delay! If it turns out that you are having a TIA, ask your doctor whether the dual clopidogrel-plus-aspirin therapy is right for you. Remember, the sooner you get started on the treatment, the better your chances of avoiding a full-blown stroke.

Heart-Rhythm Irregularities During Hospital Stays Could Mean Stroke Risk

Stroke risk doubles after surgery among people who develop irregular heart rhythms during their hospital stays. Heart flutters and fibrillations may result from the short-term stress associated with any surgery and may not be any cause for concern. But they also could be a sign of increased stroke risk and need to be followed up. Be sure to ask your doctor whether you have any heart-rhythm irregularities after surgery.

Hooman Kamel, MD, neurologist at the Brain and Mind Research Institute, Weill Cornell Medical College, New York City, and coauthor of a study of more than 1.7 million people, published in *The Journal of the American Medical Association.*

Do-It-Yourself Stroke Rehab

Pamela Woods Duncan, PhD, PT, professor of physical therapy, Duke University School of Medicine, Durham, North Carolina.

While many people survive strokes and manage to keep their own "selves" very much intact, for others the remnant physical or mental damage of the stroke goes on and on. Careers and relationships suffer when a formerly vibrant, independent person is transformed into one who is in need of assistance for everything from driving to dialing the phone to showering and dressing.

Since 1995, survival rates for stroke patients have been boosted by nearly 30% —but, sadly, many of those patients have remained deeply impaired. They have trouble walking and they are at high risk for falls. Innovative therapies have been developed for physical therapy to aid in recovery. While helpful, much of this technology is expensive to develop, costly to purchase and must be administered by a trained specialist as part of a structured exercise program, putting it out of reach for many patients.

Now a study from Duke University has taken the results of patients doing intensive, center-based rehab with high-tech equipment and

Better Time to Take Preventive Aspirin

Adults with a history of stroke or heart disease who took a 100-mg aspirin tablet at bedtime had less of the blood stickiness that is associated with heart attack than when aspirin was taken in the morning. Because blood stickiness tends to peak in the morning, taking a nighttime aspirin allows for adequate time for absorption.

Tobias Bonten, MD, researcher, Leiden University Medical Center, The Netherlands.

compared them with the results of people who work at home with a visiting physical therapist. The researchers also investigated whether rehab started long after a stroke—as much as six months later—still can be helpful.

Exciting, Unexpected Results

The study examined the progress of 408 stroke survivors, all of whom had their strokes either two months or six months earlier. Some of the patients who had suffered strokes six months previously were wait-listed to begin therapy at a center and so had not received any rehab. All of the patients were divided into three groups. Those who had strokes two months previously either underwent therapy in a center for high-tech rehab (group one)…or had home-based rehab with a therapist (group two), emphasizing progressive strength, balance and walking exercises. The third group of patients—those who were wait-listed—also started the high-tech program. Rehab for all groups took place in three weekly sessions over 12 weeks.

We spoke with the study author, Pamela Woods Duncan, PhD, PT, professor of physical therapy at Duke University School of Medicine. She explained that the goal of the study was to determine how well patients functioned one year after a stroke with different therapy protocols—and that the research yielded two excellent findings…

First, while the researchers had anticipated that high-tech rehab would be more effective, much to their surprise that was not the case. "Using technology was not superior to working with patients at home in function, balance and walking exercises," Dr. Duncan said.

Furthermore, the study put to rest the belief that only early rehab works. The results were the same in all three groups including the late starters—52% of all patients showed significant improvement, walking well in the home and walking more in their communities.

On Your Own?

Stroke patients absolutely need rehabilitation and regular exercise, Dr. Duncan said, but added that it would be a grave mistake to misinterpret these findings to mean that stroke patients can do well simply by exercising on their own at home. Stroke patients need careful cardiovascular monitoring and a trained therapist to design and conduct a program that is in keeping with their progress. Safety is an issue, especially early on in rehab when the risk of falling is high—so using professional therapists, at least initially, is critical. That said, in-home therapy uses less expensive equipment (such as elastic bands), requires less training for therapists and needs fewer clinical staff members than inpatient care. And, physical therapy for stroke patients is not just a 12-week endeavor—it must be a lifelong habit in order to keep the muscles strong and supple. Developing an at-home therapy plan that can be administered by family members can be cost-effective and also very helpful at maintaining and even continuing to improve the physical function of the patient.

Stroke Survivors Need Close Follow-up

Stroke survivors remain at high risk for another stroke and other medical problems for at least five years. Within the year following a stroke, 9.3% of survivors died…had another stroke, ministroke or heart attack…or were admitted to long-term care. After the first year, risk for these events remained at 5% for four more years.

Self-defense: Check with your doctor about closer follow-up.

Study of 24,000 stroke survivors by researchers in the Stroke Program at University of Toronto, Canada, reported by Heart and Stroke Foundation of Canada and presented at the Canadian Stroke Congress in Vancouver.

Yoga Boosts Balance Long After Stroke

Arlene A. Schmid, PhD, OTR (occupational therapist registered), assistant professor in the department of occupational therapy at Indiana University and a rehabilitation research scientist at Roudebush VA Medical Center, both in Indianapolis. She is the lead author of a study on yoga and balance published in *Stroke*.

Many people think of yoga as exercise for the limber-limbed young. So you may be happily surprised to learn that yoga can help stroke survivors improve their balance and become more active—even if they start practicing yoga long after their strokes occurred.

This news from a small but encouraging study is important because stroke victims often are left with long-term balance problems that contribute to disability and increase the risk for potentially fatal falls. What's more, the study results challenge the discouraging yet common notion that significant improvement in motor skills is unlikely when more than six months have passed since a patient's stroke.

Study scoop: Participants included 47 adults, average age 63, who had suffered strokes anywhere from six months to more than 11 years earlier. All had finished their stroke rehabilitation programs...could stand on their own or with a device...and continued to receive usual medical care throughout the study. For eight weeks, one group of participants attended twice-weekly hour-long group classes involving modified yoga postures, breathing techniques and meditation, with classes growing more challenging over time. A second "yoga-plus" group took the same yoga classes and also received an audio recording of yoga/relaxation techniques to use three times weekly at home. A third group, which served as a control, received no yoga instruction. All participants completed tests of balance, independence and quality of life at the start and end of the study.

DIY Test to Prevent a Second Stroke

About 25% to 35% of stroke survivors experience atrial fibrillation (AF)—a type of irregular heartbeat that is associated with increased stroke risk. Patients and their relatives can be trained to detect an irregular rhythm by taking a wrist pulse. If an irregularity is detected and AF confirmed, physicians may prescribe medication or other treatment to decrease stroke risk.

Bernd Kallmünzer, MD, neurologist with the stroke unit at University Medical Center, Erlangen, Germany. He is lead author of a study of 256 stroke patients, published in Neurology.

Results: No significant changes were seen in the control group. In contrast, members of both the yoga and yoga-plus groups experienced significant improvement in their ability to balance and raised their scores on tests of independence and quality of life. Yoga participants also felt less afraid of falling and reported attempting more challenging activities because of their improved balance—for instance, they talked about walking through a grocery store instead of using a motorized scooter...being able to take a shower...and feeling inspired to visit friends. (Comparing the two yoga groups, the addition of the audio recording did not change the results significantly, though the yoga-plus people did report enjoying listening to it.)

How does yoga work its magic? Researchers suggested that yoga's mind-body connection may make it more therapeutic than traditional exercise...and that yoga is especially effective in improving poststroke function because it promotes coordination of complex movements, balance, strengthening and breathing.

Stroke patients: Ask your doctor or occupational therapist whether yoga is appropriate for you. If so, request a referral to a registered yoga therapist who is experienced in working with stroke survivors.

Chapter 4

KEEP YOUR LUNGS HEALTHY FOR LIFE

How Cooking Oil with the Right Vitamin E Can Help You Breathe

Many plant oils are rich in vitamin E—but the term vitamin E is actually a catchall for eight different chemical compounds, each with its own antioxidant profile. And the problem is that we may be getting way too much of one certain type of vitamin E that's not good for us.

What's in Your Oil?

We know from animal experiments that a type of vitamin E called D-alpha tocopherol and another type called D-gamma tocopherol have completely opposite effects on lung function...one good, the other bad. Never mind animals...what about the effects in people? A team of researchers from the Feinberg School of Medicine at Northwestern University in Chicago and other universities compared blood levels of vitamin E against the results of lung-function tests (which measure how much air a person can exhale in one big breath) of more than 4,500 people. And the researchers confirmed that these two different vitamin Es—D-alpha tocoph-

erol and D-gamma tocopherol—have the different effects...

- **D-gamma tocopherol** was associated with worse lung function for everyone, and the higher the level, the worse the lung function.

- **D-alpha tocopherol** was associated with better lung function for everyone. The study also showed that increases in D-alpha tocopherol could counteract the effects of D-gamma tocopherol.

What's behind this? It seems that D-alpha tocopherol inhibits allergic inflammation—that is, inflammation that is set off by allergies—while D-gamma tocopherol promotes allergic inflammation. Sometimes your body wants and needs temporary inflammation, for example, to help isolate causes of tissue injury, such as bacteria and toxins. But a steady diet (literally!) of a substance that enhances inflammation—even if it is a vitamin—is going to hurt you. Another recent study found that too much D-gamma tocopherol in the body can aggravate osteoarthritis—so its effects aren't limited to the lungs

Joan M. Cook-Mills, PhD, professor of medicine, department of allergy/immunology, Feinberg School of Medicine, Northwestern University, Chicago. Her study was published in *Respiratory Research*.

but, in all likelihood, extend anywhere that inflammation can develop.

Breathing Easier

You are what you eat, they say, and it's becoming clearer that Europeans, for example, may breathe easier than Americans in part because they have two to six times less D-gamma tocopherol in their bodies than American adults do—and the main reason is that Europeans use more olive oil or safflower oil, which are low in D-gamma tocopherol and high in D-alpha tocopherol. Americans, on the other hand, consume more soy, corn and canola oils, which are very high in D-gamma tocopherol.

The evidence suggests that you can help your lungs be healthier and stronger and naturally breathe better by making some very simple food choices.

How to Go For More D-alpha

Cooking oils that are richer in D-alpha than D-gamma tocopherol include olive, sunflower and safflower, which can replace soy, corn and canola oils. Sunflower seeds, hazelnuts, almonds and wheat germ are also rich in D-alpha tocopherol. What about vitamin E supplements? Some contain only D-alpha tocopherol, some only D-gamma tocopherol, and some a mixture of the two types. If you want to take a supplement, consult with a doctor specifically trained in nutrition (a naturopathic doctor or a chiropractic doctor)—or a nutrition specialist (registered dietician).

4 Secrets to Easier Breathing

Gerard J. Criner, MD, professor of medicine and director of pulmonary and critical care medicine at Temple Lung Center at Temple University School of Medicine in Philadelphia.

If you can't catch your breath, walking, climbing stairs or simply carrying on a conversation can be a challenge.

When breathing is a struggle, you wouldn't think that exercise is the answer. But it can be a solution for people with chronic obstructive pulmonary disease (COPD) or heart failure or even for healthy people who occasionally become short of breath.*

Four better-breathing techniques that really help…

Pursed-Lip Breathing

When you're feeling short of breath, inhale through your nose for two seconds, then pucker your lips as if you were going to whistle or blow out a candle. Exhale through pursed lips for four seconds.

How it helps: It prolongs the respiratory cycle and gives you more time to empty your lungs. This is particularly important if you have emphysema. With emphysema, air gets trapped in the lungs. The trapped air causes the lungs to overinflate, which reduces the amount of force that they're able to generate. This results in a buildup of carbon dioxide that makes it difficult to breathe.

You may need to do this only when you're more active than usual and short of breath. Or you may breathe better when you do it often.

Changing Positions

Simply changing how you stand or sit can improve breathing when you're feeling winded.

How it helps: Certain positions (see below) help muscles around the diaphragm work more efficiently to promote easier breathing.

Examples: While sitting, lean your chest forward…rest your elbows on your knees… and relax your upper-body muscles. When standing, bend forward at the waist and rest your hands on a table or the back of a chair. Or back up to a wall…support yourself with your hips…and lean forward and put your hands on your thighs.

*If you don't have COPD, you should see a doctor if you have shortness of breath after only slightly activity or while resting, or if shortness of breath wakes you up at night or requires you to sleep propped up to breathe.

Controlled Coughing

Your lungs produce excessive mucus when you have COPD. The congestion makes it harder to breathe. It also increases the risk for pneumonia and other lung infections. A normal, explosive cough is not effective at removing mucus. In fact, out-of-control coughing can cause airways to collapse and trap even more mucus. A controlled cough is more effective (and requires less oxygen and energy). You also can use this technique to help clear mucus from the lungs when you have a cold.

How to do it: Sit on a chair or the edge of your bed with both feet on the floor. Fold your arms around your midsection…breathe in slowly through your nose…then lean forward while pressing your arms against your abdomen. Lightly cough two or three times. Repeat as needed.

Important: Taking slow, gentle breaths through your nose while using this technique will prevent mucus from moving back into the airways.

Cold-Air Assistance

This is a quick way to breathe better. When you are short of breath—or doing an activity that you know will lead to breathlessness, such as walking on a treadmill—position a fan so that it blows cool air on your face. You also can splash your face with cold water if you become short of breath.

How it helps: Cool air and water stimulate the trigeminal nerve in the face, which slows respiration and helps ease shortness of breath. That's why the treadmills and exercise bikes used in respiratory-rehabilitation facilities are often equipped with small fans.

When to Get Breathing Help from a Professional

You can do many breathing exercises on your own without the help of a health professional. For the techniques below, however, it's best to first consult a respiratory therapist (ask your doctor for a referral) to ensure that you know how to do the exercise properly. You can then continue on your own.

•**Paced breathing for endurance.** This technique is useful for people who have COPD and/or heart failure, since it improves lung capacity and heart function.

How it helps: With practice, this technique can increase your cardiorespiratory endurance by 30% to 40%. To perform the exercise, a metronome is set at a rate that's faster than your usual respiratory rate. Your therapist will encourage you to breathe as hard and as fast as you can for, say, about 15 minutes. (Beginners might do it for only a few minutes at a time.)

Example: The metronome may be set for 20 breaths per minute to start, and you may eventually work up to 40 breaths per minute.

You'll notice that breathing becomes easier when you're doing various activities—for instance, when you're exercising, climbing stairs or taking brisk walks.

•**Inspiratory muscle training.** Think of this as a workout for your breathing muscles. It is especially helpful for people with COPD or other lung diseases and those recovering from respiratory failure. People who strengthen these muscles can improve their breathing efficiency by 25% to 30%.

How it helps: For this breathing exercise, you'll use a device known as an inspiratory muscle trainer, which includes a mouthpiece, a one-way valve and resistance settings. When you inhale, the one-way valve closes. You're forced to use effort to breathe against resistance. Then, the valve opens so that you can exhale normally. This breathing exercise is typically performed for 15 minutes twice a day. You can buy these devices online.

Good choice: The Threshold Inspiratory Muscle Trainer, available at *FitnessMart.com* for $47.50.

Get Help to Quit

Medicare previously covered tobacco counseling only when patients were diagnosed with, or had symptoms of, a smoking-related disease, such as chronic obstructive pulmonary disease (COPD) or lung cancer.

New rule: Medicare now covers preventive-care services, including 100% of smoking-cessation counseling for smokers without smoking-related diseases. Coverage includes two tries at tobacco counseling a year—up to four sessions each. Medications to help with smoking cessation may be covered under some Part D plans.

To find a program: Contact your local National Cancer Institute–operated "Quitline" (877-448-7848, *SmokeFree.gov*).

Nathan Heggem, senior communications and policy associate, Medicare Rights Center, New York City.

Lung Fitness for Flu Season

Andrew L. Rubman, ND, founder and medical director, Southbury Clinic for Traditional Medicines, Southbury, Connecticut. *SouthburyClinic.com*

Everyone dreads getting sick in the wintertime, but some people find themselves unusually vulnerable to respiratory infections...most particularly those who have asthma or a history of bronchitis. Yes, we all know about flu shots and washing hands and avoiding crowds, but did you realize there's lots more you can do to fortify yourself—and your respiratory system in particular—even before the sick season kicks in? Andrew L. Rubman, ND, Daily Health News contributing medical editor, had advice on getting fit to fight the flu.

First and foremost, he said, remember that the better shape you and your respiratory system are in, the more you'll be able to tolerate exposure to germs without falling ill. Anything that weakens your immune system—such as eating poorly, stress or not getting enough sleep—increases your vulnerability to whatever is going around. And previous illness makes it worse. Not only does illness deplete energy, but with severe respiratory infections (and other diseases, too), there may be scarring and some tissue damage in your lungs that leaves you weaker and more vulnerable. Dr. Rubman also noted that more often than we realize, an illness may not be fully resolved, even after you feel better. "There may be underlying colonization with mold organisms in the respiratory tract as well," he said. When researchers at the Mayo Clinic cultured patients with chronic rhinosinusitis, over 90% showed positive culture for fungus, including mold. Mold infestation in respiratory tissues weakens the structure and capability of the lungs, allowing easier colonization of potentially infectious bacteria.

Strengthen Your Immune System

Emphasizing the importance of working with your own doctor for specific dosing, Dr. Rubman says the following supplements can be helpful in supporting lung health and immune health...

• **Indian Tobacco.** This botanical remedy has a history of use for conditions such as asthma, pneumonia and bronchitis. Today, he may prescribe Indian tobacco (also called lobelia, it's not really tobacco at all—the leaves have a tobacco-like taste) as a preventive to strengthen lungs and a treatment for respiratory ailments.

Note: Lobelia is potentially toxic in large doses and should be taken only under the guidance of a health-care provider with experience in botanical medicines.

• **Selenium—Nature's Inflammation Fighter.** This essential trace mineral has potent antioxidant properties to protect the body from inflammation and damage caused by free radicals. It fortifies the immune system to do battle with microorganisms. Research even suggests that a high intake of selenium is associated with a reduced risk of death from colorectal, prostate and lung cancers. While the usual dose is 200 mcg a day, Dr. Rubman frequently goes further, prescribing a daily dosage as high as 400 mcg to 500 mcg, taken in three doses, as a preventive during flu season.

•**Vitamin C—The Antioxidant Vitamin.** This antioxidant-packed nutrient remains a major player in immune system maintenance. Research demonstrates that vitamin C can significantly boost antimicrobial activity, including the activity of natural killer cells that hunt down and vanquish germs. Supplementation with up to one gram (1,000 mg) daily can be helpful and is usually well-tolerated, notes Dr. Rubman.

Note: Some studies suggest that vitamin C may not be safe for patients undergoing chemotherapy.

•**Fish Oil—A Rich Source of Omega-3 Fatty Acids.** Tuna and salmon (preferably wild) are rich sources of omega-3 fatty acids. Eat these three times a week. Look for fish oil supplements with the highest levels of docosahexaenoic acid (DHA) and eicosapentaenoic acid (EPA), which ideally should make up more than 50% of the total dosage. (*Caution*: If you take a blood-thinning medication such as *warfarin*, speak with your doctor before taking fish oil supplements.)

•**Mullein—A Velvety Smooth Throat Soother.** When patients complain of a scratchy throat or congestion and sense a respiratory problem coming on, Dr. Rubman often prescribes mullein. This herb contains mucilage, a substance that soothes irritated respiratory passages, along with saponins that help loosen mucus. Laboratory studies have shown that mullein can kill many viruses on contact. To make a cup of mullein tea, add one to two teaspoons of dried leaves and flowers to boiling water and steep for 10 minutes. Strain before drinking.

•**N-acetyl Cysteine and L-theanine.** New and emerging research supports using n-acetyl cysteine and L-theanine to strengthen lung function. "Discuss with your doctor whether either or both are appropriate for you, and, if they are, what the dosage should be," Dr. Rubman said.

Avoid Pollutants

Respiratory disorders of all kinds, including flu and pneumonia, are more apt to develop when foreign particles are aspirated or inhaled into the lungs, including from chimneys, wood stoves and fireplaces. This causes inflammation, which leads the delicate mucous membranes lining the respiratory system to become swollen, irritated and more susceptible to infection.

It's important to make an effort to protect your lungs from this environmental assault, especially during the winter months when flu season is in full force. Consider, with your physician's oversight, taking antioxidant supplements for protection. In one study, children with asthma who took vitamins C and E were less likely to experience breathing problems from air pollution than children who did not.

Make Your Lungs Strong

Exercising the lungs may help fend off disease as well. Many tend toward "shallow breathing," failing to fully inflate the lungs with air or clear them completely, says Dr. Rubman. This limits the exchange of gases. Dr. Rubman suggests using the intentional breathing of Pranayama yoga to strengthen your lungs. *Here's how…*

•**Sit up straight, with your spine, neck and head in a straight line.** Do so cross-legged on a floor mat, small pillow or rug, or—if you find that uncomfortable—just use a chair.

•**Close your eyes and relax.** Meditate, or visualize yourself in a peaceful environment—for example, lying on the beach, listening to the sound of the waves.

•**Take a full, deep, intentional breath, filling lungs from the bottom up.** To make sure you are doing this correctly, place your hand on your stomach and feel this area (which is above and behind the diaphragm,

Thirdhand Smoke Danger

Carcinogenic tobacco chemicals linger in rooms, on clothing and in cars long after a cigarette has been smoked.

New finding: The danger is most intense a few hours after smoking but can remain significant for more than 18 hours.

Beware: If you can smell smoke, you're inhaling harmful compounds.

Hugo Destaillats, PhD, staff scientist, Indoor Environment Group, Lawrence Berkeley National Laboratory, Berkeley, California.

a vital muscle for respiration) expand before air fills the upper chest.

• **Inhale for a count of three…exhale for a count of six.** As time goes on, with practice you will be able to gradually increase these counts (ideally, at the same one-to-two ratio).

• **Do this for 10 minutes once or twice a day.**

Note: We asked Dr. Rubman about the various breathing and blowing devices that promise to increase respiratory capacity. In his view, unless you have ongoing respiratory issues, these are a waste of money. Deep breathing achieves the same results, and for free.

Drink Up

Dr. Rubman said it is important to remain well-hydrated, drinking plenty of water and other fluids all year, but especially during flu season since fluids moisturize the mucous membranes and help keep nasal discharge thin. Dehydration can lead to dizziness, disorientation and even vulnerability to shock. Decaffeinated herbal teas, broth, diluted fruit juice and sparkling water are all good choices.

Recovery After Illness

Recovery should focus not only on resting so you will feel better, but also on improving your underlying function to better resist the next challenges. A professional nutritional consultant or physician formally trained in nutrition can be helpful in making certain you are completely over the illness and ensuring you get strong for the future.

Respect the Enemy

You can't reduce your risk of illness to zero, even with all these precautions. Recognize that flu and pneumonia can be serious and their complications potentially life-threatening, especially in older people. If you suspect something is wrong—for example, if you have chronic chest pain, a persistent cough, shortness of breath or green or yellow sputum—see your physician promptly for proper diagnosis and treatment.

Sweet Drink Beats Lingering Cough

A warm honey-coffee drink relieves persistent coughing better than corticosteroids or cough syrups.

To make: Mix one-half teaspoon of instant coffee granules with two-and-a-half teaspoons of honey. Stir into seven ounces of warm water. Drink three servings a day. Honey is a well-known remedy for cough, and caffeine dilates bronchi and stimulates breathing. If your cough hasn't eased after a few weeks of using this remedy, see your doctor.

Neda Raeessi, MD, researcher, Baqiyatallah University of Medical Sciences, Tehran, Iran.

Be Patient with Coughs!

Most coughs last an average of 18 days. And because most coughs are caused by viruses, they are not relieved by antibiotics. But patients often believe that a cough should last no more than a week and ask their doctors for antibiotics. Even many doctors estimate that a cough is expected to last only seven to nine days.

Study of 493 people by researchers at University of Georgia College of Public Health, Athens, published in *Annals of Family Medicine*.

Four-Part Plan Helps People Quit Smoking

The program includes counseling by a nurse…brochures on smoking cessation…referral to a quit-smoking phone hotline…and a six-week supply of nicotine patches at no charge. Patients using the program were four times more likely to quit before surgery than patients who were advised to quit but did not use the program. Thirty days after surgery, 29% of patients in the quit-smoking program said that they had not started smoking again, compared with 11% of those not in the program.

Study of 168 smokers due for elective surgery by researchers at University of Western Ontario, London, Canada, published in *Anesthesia & Analgesia*.

E-Cigs Do Not Help Smokers Quit

E-cigarettes don't make it easier to quit smoking. Smokers who had been diagnosed with cancer who used e-cigarettes to help them quit were more dependent on nicotine and no more likely to quit than those who did not use e-cigarettes.

Study by researchers at Memorial Sloan Kettering Cancer Center, New York City, published in *Cancer*.

Are Cigars Safer Than Cigarettes?

Absolutely not. There is no such thing as a "safe" tobacco product. Cigars contain the same addictive, toxic and carcinogenic compounds found in cigarettes and are not a safe alternative. In fact, a single large cigar can contain as much tobacco as an entire pack of cigarettes. Cigar smoking has similar consequences to cigarette smoking—for example, cigar smokers are four to 10 times more likely to die from oral, esophageal or laryngeal cancer than nonsmokers. You (or a loved one) can get help quitting from the Freedom From Smoking program. It offers a variety of smoking-cessation techniques. The free eight-session program is taught in small groups of eight to 10 people in most communities. It's also available in a self-paced online program (*www.FFSonline.org*). For more information, go to the American Lung Association's Web site, *www.Lung.org* (click on "Stop Smoking"). Or call the Lung HelpLine at 1-800-LUNG-USA.

Norman H. Edelman, MD, chief medical officer, American Lung Association, Washington, DC.

Relieve COPD Flare-Ups with Vitamin D

Study titled "Vitamin D3 supplementation in patients with chronic obstructive pulmonary disease (ViDiCO): a multicenter, double-blind, randomized controlled trial," from Centre for Primary Care and Public Health, Blizard Institute, Barts and London School of Medicine and Dentistry, Queen Mary University of London, published in *The Lancet Respiratory Medicine*.

Chronic obstructive pulmonary disease (COPD) is a crippling combination of chronic bronchitis and emphysema. If you have it, you're worn out by a constant cough, phlegm, shortness of breath and chest tightness. The symptoms can be managed (though never cured) by breathing exercises and physical therapy, bronchodilator and corticosteroid drugs and—worst-case scenario—being hooked up to an oxygen tank. And every so often, symptoms will flare up to an extreme.

Breakthrough news: If you or a loved one is a COPD sufferer, taking supplements of a certain essential nutrient can significantly reduce your risk of flare-ups.

D to the Rescue

Researchers from Queen Mary University of London expanded on a small study that looked at vitamin D deficiency and supplementation in people with COPD and confirmed the earlier findings—vitamin D supplements reduced risk of flare-ups.

The current study recruited 240 patients with COPD from across Britain and conducted a full-fledged placebo-controlled study.

The researchers first tested these patients' current vitamin D levels to keep track of who was low, normal or high. Then, about half the participants were treated with a 3-milligram dose (120,000 IU) of vitamin D, taken in the form of oral drops given every two months for a year. (This is a very large megadose of the vitamin that is, basically, only used in research studies and in people with severely low vitamin D levels. The average person should never take this amount of the vitamin on his or her own.) The other participants were given a placebo.

The results: Supplementation reduced the risk of COPD flares by 43% in patients who had borderline-to-low vitamin D levels to begin with (blood levels of less than 50 nanomoles per liter [nmol/L]) but did not do much for patients who already had normal or high levels of the vitamin (blood levels of 50 nmol/L or greater). But most people with COPD do have low levels of vitamin D or outright vitamin D deficiencies. In this study, 87% had insufficient-to-deficient levels.

The researchers are not yet sure exactly how vitamin D helps stop COPD flare-ups, but they think it might have to do with the vitamin's protective antimicrobial and anti-inflammatory properties. COPD flares often are caused by either infections or irritation of the respiratory system (from exposure to cigarette smoke or other pollutants, for example). Vitamin D likely helps the immune system fend off these onslaughts.

Beware Too Much D

Although no serious side effects were attributed to vitamin D in the study, more D was not better. In fact, patients who already had vitamin D blood levels of 100 nmol/L or greater were slightly more susceptible to flares. So, even though the large majority of people with COPD are low in D and could use a supplement, don't just start taking it on your own. Instead, speak to your doctor about having a blood test to know exactly what your vitamin D level is before starting a supplement.

Having too much vitamin D in your system is dangerous. It can cause itchy skin, calcium buildup in the arteries, daytime sleepiness, headaches, heart rhythm abnormalities, muscle pain, stomach issues, kidney stones, and high blood pressure.

If your vitamin D level is very low, your doctor may prescribe a very large dose of D that you take, for example, once a week or once a month—as the patients in this study did. But this is definitely not a regimen that anyone should do on his or her own without close medical supervision for the reasons explained above.

More than likely, your levels are just a bit low, and your doctor will recommend a high-quality daily supplement in a dosage that is right for you. The recommended daily allowance of vitamin D for people who are one to 70 years of age is 600 IU, and it's 800 IU for people 71 and older...but up to 4,000 IU per day has been considered safe by the US National Academy of Sciences Institute of Medicine.

DIY Test for Lung Health Could Save Your Life

David L. Katz, MD, MPH, internist and preventive medicine specialist. He is cofounder and director of the Yale-Griffin Prevention Research Center in Derby, Connecticut, and the author of *Disease-Proof: The Remarkable Truth About What Makes Us Well.*

If you're conscientious about your health, you probably see your doctor for an annual physical…or perhaps even more often if you have a chronic condition or get sick.

But if you'd like to keep tabs on your lung health between your doctor visits, there's an easy-to-do test that can help you assess basic lung and heart function.

Here is a self-test that you can do at home—repeat it once every few months, and keep track of results. See your doctor if you don't "pass" this test…*

Stairs Test

The prop you'll need: A single flight of stairs (about eight to 12 steps).

What to do: Walk up the steps at a normal pace while continuously reciting "Mary had a little lamb" or some other simple verse.

Watch out: You should be able to talk easily while climbing the stairs and when at the top—without feeling winded. If you cannot continue to talk, or if you feel discomfort or tightness in your chest at any time during this test, see your doctor as soon as possible.

Beware: If the small stress of climbing one flight of stairs causes physical problems, it could be a sign of hardening of the arteries (arteriosclerosis) or heart disease.

For some individuals, being out of breath could mean that they have asthma or bronchitis…chronic obstructive pulmonary disease (COPD), including emphysema…or even lung cancer.

*This self-test is not a substitute for a thorough physical exam from your doctor. Use it only as a way to identify potential problem areas to discuss with your physician.

An Afternoon Nap May Be Dangerous

Adults who napped every day for an hour or more had a 32% higher risk of dying from a respiratory illness, compared with those who did not take naps or nap as long. Researchers are studying whether sleeping during the day triggers inflammation in the body or signals that someone already has a lung disease, such as pneumonia, bronchitis or emphysema.

Study of more than 16,000 people by researchers at Cambridge University, England, published in *American Journal of Epidemiology.*

New Treatments for Sleep Apnea

People who have obstructive sleep apnea stop breathing for very short intervals during the night, disrupting sleep and increasing the risk for diabetes, heart attack and stroke. In addition to conventional treatments such as continuous positive airway pressure (CPAP) machines and oral mouthpieces that advance the jaw, newer treatments include Provent Sleep Apnea Therapy (*ProventTherapy.com*), which is a small disposable patch that fits over each nostril.

A central valve produces pressure in the airway so that it remains open during sleep. The Winx Sleep Therapy System (*Apnicure. com*) uses a soft mouthpiece that is connected to a small vacuum console. The device creates suction to open the throat.

David Rapoport, MD, professor of medicine and director of the Sleep Disorders Center, New York University Medical Center, New York City.

Hidden Brain Dangers of Sleep Apnea... Especially for Women

Paul M. Macey, PhD, assistant professor in residence, associate dean for information technology and innovation, School of Nursing, University of California, Los Angeles. His study was published in *PLoS ONE*.

You probably know that obstructive sleep apnea causes people to gasp, snort and snore as their sleep is interrupted by repeated stops and starts in their breathing. And you know that these mini-suffocations, which can occur dozens of times each hour, increase the risk for all kinds of serious health problems.

But you probably don't know that sleep apnea causes permanent changes to the structure of the brain and how the brain controls blood pressure. These changes create a vicious cycle that leaves apnea patients starved for oxygen not only at night, but also during the day—particularly at times when their bodies are most in need of oxygen!

Though sleep apnea often is thought of as a "man's problem," women develop it, too... and women are at especially high risk for the dangerous nervous system changes, a recent study reveals. *Male or female, if you (or a loved one) have or may have sleep apnea, you need to know about this new research...*

Autonomic Glitch

Participants in the new study included male and female patients who recently had been diagnosed with sleep apnea and were not receiving treatment, plus some healthy "controls" (people without sleep apnea who served as a basis of comparison).

The point of the experiment was to see how people's bodies respond to various physical "challenges" that use different nervous system pathways to signal increased cardiovascular demand. These challenges mimic day-to-day activities, such as straining, lifting and touching something cold. Normally such challenges, like many everyday activities, cause heart rate to speed up. This is a protective response of the autonomic regulatory system (the part of the central nervous system that regulates heart rate, blood pressure, breathing, etc. without you having to think about it), sending extra blood and oxygen to cells that are in greater need.

The challenges in the experiment included a hand-grip task (squeezing an inflatable bag with one hand as hard as possible for 16 seconds)...keeping a foot in icy water for one minute...and breathing out hard with the mouth closed and nose pinched shut (similar to what happens when a person is straining over a bowel movement!).

Results: For all three challenges, compared with the healthy controls, the sleep apnea patients showed an impaired response—meaning that they had heart rate increases that were less pronounced and slower to kick in.

Also, in comparing male sleep apnea patients with female sleep apnea patients, the researchers found that the degree of impairment was worse in women. Take the bag-squeezing test, for example. The heart rate of women with apnea increased just 3.3% and returned to normal very quickly, whereas in healthy women, heart rate increased 5.8% and remained elevated significantly longer. For men, however, the differences between those with and without apnea were much less pronounced. Heart rate increased 7.4% in apnea patients, compared with 8.6% in healthy men...and there was only a small difference in how long it remained elevated in the two male groups.

Why such an impaired response is dangerous: An impaired response means that tissues, including sensitive brain cells, are being starved of oxygen because blood flow is inadequate. Obviously, sleep apnea patients are oxygen-deprived whenever they stop breathing during sleep—but this study shows that people with sleep apnea also often are deprived of oxygen when they are awake and during daily physical tasks, when oxygen is needed most. That's because their nervous systems don't do a good job of increasing heart rate as needed to meet demands at times when the body is physiologically challenged.

What's more, this impaired response creates a vicious cycle—impaired blood flow leads to structural changes in the brain and cardiovascular system, which leads to further impaired blood flow—and so on. The worse this gets, the greater the risk may be for heart disease, high blood pressure and other chronic illnesses associated with autonomic dysfunction, the study researchers noted. While both male and female sleep apnea patients are at risk, the dangers for women may be particularly high, given their greater magnitude of autonomic response impairment and the fact that they are less likely to be properly diagnosed in the first place.

Self-defense for women and men: Sleep apnea affects an estimated 28 million adults in the US, more than 80% of whom do not realize that they have the disorder. If you have been told that you snore, gasp or grunt as you sleep, or if you often feel groggy during the day even after a full night's rest, ask your doctor about being tested for sleep apnea. Early detection and treatment can help protect against damage to the brain, cardiovascular system and other organs...and allow you to sleep better and feel better, too.

Sleep Device Bonus

When a person with sleep apnea begins treatment with a continuous positive airway pressure (CPAP) device, which forces air into the lungs during sleep, the person's resistance to insulin (a hallmark of diabetes) improves dramatically.

If you have sleep apnea: Treatment with a CPAP device may not only improve your sleep but also help lower diabetes risk.

Imran H. Iftikhar, MD, assistant professor of internal medicine, University of South Carolina, Columbia.

How to Cure Snoring with a Song

Murray Grossan, MD, otolaryngologist and head-and-neck surgeon with the Tower Ear, Nose & Throat Clinic at Cedars-Sinai Medical Center in Los Angeles. He is author of *Free Yourself from Sinus and Allergy Problems Permanently. GrossanInstitute.com*

If your spouse complains about your early-morning habit of singing O Sole Mio in the shower, just explain that it's better than an all-night concert of wall-shaking snores.

Nearly half of all adults snore occasionally, and about 25% do it all the time when they're sleeping.

What happens: Air passages in the back of the throat tend to sag when you sleep. The movement of air through the narrowed openings triggers vibrations that are heard as snoring.

Anyone can snore, but it tends to be worst in elderly or overweight men.

Singing exercises strengthen and tighten tissues in the throat and soft palate (the area at the back of the roof of the mouth), just as weight lifting tightens flabby arms. British researchers found that people who practiced singing exercises daily for three months slept better and had a reduction in the frequency, severity and loudness of snoring.

The Stop-Snoring Workout

Follow these steps, which include tongue exercises, singing and humming. They can help reduce snoring and obstructive sleep apnea, interruptions in nighttime breathing caused by blocked airways. Do these exercises even if you snore only occasionally because occasional snoring can develop into sleep apnea over time.

•**Press the tongue firmly (and repeatedly) against the hard palate (the roof of the mouth behind the front teeth).** Then press as much of the tongue as possible against the middle of the roof of the mouth...and then against the back. Keep pressing and moving your tongue for about three minutes.

• **Press the tip of your tongue firmly behind the front teeth while simultaneously pressing the back of the tongue against the floor of the mouth.** This is difficult to do, but just trying to do it is helpful.

• **While holding the tongue against the hard palate, sing each of the vowel sounds—"Aaaa"..."Eeee"..."Iiii"..."Oooo"... and "Uuuu"—for three minutes at a time.** While singing the vowel sounds, vary the pitch from high to low. Changes in pitch cause variations in vibration that exercise the tissues more completely. Just plain singing (that song in the shower!) helps, too.

• **Hum.** You can do this for a few minutes throughout the day—for example, when you're driving or working around the house.

• **Whenever you swallow, try to keep the tongue pressed against the roof of the mouth.** You'll feel tension at the back of your throat.

Forceful Blowing

This is another technique that reduces snoring and sleep apnea.

A few times a day, blow up balloons. Breathe in deeply through your nose, then blow out hard to fill the balloons.

If you're musically inclined—or would enjoy giving it a try—play a wind instrument, such as a trumpet, kazoo or didgeridoo (an Australian wind instrument). A study published in *British Medical Journal* found that people who played the didgeridoo for 15 to 30 minutes daily snored less and also had improvements in sleep apnea and daytime sleepiness.

Important: Be aware that these steps will take at least a few months to work, but the results can be dramatic. I advise patients who struggle with snoring and sleep apnea to do the exercises before considering surgery or other treatments. You can stop doing the exercises when there's no more snoring.

CART: A Better Way to Catch Your Breath If You Have Asthma

Study titled "Controlling asthma by training of Capnometry-Assisted Hypoventilation (CATCH) vs slow breathing: a randomized controlled trial," by researchers in the department of psychology and the Anxiety and Depression Research Center at Southern Methodist University, Dallas, published in *Chest*.

Asthma. The very mention of the word can make you feel like you have a boa constrictor wrapped around your chest. If you have asthma, chances are that when you feel that squeezing, suffocating feeling of an attack, you take deep breaths—gasping for air—but this is actually wrong. Or maybe you have heard that taking deep, slow and paced breaths is the right way to go. But the latest research shows that there really is a much better way to catch your breath.

When Less Is More

In an attempt to catch their breaths, asthmatics gulp air and breathe too rapidly during an attack. It's a natural reaction, but this can cause a decrease in the body's level of carbon dioxide (CO_2), resulting in hyperventilation and its characteristic symptoms of dizziness, breathlessness and pins and needles. The lungs become hyper-reactive, stuffy and dry, making the asthma attack far worse and scarier than it needs to be.

Now consider this: Shallow breathing does the opposite...it increases CO_2 levels. Knowing this and knowing that shallow breathing helps people with panic disorder (who also tend to hyperventilate), researchers from Southern Methodist University in Dallas decided to test the effectiveness of a shallow-breathing technique, successfully used in people with panic disorder, in adults with asthma.

They randomly assigned 120 asthma sufferers to receive either a standard breathing therapy called slow-breathing and awareness training (SLOW) or a therapy called capnometry-assisted respiratory training (CART). SLOW teaches asthmatics to take slow, full breaths through awareness and control of their respiratory rate (the number of breaths they take per minute). CART also trains its users to control their respiratory rate but encourages shallow breathing and control of CO_2 levels through use of a device called a capnometer. The capnometer provides feedback about CO_2 levels so that a person can practice how to breathe to prevent CO_2 from dipping too low.

The study participants practiced their therapies for four weeks on their own and with respiratory therapists and used their asthma medications as needed. The researchers monitored asthma attacks, need for medication and various aspects of respiratory function during this time and for six months' followup—and patients kept journals of the impact of SLOW or CART therapy on their asthma.

The results? Whereas both techniques resulted in an 81% improvement in lung function, the CART group was in better shape six months down the road than the other group. Their airways had become more widened and their CO_2 levels were more normalized than those of patients practicing SLOW, and that difference remained consistent throughout further follow-up. Patients practicing CART also coped better when under the stress of an acute asthma attack because they felt more in control of their symptoms and what exactly was happening in their bodies during attacks.

Learning to Breathe

If you have (or know someone who has) asthma and are unfamiliar with breath retraining therapies, such as SLOW and CART, it's a good idea to ask your doctor for a referral to a respiratory therapist—especially someone who knows about CART. These therapies are not a substitute for asthma medication, but they clearly work as add-ons and can help you improve lung function so that you can possibly rely less on medication. As for which therapy is better for long-term improvement, this study, at least, points to CART.

Why Your Asthma Treatment May Not Be Working

John V. Fahy, MD, professor of medicine and director, Airway Clinical Research Center (ACRN) of the University of California, San Francisco.

If you have asthma and feel that your steroid medication just doesn't help you much, there's a bit of good news for you. Researchers seem to have discovered why steroids don't do the trick for so many asthma sufferers.

The research was conducted at the Airway Clinical Research Center of the University of California, San Francisco, and published in *American Journal of Respiratory and Critical Care Medicine*. To find out more, we spoke with the senior author of the study, center director John V. Fahy, MD.

Why Steroids Don't Always Cut It

Over a period of six weeks, senior author of the study, center director John V. Fahy, MD and his colleagues analyzed sputum (mucus from the lungs) from 995 people with mild-to-moderate persistent asthma. Researchers were looking for the presence of white blood cells called *eosinophils*. Eosinophils are immune cells that release toxins to kill off parasites, but in some asthmatics they fire off toxins inappropriately, causing inflammation. For years, scientists had assumed that asthma was caused by the collection of these cells in the airways, and so asthma treatments have focused on controlling them. But since not everyone responds to certain asthma treatments in the same way, Dr. Fahy and his colleagues suspected that not all asthmatics have these types of cells in their sputum.

Here's what they discovered...

•**22% of the asthma patients persistently had eosinophils in their sputum** on every occasion and thus were categorized as having persistent eosinophilia.

• **31% of subjects had eosinophils in their sputum** on at least one occasion and were categorized as having intermittent eosinophilia.

• **But a whopping 47%—nearly half!—of subjects had no eosinophils on any occasion** and were categorized as having persistent non-eosinophilia.

So what does this mean for asthma patients? Well, if you have the type with no eosinophils (and there seems to be about a 50-50 chance of that), it means that one or more of the treatments that you have likely been using for years may not be working that well. *And that is what the researchers confirmed next...*

Treating Asthma Properly

Dr. Fahy noted that treatment for asthma is typically two-pronged. The first—and mainstay—treatment is to reduce inflammation caused by eosinophils through the long-term use of oral or inhaled corticosteroids. The second approach generally consists of a bronchodilator with albuterol (a beta agonist drug) that relaxes bronchial muscles and provides on-the-spot symptom relief.

So, during "part two" of the study, Dr. Fahy and his colleagues tested one measure of medication efficacy—lung function (a measure of how much air your lungs can hold and how quickly you can move air in and out of your lungs). They found that the corticosteroid medications improved lung function only in subjects with persistent or intermittent eosinophilia, and there was no effect in patients with persistent non-eosinpohilia. In contrast, the albuterol bronchodilator improved lung function in all three types of patients.

Dr. Fahy told me that in the past, it was thought that some genetic defect was the reason some asthmatics responded poorly to corticosteroid medication. And that may be true for some, but for most, the reason now seems to be that they have no eosinophils in their lungs.

How These Findings Affect Asthmatics

So does this mean that all asthmatics should get tested to see if they have eosinophils in their airways—and if they don't, then they should stop taking corticosteroids? Unfortunately, the answer to both questions is no—because right now, identifying whether you have eosinophilia or not won't do you any good.

Corticosteroids may not help those with non-eosinophilia improve their lung function, specifically, but according to Dr. Fahy, they are still the best treatment currently available for asthma and they do help those particular asthmatics at least a little bit in other ways. For example, studies by other researchers have shown that these steroids can reduce the rate of asthma attacks, lessen swelling in the airways and decrease the lungs' responses to irritants.

So all asthmatics on corticosteroids should continue taking them unless their doctors advise otherwise. The good news is that knowing why steroids aren't as effective as they could be is likely to help scientists develop new treatments that are more effective.

Keep a Cold Out of Your Lungs—Extra Defense for Asthmatics

Richard Firshein, DO, director and founder, The Firshein Center for Integrative Medicine, New York City.

If you have asthma, you especially want to guard against chest colds. The combination of swelling and mucus production from a chest cold makes breathing even more difficult. It can also bring on dangerous—and deadly—constriction of the airways (bronchospasms).

As soon as you feel the first symptoms of a cold coming on, take vitamin C and zinc. This regimen is not a cure-all, but it will help shorten the duration of the problem, and, for many people, it will keep the immune system healthy enough to get through the head cold without it turning into a chest cold.

I recommend at least 500 milligrams (mg) per day of vitamin C, taken in a split dose (250 mg twice per day) for three to five days. Don't take more than 1,500 mg daily or else you will risk side effects, such as painful kidney stones and soft stools or full-blown diarrhea. As for zinc, whether in lozenge or tablet form, take a dosage of 10 mg to 25 mg twice a day until symptoms clear. Be aware, though, that zinc lozenges and tablets can cause upset stomach or a metallic taste. Most people will do fine with these vitamins, but some people, especially those with ashma, might need an extra boost from supplements, such as…

•**Echinacea.** This herb, from the daisy family, has antioxidant and antiviral properties and fortifies the immune system against bacterial attack. In all, it can reduce the length and severity of colds. I prefer a liquid extract dispensed by dropper and recommends formulations marketed by Herbs Pharm and Gaia.

•**Cordyceps.** Cordyceps is a potent immune-strengthening nutrient derived from a fungus that grows inside caterpillars that live high in the Himalayan mountains. It's expensive…and natural cordyceps supplements can be hard to find. I recommend these brands—Host Defense and Jarrow Formulas. Start with a dosage of two 500-mg capsules once per day.

People with asthma have to be more vigilant. They should use all of the vitamins and supplements mentioned above and fortify their immune systems with N-acetylcysteine (NAC) and magnesium.

NAC is an antioxidant that can dissolve and loosen mucus, so it will help clear the airways. Take a dosage of 250 mg twice a day. Magnesium is a natural bronchodilator, so it will also help open up the airways. Again, the dosage is 250 mg twice a day.

See a doctor if your symptoms worsen instead of improve. Also see your doctor if an asthma attack occurs during a cold, if a bad cough doesn't go away after other cold symptoms resolve or if your temperature climbs over 99.4°F.

How to Clean the Air You Breathe: The Right Air Purifier for You

Allen P. Rathey, president of The Healthy House Institute, an independent educational resource for creating healthier homes based in Boise, Idaho, *HealthyHouseInstitute.com*. He has written articles for numerous trade and consumer magazines.

It might not be pleasant to think about, but the air we breathe is full of contaminants…dust, pollen and mold, to name just a few…as well as noxious gases, such as formaldehyde.

Surprising fact: Air is actually the number-one way that our bodies are exposed to contaminants in the home—in fact, we inhale about 35 pounds of air per day.

Unfortunately, dirty air can have significant effects on your health. For example, several studies have strongly linked air pollution to heart disease, asthma and depression.

While you can't eliminate all airborne pollutants, its always wise to take basic steps to improve your indoor-air quality. These include frequent vacuuming and dusting…as well as efforts to ventilate your home, such as opening windows and using a kitchen range hood and bathroom exhaust fans.

Air purifiers can also help. What's more, these devices can be especially beneficial for people with allergies or chemical sensitivities. What's right for you?

Choosing the Right Air Purifier

Air purifiers are available in portable devices designed for individual rooms or whole-house units that are built into your central air-conditioning or forced-air heating system. If you want air purification in your entire home, it may be cost-effective if the air ductwork is built in. However, most people get good results in the areas where they spend the most time with one or more portable units.

Important: Because there are so many options when buying a portable air purifier, it's easy to make mistakes that end up costing you money and/or prevent you from getting the pollution-fighting features you really need...

Mistake 1: Getting the wrong type of air purifier. There are two main types of air purifiers—units that remove particles (such as dust, pollen, mold and pet dander) and those that remove gases/odors (such as paint fumes and formaldehyde from glue in wood furniture). Some units remove both particles and gases/odors.

To determine which type of air purifier you need, ask yourself, *What am I trying to get rid of?*

Allergy and asthma sufferers often will want an air purifier that removes particles... someone who is chemically sensitive will want to eliminate gases and odors.

Air-cleaning devices designed to capture tiny particles from the air typically use high-efficiency particulate air (HEPA) technology. HEPA filters remove 99.97% of particles as small as 0.3 microns. For reference, a single hair is about 70 microns wide.

Air purifiers designed to remove gases and odors typically use activated charcoal or other material that binds to the pollutants. If you want to get rid of particles and gases, look for a purifier with both HEPA technology and a material such as activated carbon.

Important: If germs are your concern—for example, if you live with a person who is chronically ill or who has a compromised immune system—you might opt for an air purifier that uses ultraviolet (UV-C) light technology. This type of air purifier is frequently used in hospitals and destroys germs such as certain types of viruses and bacteria. The C stands for the frequency of UV light that kills germs.

Mistake 2: Not checking a unit's efficiency and certification. A critical factor when selecting an air purifier is the device's Clean Air Delivery Rate (CADR), established by the Association of Home Appliance Manufacturers (AHAM). This numerical rating measures how quickly a portable air purifier can remove pollen, dust and tobacco smoke from a certain square-foot dimension. Specifically, it measures how much air is moving through the filter and the volume of filtered air delivered by an air purifier.

The higher the number, the better. Maximum CADR values are 450 for pollen and smoke and 400 for dust. For a list of certified air purifiers with their CADR values, visit the AHAM website, *www.cadr.org*.

Your room size helps determine the most appropriate CADR. If there's, say, a smoker in the home, the AHAM recommends looking for a unit with a "tobacco smoke CADR" of at least two-thirds of your room's area. For example, a 10-foot by 12-foot room (120 square feet) would require a CADR of at least 80.

If you're older, have a compromised immune system or are particularly sensitive to chemicals, be sure to look for a bigger filter, more powerful fan and a high CADR, and ask to see the filter itself. If it looks thin and flimsy, it probably won't clean the air very efficiently.

Best: The RabbitAir MinusA2 Ultra Quiet HEPA Air Purifier, *RabbitAir.com* (cost: $459.95) can be custom-designed to filter chemical gases, airborne bacteria, pet dander or tobacco smoke.

If you have allergies or asthma, you may also want to visit *AsthmaAndAllergyFriendly. com* to see whether the air purifier you're considering has been certified by the Asthma and Allergy Foundation of America (AAFA).

Job-Loss Fears Trigger Asthma

People who are very worried about losing their jobs were 60% more likely to develop new-onset asthma than those with more job security.

British Medical Journal.

Mistake 3: Not placing the air purifier in the right location. It sounds obvious, but the key to achieving the cleanest air possible is to ensure that the polluted air actually passes through the filter. Many contaminants will never reach a small device that is located, for example, in the corner of your bedroom.

For the best coverage, you may wish to purchase several air purifiers depending on how big an area they can clean—or at least shut the door to the room with the single air purifier to keep out nonfiltered air.

Mistake 4: Not changing the filter often enough. Manufacturers provide a schedule of recommended times to change the filter—carefully follow these recommendations to keep your unit running in peak condition. Dirty filters lose effectiveness over time, and this could result in higher electricity costs if the air purifier has to run for longer periods of time to clean the air.

If your air is especially dirty, you might need to replace the filter every few months (or more often)…if it's reasonably clean, once a year (or less often) may be sufficient. Many units come with filter-change sensors that alert you when they're clogged, often based on airflow reduction.

No-Stink Asthma Trigger

When asthma patients believed that an odor—even if it was neutral and contained no irritants—would worsen asthma symptoms, their symptoms did increase, according to a new study.

Journal of Psychosomatic Research.

The End of Allergy Shots

The Food and Drug Administration recently approved Oralair, an under-the-tongue medicine, for people allergic to grass pollens. The first dose is taken at a doctor's office, in case of any adverse reaction. Then patients take one pill each day at home. Oralair does not relieve symptoms immediately—it needs time to build up, just as with allergy shots.

Dean Mitchell, MD, allergist and immunologist in New York City and author of *Dr. Dean Mitchell's Allergy and Asthma Solution.*

Drug Prevents Hay Fever

A new drug actually prevents hay fever instead of just treating its symptoms, says Martha V. White, MD. Ragwitek tablets, which are available by prescription, contain ragweed pollen extract and are placed under the tongue until they dissolve. One tablet is taken daily, starting 12 weeks before ragweed season, which typically begins mid-August, and is continued throughout the season. The first dose is given in a health-care setting so that the patient can be monitored for 30 minutes.

Martha V. White, MD, cofounder and director of research at Institute for Asthma and Allergy, Wheaton, Maryland.

Natural Treatments for Allergies

Joan Wilen and Lydia Wilen, health investigators based in New York City who have spent decades collecting "cures from the cupboard," traditional remedies that have been successfully used by millions of people worldwide. Their most recent book is *Bottom Line's Treasury of Home Remedies & Natural Cures.*

Attention, hay fever sufferers, help is here! Natural remedies can reduce symptoms and/or improve the ability of your immune system to resist the seasonal (or perpetual) onslaughts.

Hay fever, also called allergic rhinitis, is a catchall term for both seasonal and perennial rhinitis—and it's the most common immune system disorder in the US, affecting about 35 million Americans. Seasonal triggers include ragweed pollen (common in the fall), tree pollen (common in the spring) and grass pollen (common in the late spring and early summer). Year-round hay fever triggers include dust mites and cockroaches, spores from fungi and molds, and dander from pets.

Symptoms include runny nose, watery/itchy eyes, sneezing and/or coughing. You can treat the symptoms with antihistamines or other medications, but they're often expensive and may cause side effects.

Here are our favorite natural remedies. Try one or two at a time to see which one(s) work for you.

Caution: Always check with your doctor before starting or stopping any medications or supplements.

Bee Pollen

Research has shown that bee pollen (which is made by honeybees and is the food of the young bee) may inhibit the activity of mast cells, a class of immune system cells that release histamine, the substance that causes itchy eyes, nasal congestion and other allergy symptoms.

To use: Start taking bee pollen about four months before the start of your typical hay fever season. For the first few days, take just a few granules at a time. Then slowly increase the amount every day for a month, until you're taking about one teaspoon a day. Follow the same slow progression for the second and third months, until you're taking a total of three teaspoons a day. You have to go slowly because taking too much bee pollen too quickly could cause an allergic reaction of its own, with symptoms such as stomach pain, hives and a fast heart rate.

Caution: If you have an insect allergy—especially to bees—steer clear of bee pollen, which can contain bee saliva.

Fenugreek Tea

Fenugreek is the herb that gives curries their slightly peppery flavor. As with bee pollen, you can use it to desensitize your immune system prior to allergy season. It's also a mucolytic that naturally loosens phlegm and reduces coughing and sneezing.

To use: About three months before your allergy season, start drinking a daily cup of fenugreek tea. You can buy bags of this tea in health-food stores. Or you can buy the whole seeds...put about one teaspoon in a tea strainer...cover with just-boiled water... and steep for 10 to 15 minutes. Continue to drink it throughout your allergy season.

Honeycomb

Honeycomb is a natural antihistamine. When hay fever is flaring, chew a one-inch square of honeycomb. Swallow the honey, and keep chewing the waxy portion for about 10 minutes, then spit it out and discard. You probably will notice the difference right away.

You can buy honeycomb in most health-food stores, but try to find honeycomb that is produced in your area. You want it to contain trace amounts of the same pollens that, in larger amounts, trigger your symptoms.

Caution: If you are allergic to bees, stay away from honeycomb.

Garlic and Horseradish

Potent chemical compounds in both garlic and horseradish thin mucus and make it more watery. They will help reduce sneezing, congestion and other hay fever symptoms.

To use: Finely mince a clove of raw garlic, and add it to water, orange juice or applesauce. Then add one-quarter teaspoon of horseradish to vegetable juice—or sprinkle it on a salad—and consume that. Both the aromas and the strong flavors of these pungent herbs will clear nasal congestion in seconds.

To prevent nausea, make sure that you have food in your stomach before swallowing raw garlic.

Thank You, Fido!

Dogs may help protect babies against allergies and asthma. When mice were exposed to dust from households with dogs that were allowed outdoors, the mice's gut microbes changed significantly and they had reduced allergic responses to well-known allergy triggers.

Theory: Children in homes with dogs that are allowed outside develop intestinal bacteria that provide better immunity against many allergens.

Animal study by researchers at University of California, San Francisco, published in *Proceedings of the National Academy of Sciences.*

Nettle

Also known as stinging nettle (because the leaves and stems have hairlike barbs that sting the skin), it's a traditional allergy remedy. When taken orally, it blocks the body's production of histamine and reduces inflammation and congestion.

To use: You can drink a tea made from nettle, but it is easier to take a freeze-dried extract. The typical dose is one or two capsules every two to four hours during allergy flare-ups.

Lavender Oil

Lavender can be used as aromatherapy to relieve congestion and other allergy symptoms. The scent-filled molecules act as natural antihistamines and reduce inflammation and congestion in the nasal passages.

To use: Put a drop or two of lavender oil on a handkerchief. Take a deep sniff every few minutes when your allergies are flaring.

Quercetin

Every time you eat an apple or add onion to a recipe, you're getting small amounts of quercetin, a bioflavonoid that reduces inflammation. In large enough doses, it inhibits the effects of histamine and reduces nasal congestion. But you can't get adequate amounts of quercetin from foods to control allergies.

To use: When you are having allergy symptoms, take 300 milligrams (mg) to 600 mg of a quercetin supplement daily.

Fish Oil

The omega-3 fatty acids in fish and fish oil have been shown to reduce inflammation throughout the body. Cardiologists often recommend fish oil to lower triglycerides and prevent heart disease and stroke. It also can lessen allergy symptoms by reducing inflammation and swelling in the nasal passages.

To use: Take 2,000 mg daily.

Look for a fish-oil product that says "purified" or "mercury-free" on the label. It should contain at least 500 mg of EPA and 250 mg of DHA per capsule. You can find the capsules online or in health-food stores.

Caution: Check with your doctor, especially if you also are taking a blood-thinning medication such as warfarin. Using both together could increase the risk of bleeding.

Better Care for Allergies

Stress doesn't cause allergy attacks, but it can make them worse, a recent study reports.

Details: Among 179 allergy patients, those who had higher stress levels (as measured by daily online diaries) had more frequent flare-ups.

Why: Stress can disrupt the endocrine and immune systems, which could contribute to allergy episodes.

To reduce stress: Try positive thinking… eat right…get plenty of sleep…exercise regularly—and see a therapist, if necessary.

William Malarkey, MD, associate director, Institute for Behavioral Medicine Research, The Ohio State University, Columbus.

Is It Really Sinusitis?

Murray Grossan, MD, otolaryngologist and head-and-neck surgeon with the Tower Ear, Nose and Throat Clinic at Cedars-Sinai Medical Center in Los Angeles. He is author of *Free Yourself from Sinus and Allergy Problems Permanently*. GrossanInstitute.com

D on't assume that it's merely a bad cold when you're stuffed up and feeling lousy for more than the usual seven to 10 days. It could be something worse—and much harder to get rid of. It could be sinusitis.

Sinusitis is a condition where the nasal passages become inflamed and swollen. It's usually caused by a cold, but it could be triggered by allergies or a bacterial or fungal infection.

Here's how to tell if you have sinusitis and what to do about it if you do...

Step 1: Make the Diagnosis

Long-lasting congestion, accompanied by tenderness around the eyes, forehead and/or cheeks, is the hallmark of sinusitis. Mucus will probably be yellow or greenish rather than clear.

Sinusitis can persist for weeks, months or even years. Colds never last that long. Another hint is when you get sick. If your symptoms are predictable—they occur only in the spring or summer, for example, or when you eat certain foods—you might have sinusitis triggered by allergies.

Most people with sinusitis have slow-moving cilia, microscopic filaments in the respiratory tract that propel mucus out through the nose or down the back of the throat. After an allergy or a cold, the cilia slow down. Also, some people with certain conditions such as cystic fibrosis have chronic slow-moving cilia. Impaired mucus transport is what causes congestion, which can become a breeding ground for infection.

Step 2: Irrigate the Nasal Cavities

Irrigation is the best treatment for congestion-related problems, including sinusitis, colds and allergies. It thins and flushes away mucus and helps the sinuses drain. It also washes out allergens and infection-causing bacteria.

Mix about one teaspoon of salt and one-half teaspoon of baking soda in two cups of warm sterile water. Pour it into a squeeze bottle or another type of nasal-irrigation device. (Or you could try a system I invented called the Hydro Pulse Sinus System, available online—it applies the low, steady pressure needed to create suction and pull out mucus.)

Keeping the head centered, put the solution into one nostril. Keep it flowing until the solution begins to flow out the other nostril. Gently blow your nose, then repeat on the other side.

Caution: If you're using a squeeze bottle, try to maintain steady pressure. A University of Pennsylvania study found that infected mucus can backflow into squeeze bottles and cause a reinfection.

Step 3: Shrink the Swelling

Much of the discomfort of sinusitis comes from swollen mucous membranes. To reduce swelling, apply moist heat to the sinus area. Soak a washcloth in warm-to-hot water, and drape it over the nose and cheeks. When it cools, resoak and reapply it several times a day.

Another way to reduce swelling and congestion is to lift the tip of your nose. It sounds (and looks) silly, but it works because a downward-dipping nose (common in older adults) can block the nasal openings. At night, loop a piece of one-half-inch-wide medical-grade tape under the end of the nose...pull the ends slightly upward...and stick them between the eyes. It will keep the nasal passages open while you sleep.

Also helpful: My Clear-ease natural fruit enzyme tablets. Follow the label directions. Fruit-based enzymes such as bromelain and papain reduce sinus swelling.

Step 4: Clean Your Home

Pollens, molds and dust mites, along with plain old dust, can cause sinusitis.

You don't have to give your home the "white-glove treatment." But do wash bedding weekly in hot water to kill dust mites and their eggs. Also consider dust mite–proof mattress and pillow covers. Vacuum carpets once a week, preferably with a vacuum equipped with a HEPA filter. It's also a good idea to keep dogs and cats out of the bedroom to minimize nighttime exposure to dust and dander from their coats.

Step 5: More Vitamin C

Vitamin C can reduce the intensity and duration of coldlike symptoms, including congestion. It's a mild antihistamine that reduces mucus production and sinus swelling. When sinusitis flares, increase your dietary intake of vitamin C by eating plenty of salads, leafy green vegetables, citrus, etc.

Caution: Some fresh fruits such as strawberries contain high levels of natural histamines, but canned or cooked do not. If you notice an increase in congestion and/or head pain after eating certain foods, avoid them until you're feeling better.

Step 6: Use a Decongestant

I don't recommend decongestants before trying drug-free treatments. But if you've had sinusitis for a few weeks or longer, your body's defenses are probably exhausted. Using a decongestant spray once or twice will provide relief and give your natural defenses a chance to catch up.

Any decongestant spray, tablet or liquid can help, but I like Patanase Nasal Spray. It's a prescription spray that quickly clears congestion and doesn't contain a corticosteroid. Menthol inhalers such as Vicks and Benzedrex also can provide relief.

Step 7: De-Stress

Doctors have known for a long time that emotional stress can dampen immunity and increase the risk for infection. It also tends to increase the incidence (and discomfort) of colds, allergies and sinusitis.

Stress creates a cycle known as anxiety reinforcement. The more stress you experience, the more likely you are to get sick—and the more you'll notice the discomfort.

My advice: Practice biofeedback. It's easy—and effective. Once or twice a day, sit in front of a mirror. Slowly inhale for a count of four, then exhale for a count of six. As you exhale, consciously relax the muscles in the face, jaw and shoulders. It's physiologically impossible to feel anxiety when your muscles are relaxed.

People who practice this technique soon learn that they can reduce stress-related symptoms at any time, not just when they're in front of the mirror.

When to See Your Doctor

By taking the steps in this article, you might be able to avoid a trip to the doctor's office, which could save you $100 or so. However, if you still have sinusitis symptoms after several weeks, do see your doctor. He/she may recommend other treatments including an antibiotic (usually amoxicillin) if you have a bacterial infection.

Sweet Self-Test

Open a package of saccharin, and put a few of the granules inside your nostrils. See how long it takes before you taste sweetness. If you taste the saccharin in about five minutes, you probably don't have sinusitis. If it takes 20 to 30 minutes, sinusitis is likely.

Chapter 5

PRESERVE YOUR BRAIN… WHAT TO DO TO AVERT ALZHEIMER'S AND MORE

What You Need to Do Now to Prevent Alzheimer's

Alzheimer's disease is hands down one of the most feared diseases. But simply worrying that you'll develop the illness doesn't do any good. A far better approach is to take action—now!

What's new: Around the country, respected medical centers and hospitals are now creating Alzheimer's prevention programs staffed by neurologists and researchers who help people do all that they can do to avoid this devastating condition.*

Even if you're only in your 30s or 40s, it's wise to see a neurologist if you have a family history of Alzheimer's disease…or if, at any age, you're noticing mental changes (such as memory loss) that concern you. Everyone has momentary lapses—forgetting where you left your keys, for example—but those that impact your life, such as missing appointments, should be evaluated.

*To find an Alzheimer's prevention program near you, check with a local chapter of the Alzheimer's Association, *ALZ. org,* a local university or state or local agency for the aging.

What Can You Do?

An increasing number of Alzheimer's experts now believe that preventive lifestyle approaches may help preserve memory and cognitive abilities. It's best to start before any disease-related changes occur in the brain. By the time symptoms are recognizable, the disease already has a foothold and the benefits of intervention will be nominal. While you may think that you already know the main Alzheimer's prevention strategies, key recommendations from Dean Sherzai, MD, director of the Alzheimer's Disease Prevention Program at Cedars-Sinai Medical Center in Los Angeles, include specifics that really make a difference. *Steps to take…*

•**Control your blood sugar.** Most Alzheimer's patients have higher-than-normal blood sugar levels or full-blown diabetes. In a study that tracked more than 2,000 patients for roughly seven years, those with a glucose reading of 115 mg/dL, on average, had an 18% higher risk for dementia than those with levels of 100 mg/dL or lower (normal range). The higher the blood sugar levels, the greater the Alzheimer's risk. It's not yet clear why

Dean Sherzai, MD, neurologist and director of the Alzheimer's Disease Prevention Program at Cedars-Sinai Medical Center in Los Angeles.

elevated blood sugar increases cognitive risks, but it could be linked to the inflammation that accompanies blood glucose disorders.

Dr. Sherzai's advice: Avoid simple carbohydrates such as white bread and white rice that cause blood sugar to spike. Also, emerging evidence shows that eating a lot of sugar may cause Alzheimer's brain changes—so avoid sugar.

Recommended: No more than nine teaspoons of added sugars for men each day... six teaspoons for women. This may sound like a lot, but it's actually a lot less than many people get. Added sugars are in many foods—not only in such things as sweetened yogurt and fruit drinks but also in pasta sauces, breads and salad dressings. Also, get screened for diabetes at three-year intervals, starting at age 45—sooner (and more frequently) if you have diabetes risk factors such as obesity and/or a family history.

●**Consume the "Big 3."** The Mediterranean diet, which includes fish, fruit, beans, vegetables, whole grains and monounsaturated fat (such as olive oil), has been widely promoted for brain health. But which specific foods are most likely to help keep you mentally sharp? There's strong evidence for...

●**Fruit and vegetable juices, such as pomegranate, blueberry and grape.** A nine-year study of 1,836 participants found that those who drank fruit or vegetable juices at least three times a week were 76% less likely to develop Alzheimer's than those who had them less than once a week.

Possible reason: Juices have a high concentration of anti-inflammatory antioxidants—and this may help interrupt some of the brain changes (such as beta-amyloid deposits) that occur in Alzheimer's patients. A daily serving of a juiced mixture of fresh vegetables and low-sugar fruits, such as berries, lime or cantaloupe, is a good source of antioxidants and nutrients. Fruits high in sugar, such as bananas and mangoes, should be avoided, since as mentioned earlier, recent research has linked higher sugar levels with cognitive decline and dementia.

●**Fatty fish.** Researchers recently announced that people with high blood levels of omega-3 fatty acids had increased volume in the hippocampus, a part of the brain that's affected in those with cognitive decline. Other research has shown that there's less Alzheimer's in parts of the world where people eat the most fish.

One problem is that people often eat the wrong kind of fish. It must be omega-3–rich, fatty fish.

Best choices: Salmon, herring, mackerel, sardines or tuna, eaten at least twice a week. If you don't like fish, you can take a daily supplement. Lovaza is the only fish oil supplement approved by the FDA. Because it's available by prescription, it may be covered by your insurance. Alternatively, you can take an over-the-counter fish oil supplement (check with your doctor first—fish oil can raise risk for bleeding). Flaxseed, chia seeds and walnuts contain a plant-based omega-3.

●**Vegetables—and more vegetables.** With all the focus on brain-healthy fruits such as blueberries, vegetables are often forgotten. That's a mistake. In a study of more than 3,700 people, those who consumed the most vegetables (a median of 4.1 daily servings) had 38% less cognitive decline than those who ate the least. Good choices for those four or more daily servings are kale, spinach, brussels sprouts, broccoli and red bell peppers.

●**Give your mind the right kind of workout.** Crosswords and Sudoku help but less than you might think. They get easy with practice and target only some parts of the brain.

Better: Activities that challenge your brain on multiple levels—and stay challenging no matter how long you do them.

Examples: Playing a musical instrument, painting and even playing some challenging video or board games.

Also: Look for hobbies that use the hands and the mind—they require focus, memory, problem-solving, spatial visualization and other skills.

Dr. Sherzai's advice: List 10 activities that you enjoy, and try to do three or four of them daily. If one activity doesn't stimulate a part of your brain, another probably will.

●**Get more exercise—safely.** When it comes to preserving brain health, nothing beats exercise. It improves circulation and increases the amounts of glucose and oxygen that reach the brain.

Dr. Sherzai's advice: Be sure to exercise safely. An injury will deprive you of one of your strongest defenses against Alzheimer's. Outdoor exercise can increase risk for falls and other injuries. If you're not that sure-footed, go for indoor exercise using a machine such as a recumbent bicycle or elliptical trainer. Otherwise, take brisk walks outdoors. Aim for 30 minutes of moderate-to-vigorous exercise (breathing hard and fast with increased heart rate) on most days of the week, plus strength, flexibility and balance-improving activities. (Start with five-minute sessions if you're not used to it.)

A Medication Worth Trying?

High blood pressure is widely known to increase Alzheimer's risk. What you may not realize is that the type of medicine used to control high blood pressure could also affect your Alzheimer's risk.

Interesting finding: When the medical records of more than 5 million patients were reviewed, those who took blood pressure drugs called angiotensin II receptor blockers (ARBs), such as *irbesartan* (Avapro), *losartan* (Cozaar) and *azilsartan* (Edarbi), had a 35% to 40% lower risk of developing Alzheimer's or other brain diseases than those prescribed other blood pressure drugs. What makes these drugs different? It's possible that blocking the renin-angiotensin system provides neurological benefits in addition to lowering blood pressure.

The research is not definitive, so your doctor won't prescribe an ARB just to prevent Alzheimer's disease. But if you're already taking blood pressure medication, you may want to ask about trying an ARB.

Don't Let Your Brain Shrink

Exercise prevents brain shrinkage. People who have the APOE epsilon4 allele (e4 gene) are at increased risk for Alzheimer's disease.

Recent finding: After 18 months, the brain scans of people with the e4 gene who exercised moderately a few times a week showed dramatically less shrinkage in the hippocampus—which is associated with Alzheimer's—compared with people with the gene who were not physically active.

Stephen Rao, PhD, professor and director of Schey Center for Cognitive Neuroimaging, Cleveland Clinic, and leader of a study of 97 people, published in *Frontiers in Aging Neuroscience.*

It Might Not Be Alzheimer's

Jacob Teitelbaum, MD, board-certified internist and founder of Practitioners Alliance Network, an organization for health-care providers dedicated to improving communication among all branches of the healing arts. Based in Kona, Hawaii, he is author, with Bill Gottlieb, of *Real Cause, Real Cure.*

If a doctor says that you or a loved one has Alzheimer's disease, take a deep breath and get a second opinion. Studies have shown that between 30% and 50% of people diagnosed with Alzheimer's turn out not to have it.

Bottom line: The symptoms common to Alzheimer's can be caused by other reversible conditions. Problems with memory and other cognitive functions often are linked to what I call MIND—metabolism, infection or inflammation, nutrition or drug side effects—or a combination of these factors. Addressing these can markedly improve cognitive function. Even people who do have Alzheimer's will see improvements.

Metabolism

Anyone who is experiencing confusion, memory loss or other cognitive problems should have tests that look at the hormones that affect metabolism. *In particular…*

•**Thyroid hormone.** A low level of thyroid hormone often causes confusion and memory loss. It also increases the risk for Alzheimer's disease. In recent studies, thyroid levels on the low side in the normal range are associated with a 240% higher risk for dementia in women. Borderline low thyroid hormone is associated with as much as an 800% higher risk in men.

My advice: For most people with unexplained chronic confusion and memory loss, I recommend a three-month trial of desiccated thyroid (30 mg to 60 mg) to see if it helps. It is a thyroid extract containing the two key thyroid hormones. (The commonly prescribed medication Synthroid has just one of the two.) If you have risk factors for heart disease—such as high LDL cholesterol and high blood pressure—your doctor should start you with a low dose and increase it gradually.

Infections and Inflammation

You naturally will get large amounts of protective anti-inflammatory chemical compounds just by eating a healthy diet and using supplements such as fish oil and curcumin. For extra protection, take aspirin. In addition to reducing inflammation, it's among the best ways to prevent blood clots and vascular dementia, which is as common as Alzheimer's disease. In addition, infections leave us feeling mentally foggy. Have your doctor look for and treat any bladder and sinus infections.

My advice: Talk to your doctor about taking one enteric-coated low-dose (81-mg) aspirin daily to improve circulation and reduce the risk for ministrokes in the brain. Even people with Alzheimer's may have had a series of ministrokes, adding to their cognitive decline. This is especially important when mental worsening occurs in small distinct steps instead of gradually.

Nutrition

The typical American diet is just as bad for your brain and memory as it is for your heart. Too much fat, sugar and processed food increase cell-damaging inflammation throughout the body, including in the brain.

In one study, Columbia University researchers studied more than 2,100 people over the age of 65 who consumed healthy foods such as nuts, fruits, fish, chicken and leafy, dark green vegetables and who limited their consumption of meat and dairy. They were 48% less likely to be diagnosed with Alzheimer's over a four-year period.

Especially important…

•**B-12.** Millions of older adults don't get or absorb enough vitamin B-12, a nutrient that is critical for memory and other brain functions. You might be deficient even if you eat a healthful diet due to the age-related decline in stomach acid and intrinsic factor, a protein needed for B-12 absorption.

My advice: Take a multivitamin that contains 500 micrograms (mcg) of B-12 and at least 400 mcg of folic acid and 50 mg of the other B vitamins. If you test low-normal for B-12 (less than 400 ng/ml), also ask your doctor about getting a series of 10 B-12 shots.

Helpful: Have one teaspoon of apple cider vinegar with every meal. Use it in salad dressing, or mix it into eight ounces of vegetable juice or water. It will increase B-12 absorption.

Caution: Vinegar is highly caustic if you drink it straight.

• **Fish oil.** The American Heart Association advises everyone to eat fish at least twice a week. That's enough for the heart, but it won't provide all of the omega-3 fatty acids that you need for optimal brain health. Fish-oil supplements can ensure that you get enough.

My advice: I recommend three to four servings a week of fatty fish, such as salmon, tuna, herring or sardines. Or take 1,000 mg of fish oil daily. You will need more if you're already having memory/cognitive problems. Ask your doctor how much to take.

• **Curcumin.** Alzheimer's is 70% less common in India than in the US, possibly because of the large amounts of turmeric that are used in curries and other Indian dishes.

Curcumin, which gives turmeric its yellow color, reduces inflammation and improves blood flow to the brain. Animal studies show that it dissolves the amyloid plaques that are found in the brains of Alzheimer's patients.

My advice: Unless you live in India, you're not likely to get enough curcumin in your diet to help, because it is poorly absorbed. Use a special highly absorbed form of curcumin (such as BCM-95 found in CuraMed 750 mg), and take one to two capsules twice a day.

Caution: Taking curcumin with blood thinners can increase the risk for bleeding.

Too Many Drugs

Medication side effects are a very common cause of mental decline. This can occur even when you aren't taking drugs with obvious "mind-altering" effects, such as narcotic painkillers. Many drugs—antihistamines, antidepressants, incontinence meds and even simple muscle relaxants—can impair cognitive functions. The risk is higher when you're taking multiple medications and experience drug-drug interactions.

Doctors are far more likely to add medications than to subtract them. Many older adults are taking five or more medications daily.

My advice: Ask your doctor to review all of your medications. Make sure that you're taking only drugs that you absolutely need—not "leftover" medications that might have been prescribed in the past and that you no longer need. Then ask for a three-week trial off each medication that is considered necessary to see if those drugs are contributing to the dementia (substituting other medications or closer monitoring during those three weeks usually can allow this).

Peanut Butter Test for Alzheimer's

One of the first areas of the brain to be affected by Alzheimer's is the one that controls the sense of smell. People with Alzheimer's couldn't smell a teaspoon of peanut butter until it was five centimeters (about two inches) away. People without Alzheim-

---

Vitamin E Slows Mild-to-Moderate Alzheimer's

A daily dose of 2,000 IU of vitamin E delays a patient's functional decline, specifically affecting activities of daily living, such as handling finances, taking medications and preparing meals. Earlier research showed that vitamin E helps people with moderate Alzheimer's—the new study extends that to those with mild Alzheimer's.

Mary Sano, PhD, director of the Alzheimer's Disease Research Center at Mount Sinai School of Medicine, New York City, and leader of a study published in *The Journal of the American Medical Association.*

119

Brain Scans Reveal Alzheimer's Risk

•**An MRI may show Alzheimer's risk.** By using arterial spin labeling (ASL), which can be done by all modern MRI scanning machines, it may be possible to detect very subtle blood flow changes in parts of the brain linked to memory. Early detection could make it possible to start medicines to slow decline.

Sven Haller, MD, senior physician in clinical neuroradiology at Geneva University Hospital, Switzerland, and leader of a study published online in *Radiology*.

•**Brain scan detects leakage.** People at high risk for Alzheimer's should have a scan to detect leakage in the barrier between blood vessels and the brain. This barrier can become leaky with age, beginning in the hippocampus—an important learning and memory center. Identifying the leaks before Alzheimer's develops would allow treatment to start earlier and possibly slow development of the disease. Brain scans could be useful for people with symptoms of mild dementia on neuropsychological tests and people with genetic risks for Alzheimer's.

Berislav V. Zlokovic, MD, PhD, professor and chair, department of physiology and biophysics, Keck School of Medicine, University of Southern California, Los Angeles, and leader of a study published in *Neuron*.

er's could smell it when it was 17 centimeters (about seven inches) away, on average.

Study by researchers at McKnight Brain Institute Center for Smell and Taste, University of Florida, Gainesville, published in *Journal of the Neurological Sciences.*

Low Blood Pressure Alert

Having high blood pressure (above 140/90 mmHg) throughout midlife is a known major risk factor for dementia. However, blood pressure that is consistently far below the normal 120/80 in older people can signal reduced blood flow to the brain, which can raise risk for cognitive decline and dementia. Lower pressure in younger adults does not necessarily harm the brain. Older adults' brains are less able to compensate for the reduced blood flow. Similarly, new research has linked diastolic (bottom number) blood pressure under 70 in adults with cardiovascular disease to increased risk for brain atrophy, which can lead to dementia.

Majid Fotuhi, MD, PhD, author of *Boost Your Brain* and founder and chief medical officer, NeurExpand Brain Center, Lutherville, Maryland. *NeurExpand.com*

Don't Feed Your Brain Sedatives

Sedatives increase the risk for Alzheimer's. Older adults who used benzodiazepine sedatives, such as *lorazepam* (Ativan), *diazepam* (Valium) and *alprazolam* (Xanax), for more than three months within a five-year period had a 51% increased risk for Alzheimer's. These drugs often are prescribed for insomnia or anxiety, but they should not be used long term.

Better approach: The underlying cause of the anxiety or insomnia should be identified and treated without using medicines—for example, with talk therapy.

Malaz Boustani, MD, MPH, chief innovation and implementation officer at Indiana University Health and Richard M. Fairbanks Professor of Aging Research at Indiana University School of Medicine, both in Indianapolis.

Is Your Heartburn Remedy Stealing Your Vitamin B-12?

Study titled "Proton pump inhibitor and histamine 2 receptor antagonist use and vitamin B12 deficiency," published in *JAMA*.

People who have chronic heartburn can find themselves living on antacids just to stay reasonably comfortable. Whether the heartburn is caused by gastroesophageal reflux disease (GERD) or something else, we already knew that these drugs had a big downside—they can interfere with digestion, encouraging diarrhea and gassiness and even promoting food sensitivities. But it just got worse for folks who rely heavily on antacids like *omeprazole* (Prilosec), *esomeprazole* (Nexium), *lansoprazole* (Prevacid), and *famotidine* (Pepcid). A large study shows specifically that these drugs rob the body of a very important nutrient—vitamin B-12—which is essential for brain function and your body's ability to make blood cells and DNA.

Here's the scoop: Because small studies had been cropping up hinting that antacid use might have something to do with why some people have a vitamin B-12 deficiency, a team of researchers from Kaiser Permanente, a major health-care organization, went ahead and accessed 14 years of medical and pharmacy records (1997 to 2011) of the company's millions of members to look more closely for a link between antacid use and lack of vitamin B-12.

They found about 26,000 members who had been given a diagnosis of B-12 deficiency or had otherwise been prescribed a vitamin B-12 supplement. Then the team dug deep into those people's medical and pharmacy records. The team was looking to see whether prescription antacid use was common in members with B-12 deficiency. To prevent any faulty assumptions, the researchers compared each member in this group with up to 10 matched controls—that is, members in the database who didn't have B-12 deficiency but shared other key characteristics with the members who did. They also adjusted their findings to make sure that the B-12 deficiencies weren't being caused by diabetes, thyroid disorders, smoking, alcohol abuse or other factors known to cause B-12 deficiency.

A wide variety of antacids were included in the study. You're probably familiar with their commercial names—Prilosec, Nexium and Prevacid, which are proton pump inhibitors (PPIs)...and Pepcid and *ranitidine* (Zantac),

which are histamine 2 receptor antagonists (H2RAs). PPIs, which are the most effective and popular, work by blocking the enzymes that make stomach acid. H2RAs stop overproduction of acid in a more roundabout way by blocking stomach cells that produce histamine.

Who's At Risk

The results of the study were striking. Essentially, if you've been taking one of those just-mentioned PPIs daily for two years or more, there's a very good chance that you are not getting as much vitamin B-12 as your body needs. No wonder you're feeling tired, foggy or light-headed, have muscle weakness, the runs or constipation, or feel like your heart or lungs are working too hard. Although only a medical exam can confirm why you feel this way, these are symptoms of vitamin B-12 deficiency.

Although B-12 deficiency was more frequently associated with use of PPIs than with use of H2RAs, both types of antacids were implicated...

• **People in the study taking PPIs daily for two or more years were 65% more likely to be vitamin B-12 deficient than those not taking antacids daily...**people on daily H2RAs were 25% more likely to be B-12 deficient than those not taking antacids daily.

• **The higher the daily dose of a PPI, the higher the likelihood that the person was vitamin B-12 deficient after being on the PPI for two or more years.** In fact, the highest average dosage (more than 1.5 pills each day) was associated with a whopping 95% increased risk for vitamin B-12 deficiency. The lowest dosage of a PPI was associated with a 63% increased risk—still very high. In comparison, the highest dosage of H2RAs was associated with a 37% increased risk for vitamin-B deficiency.

• **The younger a person was, the more vulnerable she or he was to vitamin B-12 deficiency.** This was true if he or she was taking a PPI or a PPI plus an H2RA but not an H2RA alone. For example, B-12 deficiency

121

was eight times more likely to be diagnosed in PPI users who were age 29 or younger than in those age 80 or older. Why is a topic for further investigation.

●**Women were at higher risk than men for B-12 deficiency.** Among all people studied who had been taking PPIs or PPIs and H2RAs but not H2RAs alone for two years or more, women had an 84% higher risk of being vitamin B-12 deficient than people not taking antacids…while men had a 43% higher risk.

Why is this happening? The researchers didn't get into causality, but stomach acid is the very thing that makes your body separate out vitamins B-12 from proteins in the foods you eat, and this separation is what allows your body to absorb B-12 from your gut.

In other words, the antacids are out-and-out preventing you from digesting an incredibly important nutrient.

It's Temporary—So Get Off Them!

Fortunately, when people stop using antacids, the body's ability to break out and absorb vitamin B-12 returns to normal—but not very quickly. Although the incidence of vitamin B-12 deficiency for current antacid users and people who had gone antacid-free for about a year was about the same, the incidence was halved for former daily antacid users who had been antacid-free for at least two years.

What you can do: If you must take an antacid on a regular basis, take the lowest dose that will effectively relieve your symptoms. This may help reduce your risk of vitamin B-12 deficiency. But don't make this decision alone. Talk to your doctor. If you're using a PPI, discuss possibly switching to an H2RA or using a lower dose of the PPI. You also may consider taking a B-12 supplement. If a blood test confirms that you are vitamin B-12 deficient, though, your doctor may give you a special, high-dose prescription or even suggest that you get vitamin B-12 injections, depending on how B-12–deficient you are.

Midlife Stress Linked to Late-Life Dementia

Among 800 women tracked for nearly 40 years, those who experienced significant stress (divorce, widowhood, loss of a child or mental illness in a loved one) were 21% more likely to develop Alzheimer's disease.

Why: Stress may cause structural and functional changes in the brain, which may linger for years after a stressful event.

If you're facing midlife stress: Try psychotherapy, meditation and/or yoga.

Lena Johansson, PhD, researcher, University of Gothenburg, Mölndal, Sweden.

But your real goal is to get at the root cause of your heartburn and do away with the need for any regular antacid use. This might mean adjusting lifestyle habits such as diet, sleep and exercise. Talk to your doctor, and visit *BottomLineHealth.com/drug-free-help-for-chronic-heartburn* for more natural ways to get off these dangerous drugs.

Anemia Linked to Dementia Risk

In an 11-year study of more than 2,500 adults, those who had anemia (low levels of healthy red blood cells) were 41% more likely to develop dementia than those who were not anemic.

Theory: Anemia may reduce the amount of oxygen getting to the brain, which over time may adversely affect memory and cognitive skills.

If you have anemia: Be sure to get proper treatment, which may include iron supplementation.

Kristine Yaffe, MD, professor of psychiatry, neurology and epidemiology and biostatistics, University of California, San Francisco.

Beware of Online Tests for Alzheimer's

When 16 online Alzheimer's tests were evaluated by two panels of experts, the tests were found to be misleading and their results invalid...and some of the tests did not disclose that they were associated with companies that market products and services to people who have dementia.

Study of 16 online Alzheimer's tests by researchers at British Columbia University, Vancouver, Canada, presented at the Alzheimer's Association International Conference in Boston.

Music and Cooking Help Behavioral Problems in Alzheimer's Patients... and Ease Stress for Caregivers, Too

Pauline Narme, MD, Neuropsychology of Aging, Paris Descartes University, Boulogne-Billancourt, in collaboration with the University of Lille and the University Medical Center of Reims, all in France.

Dealing with a loved one who is agitated and aggressive is never easy—but it's especially tough when that person has Alzheimer's disease and can no longer understand what is "appropriate" behavior and what isn't. Such behavioral issues are very common in Alzheimer's patients...and medication helps little while potentially causing side effects.

This places a tremendous burden on family caregivers. In fact, behavioral problems are a primary reason why people with Alzheimer's end up in nursing homes. And even if you're just visiting your loved one in a nursing home rather than delivering around-the-clock care yourself, it's still upsetting to witness and try to deal with that person's distress.

So what can be done about these difficult behavioral issues? According to a new study, activities involving music and cooking can help patients and as their caregivers. *Here's why...*

Engaging Through Song and Food

Forty-eight nursing home residents with moderate-to-severe Alzheimer's disease were randomly assigned to one of two group-activity programs—music or cooking. The goal was to see whether either or both programs would help reduce behavioral problems in patients and ease caregiver stress.

Before beginning the programs, each resident's caregiver (the nursing home staff member assigned to that resident) completed a questionnaire. The point was to gauge the frequency and severity of the patient's problem behaviors—including aggression, agitation, delusions, disinhibition (loss of inhibitions that would normally govern behavior) and sleep abnormalities (frequent awakenings, sleeping during the day instead of at night, etc.)...and to measure how much emotional or psychological distress the patient's behavior caused for the caregiver. The higher the scores, the worse the problems. The questionnaire was repeated halfway through the programs and four weeks after the programs ended. The caregivers did not know which program the residents were enrolled in. (Though this study looked at professional caregivers, it's reasonable to suppose that family caregivers—who typically would have less caregiving training and a deeper emotional attachment—would experience even greater stress when trying to manage a loved one's behavioral problems.)

Two one-hour sessions were held each week for four weeks. In the music group, CDs were played featuring classical music and popular songs from the 1950s through 1980s. Participants were encouraged to listen, sing along and/or keep the beat on a small drum. In the cooking group, all participants cooperated in preparing various foods—for instance, by measuring, mixing, etc.—depending on their capabilities. Participants were invited to express their feelings and to recall memories that were evoked by the music or the food preparation.

The results were encouraging. Both programs helped reduce the severity of behavioral disorders and caregiver distress, with the music program being especially effective. Specifically, in terms of…

Severity of patients' behavioral problems: In the music group, patients' average score improved by 74% during the program… and four weeks after the program ended, there was still a 37% improvement. In the cooking group, the patients' average behavioral score improved by 57%…and four weeks after the program ended, there was still a 32% improvement.

Caregiver distress levels: Among caregivers of patients in the music group, the average distress score improved by 78% during the program…and four weeks after the program ended, there was still a 44% improvement. In the cooking group, caregivers' average distress score improved by 65% during the program…and four weeks after the program ended, there was still a 34% improvement.

Music to Their Ears

According to the Alzheimer's Foundation of America, music has the power to improve patients' mood and cognitive function and to stimulate positive interaction because the part of the brain that responds to auditory cues requires little cognitive functioning. That's why, even in advanced dementia, the ability to engage in music by singing along may remain intact.

Although this study showed greater benefits from music than from cooking, the benefits from the cooking were significant…and it's possible that a patient who had a lifelong interest in cooking would respond more positively to a cooking activity than to a music activity.

Advice for caregivers: Why not try re-creating the programs' positive effects yourself when you're with the Alzheimer's patient you care for?

For instance, play some CDs when you're together, choosing a style of music that is familiar and soothing, and encourage your loved one to sing, clap or drum along to the tune. Or spend time together in the kitchen, preparing a simple recipe (such as pancakes) and inviting your loved one to handle safe and easy tasks, such as measuring, mixing and pouring. You might include other family members, too, to more closely duplicate the social aspect of the study's group activities. You may end up doing everyone involved a world of good.

Watch This Vitamin Level

Alzheimer's is linked to low vitamin D levels. In a study led by University of Exeter, England, adults over age 65 with very low levels of vitamin D were more than twice as likely to have Alzheimer's as those with normal levels. Vitamin D levels can be boosted with supplements, sun exposure and/or dietary changes, such as eating more salmon and other fatty fish and fortified dairy products.

Heather M. Snyder, PhD, director of medical and scientific operations at the Alzheimer's Association, Chicago. *ALZ.org*

Best New Brain Boosters—Your Brain Can Improve at Any Age

Sandra Bond Chapman, PhD, a cognitive neuroscientist, founder and chief director of the Center for BrainHealth and the Dee Wyly Distinguished University Chair at The University of Texas at Dallas. She is coauthor, with Shelly Kirkland, of *Make Your Brain Smarter: Increase Your Brain's Creativity, Energy, and Focus. BrainHealth.utdallas.edu*

Expecting crossword puzzles or any particular activity to give your brain a full workout is a bit like expecting biceps curls to tone your entire body. Our bodies need specific types of exercise to optimize results—and so do our brains.

Newest thinking: One of the most effective ways to maintain (or even improve) your brainpower is to tailor specific workouts to your age.

Don't Dwell on Your Memory

When I talk to people about mental fitness, they almost always say that their main goal is to improve their memory. But virtually everyone is surprised to learn that the ability to remember facts has almost nothing to do with brain efficiency.

The ability to understand big ideas, extrapolate meaning and make sound decisions in real-life contexts is far more vital to effective brain performance than maintaining a repository of data. Unnecessary memorization wastes brain energy, depleting reserves better served for higher-order thinking. Fortunately, increasing higher-order thinking ability may naturally help improve your memory.

Mental Fitness for Life

What exactly can you do to improve your mental fitness? Here are some regimens that are geared toward the changes your brain is undergoing as it ages.

Ages 46 to 65

Beginning in one's mid-40s, it's common to start losing the capacity to quickly process new information and store and retrieve data (such as a person's name). However, most people in the 46-to-65 age group are more adept at sorting through information efficiently and accurately discerning critical points to more quickly weigh facts than younger counterparts.

Best brain-boosting strategies if you're age 46 to 65...

•**Narrow your focus.** Multitasking isn't recommended for anyone, but particularly not for people in this age group. As you age, the capacity to rapidly switch from task to task (as occurs with multitasking) slows, adding to brain fatigue and reducing efficiency.

To keep the mind sharp: Pick one job—such as answering e-mails or planning a report—and take your time doing it. Making an effort to create meaningful responses and original content not only increases work quality and productivity but also flexes your brain.

•**Synthesize.** Not every detail is important, so don't let yourself get lost in a sea of information.

To keep the mind sharp: Gather enough information for the task at hand, then focus mainly on the key meanings. Applying internally generated novel ideas to affect an outcome boosts brain health.

Note: Don't feel insecure because your grasp of details may not be what it used to be. This can be a strength—it means that you're more likely to see the bigger picture.

Ages 66 and older

You may notice increasing incidences of memory glitches, but it is probably not as dramatic as you think. People tend to notice when they forget a few minor details, such as the name of the movie they saw last month. They don't consider the tens of thousands of details that they didn't forget.*

Try to nourish your brain by putting accumulated knowledge and wisdom to work. Deep thinking and disciplined use of brainpower helps fine-tune brain resources for optimal performance.

Best brain-boosting strategies if you're age 66 or older...

•**Get off autopilot.** At this age, you are especially at risk for slipping into autopilot—a dangerous state, since a bored brain is going backward.

To keep the mind sharp: Continue to push yourself to learn something new, especially if it's related to technology, which can help build new connections in the brain. You

*If problems with memory or decision-making begin to interfere with daily life, such as completing household tasks, consult your doctor.

will feel energized as you go from being a novice to an expert in an area of interest.

•**Stay challenged.** The problem with crossword puzzles and other brain teasers is that they get easier with practice. People who do crosswords get better mainly at crosswords, and the gains generally don't translate into other high-level mental areas.

To keep the mind sharp: Take on real challenges that you are motivated to master. Forcing yourself to learn a new language just to exercise your brain will not produce the same far-reaching cognitive benefits as honing a foreign language for practical use, such as for a trip. The brain expands and develops new pathways when it's pushed to explore unfamiliar areas.

Fortifying Younger Brains

Adults who are under age 45 tend to be very comfortable with collecting facts—but they often are less confident than they could be when dealing with abstract concepts and making decisions. *How people in this age group can improve their brain performance…*

•**Don't get distracted.** Younger adults have a tremendous ability to memorize, but they're typically poor at choosing what they need to remember. Most people will function just fine if they ignore about 50% of the information that comes their way.

Helpful: Focus on accomplishing your top two or three priorities for the day without letting distractions, such as constant text, e-mail and social-media alerts, disrupt your progress.

•**Zoom out.** When every fact in the world is a click away, our brains often get stuck regurgitating facts and blindly following directions.

Helpful: When you're reading for knowledge (not for entertainment), skim the material quickly…find the takeaway message…and then condense it to a succinct thought. Translating new information into your own words increases comprehension and helps you achieve new perspectives that can inspire your brain to generate new ideas and solutions.

The Nutrient That Boosts Brain Power

Erin McGlade, PhD, clinical psychologist at the University of Utah Brain Institute and University of Utah Department of Psychiatry in Salt Lake City. Her research includes the effects of citicoline supplementation on healthy adults and adolescents.

Many of us may feel like our to-do lists are growing faster than Jack's bean stalk. The longer those lists get—and the older we get—the tougher it is to focus and get things done. It's annoying to feel overwhelmed and scatterbrained when we want to keep our wits sharp.

If that frustration sounds familiar, you'll want to read on about a nutrient called citicoline that helps us pay attention, according to a recent study.

Citicoline is a naturally occurring chemical found in cells, including brain cells. Earlier studies showed that citicoline (also called CDP-choline) improved memory and attention in seniors with mild-to-moderate memory loss. It also helped individuals with dementia caused by small strokes to recover some cognitive functions. This recent study, though, is thought to be the first to examine the compound's effects on healthy middle-aged people.

Published in *Food and Nutrition Sciences*, the recent study included 60 healthy women ages 40 to 60. For 28 days, participants took either 250 mg of citicoline daily…500 mg of citicoline daily…or a placebo. Neither the women nor the investigators were told which participants had been assigned to which regimen until the study was over. On day 28, each participant completed a 14-minute computerized version of a standard test often used to gauge sustained attention and focus. Specifically, they were asked to pay close attention as individual letters flashed on a

Brain Spice?

When mice consumed cinnamon, it was converted into sodium benzoate, a compound that may improve motor functions and reverse brain damage caused by Parkinson's disease.

Journal of Neuroimmune Pharmacology.

computer screen for one-quarter of a second each and to press the keyboard's space bar whenever any letter other than X appeared. Mistakes were either by commission (hitting the bar when an X flashed by) or omission (not hitting the bar when another letter appeared).

Impressive results: Women who had taken citicoline at either dosage made fewer errors of both commission and omission than women who had taken a placebo. Interestingly, the lower-dose citicoline group performed best of all.

The study's lead author, Erin McGlade, PhD, a clinical psychologist at the University of Utah Brain Institute in Salt Lake City, explained, "This study suggests that citicoline helps with what I call the 'spacing out' that can accompany aging. For example, if I'm at work trying to read article after article, instead of my mind wandering to, 'Where am I going tonight?' the citicoline helps me focus on what I need to do at that moment."

Why it works: Researchers theorize that citicoline increases brain levels of dopamine, a neurotransmitter that is closely linked to our ability to focus. As we get older, it becomes harder to rein in our focus, a phenomenon that has been linked to having fewer available dopamine receptors, Dr. McGlade said. Citicoline may boost dopamine to help us pay attention to the task at hand. The nutrient also helps keep brain cell membranes healthy.

If you want to give citicoline a try: Unless you're fond of organ meats such as liver and brains, you're unlikely to get a substantial amount of citicoline in your diet. Because the nutrient appears in only small quantities in other foods, taking supplements of citicoline may be the easiest way to be sure of

getting a therapeutic dosage. Remember, the current study found that a dose as low as 250 mg resulted in increased attention (the brand used in the study was Cognizin). Certain energy drinks also have citicoline—but these typically do not contain the efficacious amount, Dr. McGlade noted, so be sure to check product labels.

Though long-term studies of the potential side effects of citicoline have yet to be done, side effects appear to occur only occasionally and mostly involve mild gastrointestinal upset. As a general precaution, citicoline should not be used by women who are pregnant or breast-feeding.

Exercise May Tone Up Women's Bodies and Minds

Liana Machado, PhD, senior lecturer, psychology, University of Otago, Dunedin, New Zealand.

Sandra Bond Chapman, PhD, chief director, Center for BrainHealth, University of Texas at Dallas.

Psychophysiology online.

Young women who regularly exercise may have more oxygen circulating in their brains—and possibly sharper minds, a small study suggests.

The findings, from a study of 52 healthy young women, don't prove that exercise makes you smarter, researchers said.

On the other hand, it's "reasonable" to conclude that exercise likely boosts mental prowess even when people are young and healthy, said Liana Machado, PhD, of the University of Otago in New Zealand, the lead researcher on the study.

Previous studies have found that older adults who exercise tend to have better blood flow in the brain, and do better on tests of memory and other mental skills, versus sedentary people of the same age, the authors point out.

But few studies have focused on young adults, they said. The women in this study were between 18 and 30.

The "predominant view" has been that young adults' brains are operating at their lifetime peak, no matter what their exercise level, the researchers write in the journal *Psychophysiology*.

But in this study, brain imaging showed that the oxygen supply in young women's brains did vary depending on their exercise habits.

Compared with their less-active peers, women who exercised most days of the week had more oxygen circulating in the frontal lobe during a battery of mental tasks, the study found.

The frontal lobe governs some vital functions, including the ability to plan, make decisions and retain memories longer-term.

Work for Your Brain

●**Delaying retirement may protect your brain.** For each additional year that a person worked before retiring, dementia risk dropped by 3%. That means someone who retired at age 60 had a 15% greater chance of developing dementia, on average, than someone who retired at 65.

Theory: The mental stimulation and social connections at work may keep the brain healthy.

Analysis of the records of more than 400,000 retired workers in France by researchers at National Institute of Health and Medical Research, Paris, presented at the 2013 Alzheimer's Association International Conference.

●**The right job for your brain.** Individuals with complex and/or people-oriented jobs—such as architects, lawyers, social workers and teachers—do better on later-life memory tests than those with less stimulating occupations.

Neurology.

Dr. Machado's team found that active women did particularly well on tasks that measured "cognitive inhibitory control."

"That refers to the ability to suppress reflexive responses and instead respond strategically, using self-control," Dr. Machado explained.

That skill turns up a lot in daily life, she noted, whether in playing a video game or driving a car.

Similarly, the researchers found a link between higher brain oxygen levels and women's performance on the toughest test in the battery—where the challenge was to combine inhibitory control with multitasking.

None of that proves cause-and-effect, Dr. Machado said.

But, she added, "it seems reasonable to deduce that a causal relationship likely exists—where regular physical activity increases oxygen availability in the brain, which in turn supports better cognitive performance, particularly for more challenging tasks."

Expert Response

Another researcher said that when it comes to exercise and brain health, there is always a "chicken-or-egg" question.

It's possible that the young women who did better on the mental tasks were more likely to choose healthy habits because the frontal lobe is involved in "orchestrating a plan," said Sandra Bond Chapman, PhD, chief director of the Center for BrainHealth at the University of Texas at Dallas.

Dr. Chapman, who was not involved in the study, said it would be helpful for researchers to follow groups of people long-term to see whether those who adopt healthy habits end up sharpening their mental skills.

That said, Dr. Chapman encouraged people to lace up their sneakers and "get moving."

"There is growing scientific evidence that physical exercise is good for the body and the brain, no matter the age," she said.

How Much Exercise Boosts The Brain

And how much exercise would be enough to benefit a young person's brain? It's not clear, said Dr. Machado.

Women in this study were considered to be meeting guidelines on regular exercise if they got at least 30 minutes of moderate activity (such as brisk walking) or 15 minutes of vigorous activity (such as running) at least five days a week.

So the findings suggest that moderate amounts of exercise would "suffice," Dr. Machado said. "But it will be important to test whether more vigorous exercise affords greater benefits," she added.

Future studies should also focus on young men, Dr. Machado said, since women and men differ in the way the brain's vasculature (system of blood vessels) functions.

"It can't be assumed that similar findings will arise in men," she said.

The Society for Neuroscience has more on exercise and the brain at *http://www.brainfacts. org* (search "exercise beefs up the brain").

Yoga Makes You Smarter!

In a recent eight-week study, adults over age 55 who took an hour-long class of hatha yoga (the most commonly practiced form of yoga worldwide) three times a week had significantly better memory and attention than adults who simply did stretching and toning exercises.

Possible reason: The focus required to hold poses and control breathing during yoga may result in better attention to mental tasks as well.

Neha Gothe, PhD, assistant professor of kinesiology, Wayne State University, Detroit.

For Mild Cognitive Impairment, Dementia Drugs Don't Help...and May Hurt

Sharon E. Straus, MD, physician, St. Michael's Hospital, Toronto, and professor, department of medicine, and director, geriatric medicine, University of Toronto, Canada. Her study was published in *CMAJ*.

It's very scary to feel like your memory is slipping and you can't think as clearly as you once did...and to wonder whether you've started down the path toward dementia. This condition is called mild cognitive impairment (MCI). And unfortunately, within two years of an MCI diagnosis, an estimated 11% to 33% of patients do progress to full-blown dementia.

So it's no wonder that a growing number of people with MCI are asking for prescription drugs in an attempt to keep their minds sharp. These drugs, called cognitive enhancers, support the production and performance of memory-related neurotransmitters, and they sometimes help patients who already have dementia. And doctors in some countries, including the US and Canada, are giving these drugs to patients who don't have dementia.

The hope is that the medications might help MCI patients in the short term by enhancing memory...and in the long term by reducing dementia risk.

Is the strategy working? Or are the drugs doing more harm than good for patients with MCI? *A new study has the answer...*

Examining the Evidence

Researchers from Canada examined existing studies that involved a total of more than 4,500 patients with MCI who were given either a placebo or one of the cognitive-enhancing drugs. They identified eight high-quality studies that were conducted between 1999 and 2007 in various parts of the world.

The goal was to gauge the safety and effectiveness of four medications—*donepezil* (Aricept), *rivastigmine* (Exelon), *galantamine*

(Razadyne) and *memantine* (Namenda). These drugs are widely prescribed for dementia patients to improve mental functioning—memory, attention, mood, reasoning, language and ability to perform activities of daily living. The drugs work by increasing the amount of naturally occurring neurotransmitters in the brain or by decreasing abnormal brain activity.

Disheartening results: Not a single one of the medications brought about significant improvement in short-term cognitive performance for MCI patients...nor did any of the drugs help in the long term to help stave off the progression to full-blown dementia. What the drugs did do was cause unpleasant side effects, including diarrhea, nausea, vomiting and headaches. Worse, the researchers found a link between the medications and an elevated risk for cardiac problems—specifically, the drug galantamine was associated with a higher incidence of bradycardia (slow heart rate), which can be dangerous.

Bottom line: It's understandable that people with MCI would be desperate to try just about anything that might reduce their risk of progressing to full-blown dementia...but this study shows that taking what are essentially Alzheimer's drugs is not the answer, because they don't help with MCI and can cause harm.

What does help: Anyone who wants to reduce dementia risk is best off living a healthy lifestyle—eating properly, exercising, and staying mentally and socially active. A plethora of studies show that these measures really can help keep us fit in both body and mind.

Unusual Memory Trouble

Louis R. Caplan, MD, professor of neurology, Harvard Medical School, Boston.

If you suddenly cannot remember where you are or how you got there, then your memory comes back, what could be happening?

One possibility is that you had a condition called transient global amnesia (TGA). It is a temporary loss of memory that typically lasts for six to 12 hours. People who have TGA can perform physical tasks, such as driving, and can recognize familiar people, but they are unable to remember recent events. They often ask the same questions repeatedly even after those questions have been answered.

Neurologists don't know exactly what triggers TGA, but many believe it to be a type of migraine headache. It usually is a onetime event. Even though TGA is disturbing, it is a fairly benign condition. However, if this happens to you or someone you know, a neurological exam should be administered to rule out anything more serious, such as a stroke.

Sleep and Alzheimer's

A long-term study of initially healthy 65-year-olds found that those who slept the least (about five hours or less without waking) tended to have fewer neurons (brain cells) in a part of the brain that controls sleep.

Also: Many in the study who developed Alzheimer's disease were those who had fewer neurons and less sleep.

To protect your brain: Keep neurons healthy with good sleep habits, and seek treatment if you suspect you may have a sleep disorder.

Andrew Lim, MD, assistant professor of neurology, University of Toronto, Canada.

REM Sleep Disorder Is a Warning Sign for Dementia

Study titled "Breakdown in REM sleep circuitry underlies REM sleep behavior disorder," published in *Trends in Neuroscience*.

Do you sleep next to (or barely sleep because of) someone who acts out dreams—or has your bed partner told you that you're the nasty bump in the night? If a nightly "wrestlemania" is just starting or getting worse over time, you may be chalking it up to aging. Don't do that! Restless dreaming—that is, lots of physical movement, including sleep walking, during rapid eye movement (REM) sleep—is not a natural part of aging. It may be REM sleep behavior disorder, which researchers are now learning is a warning sign that dementia, Parkinson's or another neurological disease may be coming to get you.

Consider this...a neurodegenerative disease will be diagnosed in 50% of people with REM sleep behavior disorder within five years and 80% within 15 years, according to a recent University of Toronto study. Within the years between diagnosis of REM sleep behavior disorder and a full-fledged neuro problem, subtle yet growing signs of neurodegeneration, such as difficulty recognizing smells and colors and not being able to think or walk straight, are likely to crop up. This might sound like a nightmare, but it might be a boon in more than one respect. It means scientists can even more fully study how neurodegenerative diseases begin and progress in people—and that means getting closer to cures for Alzheimer's disease, Lewy body dementia, and Parkinson's and Lou Gehrig's diseases. It also means that, until a cure is found, you and an informed and forward-thinking doctor can take action to quickly recognize and slow down a neurodegenerative disease before it sets in.

What to Do

First, know what REM sleep behavior disorder is. It's a condition in which the body's safety catch that keeps us from physically acting out dreams doesn't kick in properly. People with this disorder risk seriously hurting themselves or their bed partners. Instead of staying still, their bodies act out whatever they are doing in their dreams—be it picking flowers, fighting dragons or making love. So this is just another important reason not to ignore this annoyance if it is happening to you or someone dear to you. And given

what we now know—that restless dreaming is closely tied to dementia and other neurological diseases—it is even more crucial not to delay getting a diagnosis for REM sleep behavior disorder.

If you know or suspect that you experience restless dreaming, your first step is to discuss it with a primary care physician, who will most likely refer you to a neurologist. The neurologist will set up a sleep study at a hospital or sleep disorders clinic. The essentials of a sleep study are a video polysomnogram, which videotapes you sleeping and records your brain waves, and an electromyogram, which records the electrical activity of your muscles to see whether the movements you make are consistent with those of REM sleep behavior disorder.

If it turns out that the neurologist says, yes, you have REM sleep behavior disorder, he or she may suggest a treatment that will reduce the symptoms, such as the antiseizure medication *clonazepam* or the sleep aid melatonin. If your neurologist doesn't bring up the link between this sleep disorder and the very high risk of neurodegenerative disease down the road, you must bring up this link and make a plan with this neurologist—or another one you have confidence in, if necessary—for monitoring and staving off symptoms of neurodegeneration.

To learn more about REM sleep behavior disorder and other sleep disorders, visit the website of the National Sleep Foundation.

Watch Out for Apathy

Apathy may mean your brain is changing. Older adults who show a lack of interest, energy and emotion and drop activities to stay at home have less brain volume than their active peers. That was the finding in a recent study of more than 4,000 healthy adults (average age 76) who underwent MRI brain scans.

The upshot: It's normal to lose some brain volume as you age, but the larger losses found in this study could be a sign of a brain disorder, such as dementia. If you frequently feel apathetic, discuss this with your doctor.

Lenore Launer, PhD, chief of neuroepidemiology, National Institute on Aging, Bethesda, Maryland.

Supplements That Can Impair Your Brain

Cynthia Kuhn, PhD, professor of pharmacology, cancer biology, psychiatry and behavioral sciences at Duke University School of Medicine in Durham, North Carolina. Dr. Kuhn is also coauthor, with Scott Swartzwelder, PhD, and Wilkie Wilson, PhD, of *Buzzed: The Straight Facts About the Most Used and Abused Drugs from Alcohol to Ecstasy.*

It's hardly news that supplements—just like drugs—can have physical side effects.

Recent development: Researchers are now learning more and more about unwanted mental changes that can occur when taking popular supplements (such as herbs and hormones).

These supplements can be a hidden cause of depression, anxiety, mania and other mental changes because patients—and their doctors—often don't realize how these products can affect the brain.

Supplements that may cause unwanted mental changes…

Melatonin

Melatonin is among the most popular supplements for treating insomnia, jet lag and other sleep disorders. Melatonin is a natural hormone that's released by the pineal gland at night and readily enters the brain. Unlike many sleep aids, it doesn't render you unconscious or put you to sleep—it causes subtle brain changes that make you "ready" for sleep.

Studies have shown that people who take melatonin in the late afternoon or early evening tend to fall asleep more quickly when they go to bed. The amount of melatonin used in scientific studies ranges from 0.1 mg

Do You Have an Accurate Memory?

It may depend on how well you slept the night before.

New research: People who are sleep-deprived are more likely to develop false memories, a finding that could call into question the reliability of crime eyewitnesses.

Psychological Science.

to 0.5 mg. However, the products in health-food stores typically contain much higher doses—usually 1 mg to 5 mg. Supplemental melatonin also may become less effective over time, which encourages people to increase the doses even more.

Effects on the brain: In people with depression, melatonin may improve sleep, but it may worsen their depression symptoms, according to the National Institutes of Health.

What to do: Melatonin can help when used short term for such problems as jet lag. It is not particularly effective as a long-term solution for other causes of insomnia.

St. John's Wort

St. John's wort is probably the most studied herb for treating depression. Researchers who analyzed data from 29 international studies recently concluded that St. John's wort was as effective as prescription antidepressants for treating minor to moderate depression.

St. John's wort appears to be safe, particularly when it's used under the supervision of a physician. However, it can cause unwanted mental changes.

Effects on the brain: St. John's wort may increase brain levels of "feel good" neurotransmitters, including serotonin and dopamine. But unwanted mental changes that may occur in anyone taking St. John's wort include anxiety, irritability and vivid dreams. It may also lead to mania (a condition characterized by periods of overactivity, excessive excitement and lack of inhibitions)—especially in individuals who are also using anti-psychotic drugs.

Caution: This supplement should never be combined with a prescription selective serotonin reuptake inhibitor (SSRI) antidepressant, such as *sertraline* (Zoloft) or *paroxetine* (Paxil). Taking St. John's wort with an SSRI can cause serotonin syndrome, excessive brain levels of serotonin that can increase body temperature, heart rate and blood pressure—conditions that are all potentially fatal. It also can interact with certain drugs such as oral contraceptives and immunosuppressant medications.

What to do: If you have depression, do not self-medicate with St. John's wort. Always talk to your doctor first if you are interested in trying this supplement.

Weight-Loss Supplements

Two ingredients that are commonly used in weight-loss supplements, *beta-phenylethylamine* (PEA) and *P-synephrine*, are said to increase energy and metabolism and burn extra calories.

Effects on the brain: Both PEA and P-synephrine (a compound found in supplements made from bitter orange) can make you feel jittery and anxious, particularly when they are combined with stimulants such as caffeine.

Many weight-loss and "energy" products are complicated cocktails of active ingredients that haven't been adequately studied—nor have they been approved by the FDA. They're risky because they've been linked to dangerous increases in blood pressure.

Important: There is little evidence that any of these products is particularly effective as a weight-loss aid.

What to do: Don't rely on weight-loss supplements. To lose weight, you need to decrease your food intake and increase your exercise levels—no supplement can accomplish that!

Stay Away from Toxins

The brain may never recover from chemical fumes. In a study of more than 2,000 retired industrial workers, those who had high exposure to benzene, petroleum, paint, glue, chlorinated solvents and other chemicals scored worse on tests for cognitive functioning—and impairment was detected in people whose exposure dated back 50 years.

Explanation: Industrial solvents may permanently damage brain cells, so if you're around them, be sure to wear a face mask and keep the area ventilated.

Erika Sabbath, ScD, assistant professor, Boston College Graduate School of Social Work, Chestnut Hill, Massachusetts.

What If It's a Brain Tumor?

Alessandro Olivi, MD, a professor of neurosurgery and oncology and director of neurological oncology at Johns Hopkins University School of Medicine and chairman of neurosurgery at Johns Hopkins Bayview Medical Center, both in Baltimore.

No one wants to hear a doctor say, "It's a brain tumor." But what most of us don't realize is that for the majority of people who hear these words, the diagnosis is not a death sentence.

Meningioma is the most common kind of brain tumor—and the majority of these, 85%, are benign. This does not mean that these tumors are not harmful or do not cause serious problems. But understanding of these tumors has advanced, and research is ongoing to determine why these tumors occur and in whom—and this has produced new detection and treatment options.

New findings you should know about...

What Are Meningiomas?

Meningiomas are tumors that do not grow within the brain tissue itself, but on the meninges, the membrane that covers the brain and lines the spinal cord. Commonly, meningiomas develop between the upper surface of the brain and the skull.

Meningiomas also can occur on the skull base—including forming in the bones at the bottom of the skull and the bony ridge in the back of the eyes.

Symptoms can occur as the meningioma grows large enough to exert pressure on the brain or if it irritates the surrounding areas. Depending on its location and which brain areas and nerves are disrupted, symptoms may include blurred vision, impaired hearing or sense of smell, loss of balance or facial pain or numbness. Symptoms such as headaches, seizures, muscle weakness and/or memory loss may also occur.

Who Is Affected?

Meningiomas are two to three times as common in women as in men and are found more frequently in blacks than in any other ethnic group. The higher rate among women has led scientists to wonder whether hormones might play a role—and whether hormone treatment may increase risk.

So far, the data from large population studies in both the US and Finland have found no connection between oral contraceptives and meningiomas and no more than a weak association between postmenopausal hormone-replacement therapy (HRT) and the occurrence of brain tumors.

A large 2011 study that looked at lifestyle factors suggested that the risk for meningioma after menopause rose for women who were overweight but dropped slightly for active women.

The Cause Is Unknown

Researchers are still working on what causes meningiomas. One area of interest is radiation. Several studies have shown that very large amounts of radiation appear to increase the risk for these tumors. Most susceptible are children and young adults who had high doses of radiation to treat a previous cancer. A connection between cell-phone use and meningioma has not yet been determined.

Now researchers at Brigham and Women's Hospital and Yale University are using genetic analysis to help understand why some individuals develop meningiomas after radiation exposure while other people do not.

A study that was published in the journal *Cancer* in 2012 suggested that there may be a connection between bitewing dental X-rays and meningioma, but the evidence is not definitive. For now, the best advice is simply to have dental X-rays no more often than is necessary.

Diagnosis of Meningiomas

Sometimes, meningiomas are diagnosed by accident, even before they cause symptoms—for example, in the course of examination for an unrelated problem such as head trauma.

For other patients, meningiomas are not diagnosed until they have been growing for years and reached a substantial size. Slow-growing tumors are almost always benign and rarely become cancerous.

When symptoms (such as those mentioned earlier) make physicians suspect a meningioma, they turn to computed tomography (CT) and magnetic resonance imaging (MRI), with contrast dye to better see the tumor, for diagnosis.

Recent progress: The development of powerful magnets has made MRI scans far more precise than they were in the past—and they are able to detect brain tumors that might have been missed a few years ago.

Treatment Strategies

Once found, not all meningiomas need to be treated. Physicians may opt for the "watchful waiting" approach for small, benign tumors that do not create symptoms.

Researchers are studying these benign tumors. At Johns Hopkins, they are looking at the genetic differences between benign meningiomas that stay benign and those that

Distrust Harms the Brain

People who habitually distrust others, believing that others act mainly in their own self-interest, are three times more likely to develop dementia than those who do not. That was the finding of a recent eight-year study of older adults (average age 71).

Anna-Maija Tolppanen, PhD, development director of neurology, University of Eastern Finland, Kuopio.

become malignant. This will help doctors determine which tumors need treatment and when it is safe to wait and watch a tumor.

Surgery may become necessary if symptoms develop or if periodic brain scans show that the tumor is starting to grow rapidly. The usual surgical treatment is removal of the entire tumor.

Major advances: With image-guided surgery, the surgeon uses CT or MRI as a kind of 3-D internal GPS to tell him/her just where the tumor ends and to navigate around blood vessels and neural structures.

This type of advance makes it possible to remove tumors that would previously have been considered too risky to remove, and to remove them more completely, making recurrence less likely. The use of intraoperative CT and MRI in the operating room enables surgeons to verify that the entire tumor has been removed.

Sometimes the location of the tumor makes surgery impossible. For instance, a meningioma in the middle of the skull base is likely to be surrounded by crucial nerves and blood vessels that make surgery too risky.

In cases like these, radiation therapy (also called radiotherapy) is used. Radiation therapy has also advanced. Today, stereotactic radiosurgery uses imaging and computerized programming to precisely target high-intensity radiation to the tumor while limiting damage to nearby brain tissue. Gamma Knife, CyberKnife and similar methods deliver this type of concentrated radiation. Stereotac-

tic radiosurgery usually keeps tumors from growing but only occasionally shrinks them.

One possible side effect is brain swelling, which can cause symptoms such as headaches or neurological problems such as seizures or loss of balance.

Chemotherapy plays a small role in meningioma—it is reserved for aggressively malignant or recurrent tumors that cannot be treated effectively with surgery or radiotherapy alone.

Research is ongoing to develop new drugs. At Johns Hopkins, scientists have identified a molecular pathway within meningioma cells that spurs their growth—and this could lead to the development of drugs to block their growth.

Researchers at Harvard Medical School, Memorial Sloan-Kettering Cancer Center and elsewhere also are testing medications approved for pancreatic and gastrointestinal cancers with hopes of identifying more effective chemotherapy for those meningiomas that do become aggressive or recurrent.

Alcohol Can Help Your Brain

Light-to-moderate drinking in later life may keep memory strong. Consuming up to one drink a day is associated with better episodic memory—the ability to remember specific events. Episodic memory is the type that usually diminishes in dementia.

Theory: Alcohol may help preserve the hippocampus, a brain area that shrinks in people with dementia.

Faika Zanjani, PhD, associate professor, department of behavioral and community health, University of Maryland School of Public Health, College Park, and leader of a study of 664 people, average age 75 at the end of the study, published in American Journal of Alzheimer's Disease & Other Dementias.

Chapter 6

HELP FOR FALLS AND PHYSICAL INJURY

Catch Your Balance Problem Before It's Too Late

No one expects to get seriously injured—or even die—from a fall. But it happens all the time. And while older adults are at greatest risk for falls, there are no age requirements for taking a tumble.

Surprising statistic: Even among adults in their 30s, 40s and 50s, falls are the leading cause of nonfatal injuries (more than 3 million each year) that are treated in US hospital emergency departments. For adults age 65 and older, falls are the leading cause of fatal injuries.

Certain "fall hazards" are well known—electrical cords and area rugs…slippery floors …medications such as sleeping pills and blood pressure drugs…vision problems…and even poorly fitting shoes.

What often gets overlooked: Subtle changes in the neuromuscular system (the nervous system and muscles working together), which helps keep us upright. Regardless of your age, exercising and strengthening this system before you get unsteady (or fall)

is one of the best steps you can take to protect your health. *Here's how…*

Why Our Balance Slips

Does your foot or ankle feel a little wobbly when you stand on one leg? Some of that is probably due to diminished strength and flexibility. After about age 40, we begin to lose roughly 1% of our muscle mass every year. As we age, we also become more sedentary and less flexible. These factors make the body less able to adapt to and correct a loss of balance.

The nervous system also gets less sensitive with age.

Example: Sensory receptors known as proprioceptors are found in the nerve endings of muscles, tendons, joints and the inner ear. These receptors make us aware of our bodies in space (proprioception) and can detect even the slightest variations in body positions and movements. But they don't work well in people who don't exercise them and

---

Jason Jackson, MSPT, physical therapist in the outpatient rehabilitation department at Mount Sinai Hospital in New York City, where he specializes in balance training, along with prosthetic training, manual therapy and neuromuscular disease.

these people find it harder to keep their balance.

The other danger: Muscle weakness, even when it's slight, can lead to apprehension about losing your balance. You might then start to avoid physical activities that you feel are risky—walking on uneven pavement, for example. But avoiding such challenges to your balance actually accelerates both muscle and nervous system declines.

Are You Steady?

If you're afraid of falling or have a history of falls, a professional balance assessment, done by your doctor or a physical therapist, is the best way to find out how steady you are on your feet. *The assessment usually includes tests such as the following (don't try these tests on your own if you feel unsteady)…*

•**Sit-to-stand.** Sit in a straight-backed chair. If your balance and leg strength are good, you'll be able to stand up without pushing off with your hands.

•**Stand with your feet touching.** You should be able to hold this position for 15 seconds without any wobbling.

•**The nudge test.** Ask someone to gently push on your hip while you're in a normal stance. If you stagger or throw out your hands to catch yourself, your balance is questionable. If you start to fall, your balance needs improvement.

Boost Your Balance

Balance, like strength and endurance, can be improved with simple workouts. Incorporate the exercises below into your daily routine—while at the grocery store, in the office, while watching TV, etc. Do them for about 15 minutes to 30 minutes a day, three to four days a week (daily if you have the time). *What to do…**

•**One-legged stands.** You don't have to set aside time to do this exercise. You simply

*Do these exercises next to a stable object, such as a countertop, if you feel unsteady. Also, they are more easily done while wearing shoes. When you feel comfortable doing these moves, you can perform them barefoot to add difficulty.

stand on one leg as you go about your daily activities—while waiting in line, for example. Lift your foot about six inches to 12 inches off the floor to the front, side and back. Try to hold each position for about 15 seconds, then switch legs. This strengthens the muscles in the ankles, hips and knees—all of which play a key role in one's balance.

•**Heel raises.** This move is good for balance and strength. While standing, rise up on your toes as far as you can. Drop back to the starting position, then do it again. Try for 10 repetitions. You can make this exercise more difficult by holding weights. Start with three-pound weights, gradually increasing weight as you build tolerance.

For More Benefits

Once you have become comfortable with the exercises described earlier, you can up your game with the following to keep you even safer from falling…

•**Balance on a Bosu ball.** It's a rubber-like half-ball (about two feet in diameter) that you can use for dozens of at-home workouts, including balance and abdominal exercises.

Cost: About $100, on Amazon.com and in some sporting-goods stores.

Example: With the flat side on the floor, start by standing with both feet on the ball. Your muscles and joints will make hundreds of small adjustments to keep you balanced. When you get better at it, try to stand on one leg on the ball. When you're really comfortable, have someone toss you a basketball or tennis ball while you maintain your balance.

Just for Fun

You don't always need formal balance exercises. *Try this…*

•**Walk barefoot.** Most of us spend our days in well-padded shoes that minimize the "feedback" between our feet and the ground. Walking without shoes for at least a few minutes each day strengthens the intrinsic muscles in the feet and improves stability. If you prefer to wear socks, be sure to use nonslip varieties that have treads to avoid slipping on wood or tiled floors.

Also helpful: Minimalist walking/running shoes. They're made by most major footwear companies, such as New Balance, Adidas and Nike, as well as by Vivobarefoot. Because they have a minimal amount of heel cushioning and arch support, they give the same benefits as barefoot walking but with a little extra protection.

When Your New Glasses Are Hazardous to Your Health

David B. Elliott, PhD, MCOptom, professor of clinical vision science, Bradford School of Optometry and Vision Sciences, University of Bradford, West Yorkshire, United Kingdom. His article was published in *Optometry and Vision Science.*

D o you remember playing "Pin the Tail On the Donkey" and what fun it was to watch the blindfolded kids stumble and sway as they tried to walk a straight line after being twirled? The brain needs vision to keep the body balanced. Otherwise (unless you're blind and learn to compensate), you might wander around looking a bit drunk, misjudge distances, stumble and even fall.

So you'd think that getting a new, updated prescription for eyeglasses or contacts, or surgery to remove cataracts, would make you steadier, more sure-footed and safer.

Not so fast. Studies show that updated vision correction, even if it technically improves your ability to see, is associated with a dangerous adjustment period that could land you in the hospital or worse.

Take heed—there's a right way and a wrong way to get used to vision correction, and knowing the right way could literally save your life…

A Too-Common Hazard

How can seeing better lead to a potentially fatal fall? David B. Elliott, PhD, professor of clinical vision science at University of Bradford in West Yorkshire, United Kingdom, reviewed several studies on the association between vision correction and falls in older people to find out—and look for ways that people can stay safe.

In one study of more than 28,000 men and women over age 60, risk of serious falls more than doubled after a first cataract operation. Even after cataracts in both eyes were repaired, risk of serious falls increased by more than one-third.

Another study found that, for older adults, getting a pair of glasses or other vision correction was potentially more dangerous than muddling along with bad eyesight. In this study, 300 men and women who were age 70 or older were divided into two groups—one, a treatment group and the other, a control group. The treatment group had eye exams and, if needed, got glasses or cataract surgery. The control group had no special intervention. Members of this group may have had a vision check and received new glasses on their own if they so wished, but they were not encouraged to do so as part of the study.

You would think that people who specifically had vision correction would be better off, but in the first year of the study, there were 30% more falls in the treatment group than in the control group. Almost three-quarters of people in the treatment group who had significant changes in vision correction—whether they had received glasses for the first time or had major updates to their existing eyeglass prescriptions—fell at least once, and 53% of those who had more minor changes did so as well. This suggests that falls may, in part, be attributable to vision correction that is too much too soon for older adults, according to Dr. Elliott.

What explains it? For one, older people may have challenges adapting to lens magnification. Take, for instance, the simple action of stepping off a curb or walking down stairs. The magnification of a new pair of glasses can make the step appear further away than it actually is. And when an astigmatism (a distortion in the shape of the cornea) is compensated for with glasses, it can initially be difficult to get used to the new way of seeing. Floors and walls can initially appear to be sloped, and this can naturally mess up balance.

Safety and New Glasses

No one is suggesting that you should suffer with poor eyesight as a strategy to prevent falls, but powerful new glasses aren't always the best solution. Firstly, know that folks most at risk for falls related to vision correction are seniors (people age 75 or older) and people who are otherwise frail or have medical conditions that can throw off balance, such as Parkinson's disease, stroke, arthritis, diabetes, low blood pressure, inner ear disease and dementia. People who are on sedative or antidepressant medications or who take more than four prescription medications a day are also at higher risk. *Based on the medical evidence, Dr. Elliott offers these tips about new glasses can keep you safe…*

•**New prescriptions.** If you are an older person who already is wearing glasses and feel that your vision is just fine with them, but an optometrist says you need a stronger prescription, assert your option to refuse or to request that a small, incremental improvement be made instead of a full-blown correction. The point here is, if it "ain't broke"—by your needs and standards—don't feel pressured into having to "fix it."

•**New frames.** Do you need a new pair of eyeglass frames? Choose frames that are similar in design and fit to the old pair. The more the new pair of glasses is similar to the old pair, the easier—and safer—the adjustment to the glasses will be.

•**Bifocal and progressive lenses.** If you know that you are prone to being off balance or otherwise fit into the high-risk category, avoid bifocal or progressive lenses if you've never worn these types of glasses. For safety's sake, it would be better for you to purchase both near and distance glasses. This advice even holds true for bifocal-lens wearers once they fall into the high-risk cat-

egory. Does this extra step need to be expensive? Not necessarily. Consider purchasing prescription glasses for distance and one or two pairs of less expensive, nonprescription magnifying glasses ("readers") for reading and computer use.

If you are already using bifocal or progressive lenses, get used to a new prescription first by carefully walking around and paying attention to how your surroundings look through your new glasses. This has been shown to help prevent falls. Another tip is to tuck your chin in while going up or down stairs so you look through the upper (distance) part of the lens, not the lower (near-vision) part.

Even though studies on falls and vision correction focus on older adults, taking time to get used to new glasses is smart advice for anyone of any age.

Antipsychotic Drugs Cause Deadly Falls in Older Adults

Research letter titled "Falls and fractures with atypical antipsychotic medication use: a population-based cohort study," from researchers at Western University, London, Ontario, published in *JAMA Internal Medicine.*

If you have a spouse, relative or friend who is in the later stages of Alzheimer's disease, Lewy body dementia or a neurodegenerative illness such as Parkinson's disease, he or she is probably being given an antipsychotic drug to manage behavior problems, such as agitation and aggression, and/or psychotic symptoms. Or perhaps you are caring for a person who is aging with schizophrenia or severe bipolar disorder and is on an antipsychotic drug. The medication is as much for the person's comfort as for the people taking care of him or her, but like all drugs, antipsychotics carry side effects. And now, researchers have confirmed that newer antipsychotic drugs, thought to be safer than the older drugs, are also associated with a particularly dangerous side effect in older adults—falls. Because antipsychotic drugs can weaken bones and cause osteoporosis and osteoporotic fractures, falls can easily be deadly in this population group.

Tripped Up by a Drug

The idea that antipsychotic medications and bone fractures go together is not entirely new—reports have periodically surfaced in the medical literature, and it is known that antipsychotics can weaken bones. But there wasn't enough evidence to prove a direct link between osteoporotic fractures and falls and the newest class of antipsychotic drugs, called atypicals.

Enter a team of Canadian researchers from University of Western Ontario. The team reasoned that atypicals might be likely to cause falls, resulting in fractures, in older adults because they can cause orthostatic hypotension, a sudden drop in blood pressure that causes dizziness or fainting, as well as gait and coordination difficulties and sedation.

To investigate an association between atypicals, falls and fractures, the researchers studied the medical records of a total of 200,000 Ontario residents, all 65 years old or older. They homed in on patients who had received new (first-time) prescriptions for one of three atypical antipsychotic drugs—*quetiapine* (Seroquel), *risperidone* (Risperdal) or *olanzapine* (Zyprexa). Each person was matched with a person of the same age and gender and several dozen other characteristics, such as presence of dementia or psychotic illness, diabetes or arthritis, previous fractures or falls, use of osteoporotic drugs and whether or not they lived in a nursing facility. Patients and controls were followed for the first 90 days after the patients started on the drugs.

The results: Among patients taking atypical antipsychotics, the rate of fractures associated with osteoporosis was 7% and the rate of falls was 4.4%–and if those numbers don't sound high to you, keep in mind that this was only in the first 90 days of taking the drugs. That's not much time at all! And

meanwhile, members of the control group of similar people who were not taking the drugs were only about half as likely to suffer osteoporotic fractures or falls.

And in terms of fall and fracture risk, it didn't matter which atypical antipsychotic was taken or at what dosage—all three drugs and various dosages were associated with similar heightened risk.

Take Steps to Prevent Falls

The take-home message here is pretty clear. If a doctor has prescribed an atypical antipsychotic medication for a loved one— perhaps someone under your care or in an assisted-living environment—he is at an increased risk for falls. If you believe the drug's overall benefits are worth its risks, even if this person has never had a history of unsteadiness or falling, consider taking steps to reduce risk of falls, such as improving the lighting and removing throw rugs in the living area of the patient and installing safety grab bars and raised toilet seats and bathtub benches in the bathroom. Caretakers also might want to speak to the patient's doctor about physical therapy and the value of a cane or walker to reduce risk of falls.

How to Fall Safely

Marilyn Moffat, DPT, PhD, professor of physical therapy at New York University in New York City, reported by Rebecca Shannonhouse, editor, *Bottom Line/Health*.

We've all read plenty of articles about the best ways to prevent falls, but few of them describe *how* to fall.

Sooner or later, we all encounter one of the many fall hazards—uneven sidewalks, curb grates, an unexpected step or simply tangled feet. What do you do when you know you're going down? *Try these pointers...*

If you fall forward: Don't stick out your arms to "break" the fall. The only thing that will get broken is your arm or wrist.

Instead, keep your head up and let your knees hit the ground first. If you can, briefly slap your palms on the ground to slow the fall.

If you fall sideways: Try to grab the opposite hip and roll sideways as you fall.

For a backward fall: Fold your hips and knees at the same time...land on your buttocks...and roll backward.

But how do you remember all this when you're going down? "Individuals may practice falling," says Marilyn Moffat, DPT, PhD, a professor of physical therapy at New York University in New York City. You can use soft mats to absorb any impact—but only if your bones and joints are healthy, she adds. For appropriate guidance, consult a physical therapist, since strength and balance may need to be developed first.

For helpful videos that show fall techniques, go to *TWU.edu/rm/FallingSafely.asp*.

Is It a Concussion?

Diane Roberts Stoler, EdD, neuropsychologist and board-certified health and sport psychologist with a private practice in Boxford, Massachusetts. A brain injury patient herself, she is coauthor, with Barbara Albers Hill, of *Coping with Concussion and Mild Traumatic Brain Injury. DrDiane.com*

With all the recent talk about football players suffering concussions that have caused permanent brain damage, you might think that these brain injuries occur only on sports fields.

But that's far from the truth. Anyone can suffer a concussion. More than 40% of concussions are caused by falls...and 14.3% by car accidents.

So how can you tell when a concussion might lead to permanent damage...or will simply heal on its own? *Here's what you need to know to make that call...*

Why the Brain Is Vulnerable

Most people imagine that the brain is firmly anchored inside the skull. Actually, it floats on cushions of fluid and air, with plenty of room to move. This means that if you bang your head hard enough, or if your head is "whipped" during a car accident, the brain can slam against the skull. The violent movement stretches and shears nerve fibers.

What most people don't realize: Even if your head feels fine, there might be areas of microscopic damage that impair normal brain functions and may cause headaches, dizziness, fatigue and other symptoms for weeks or longer.

Fortunately, a single concussion is unlikely to cause long-term problems, and symptoms usually begin to improve within hours. Most people recover completely within a month to six weeks.

The risk: Once you've had a concussion, you're more likely to get another one if you suffer an additional brain injury—and the brain is more susceptible to long-term damage if you do.

For example, recent studies have linked repeated concussions to Parkinson's-like symptoms, such as hand tremors and gait problems, and other cognitive problems, such as memory loss. People who have suffered repeated concussions may also experience concussion symptoms (sometimes years after the last brain injury) if they receive anesthesia or medication that affects the central nervous system, such as pain medications and steroids. Repeated concussions, such as those suffered by some football players and boxers, can even lead to progressive, life-threatening dementia.

Is It a Concussion or Not?

You may assume that you don't have a concussion if you didn't "black out." In fact, a concussion may not cause a noticeable loss of consciousness. You're more apt to be dazed...unaware of where you are...or briefly confused.

Because injuries to the brain can feel minor even when they're life-threatening, I would advise anyone who's been in a car accident that caused significant head movement, taken a hard fall or been hit hard on the head to go to a hospital emergency department.

Doctors can usually diagnose a concussion in a few minutes. You'll be given a quick, in-office neurological exam to assess the degree—and location—of brain damage.

Examples: You might be asked to recite numbers backward and forward…and/or recall what the doctor just said. You will also be given tests to check your balance, reflexes, vision and hearing.

If you have acute symptoms—for example, severe headaches and/or repeated vomiting—you may be hospitalized for further tests, such as an MRI or a CT scan, which also check for conditions that are even more serious, such as hemorrhagic (bleeding) stroke or subdural hematoma (in which blood collects on the surface of the brain).

If these tests are inconclusive and your symptoms suggest a concussion, you can ask your doctor for a specialized test called diffusion tensor imaging. It's a type of MRI that can identify extremely small areas of nerve damage, blood clots or bleeding in the brain.

However, unless you are planning a personal injury or workers' comp claim, you probably don't need to prove your diagnosis with these imaging tests. If you have symptoms of a concussion, your doctor will probably advise you just to wait it out. Symptoms usually subside within six weeks.

Let Your Brain Heal

If you suffer a concussion, getting enough rest—including mental rest—is crucial. Until you've recovered, use your television, computer and smartphone only when absolutely necessary and for no more than two hours a day for the first few weeks after a concussion.

Also important…

•**Focus on your sleep.** Many people who have had concussions complain that they sleep fitfully or sleep too little or too much.

To promote sleep: Go to bed and get up at the same time every day…avoid bright lights in your bedroom…and create a soothing atmosphere.

Helpful: Try Bach Flower Rescue Remedy, which promotes the calm and relaxation that's needed to heal the brain.

•**Soothe the inflammation.** Because the brain is inflamed after a concussion, avoid foods that promote inflammation, such as sugar and other refined carbs. Instead, eat plenty of anti-inflammatory foods, such as omega-3–rich salmon and sardines.

Also: Give up all alcohol while a concussion is healing because it can increase the severity of your symptoms.

When Symptoms Persist

Concussion symptoms may linger for three months or longer, especially if you've had multiple concussions. If you have post-concussion syndrome (PCS)—continued symptoms may include sleep problems, difficulty concentrating, memory problems, sensitivity to lights or sounds, or unexplained emotional ups and downs—see a neurologist with training in traumatic brain injury. For a referral, consult the American Academy of Neurology, *Patients.AAN.com/FindaNeurologist*, and click on "Traumatic Brain Injury" under "Subspecialty."

Women's Brains May Have Tougher Time Recovering from Concussions

Steven Broglio, PhD, brain researcher and director, NeuroSport Research Laboratory, University of Michigan, Ann Arbor.

Dave Ellemberg, PhD, MSc, associate professor, University of Montreal, Canada.

Radiology, online.

New research from Taiwan uncovers more evidence that women may have a tougher time recovering their memory after concussions.

Scientists don't know why the brains of women seem to respond to these brain injuries differently from those of men. But experts think it might have something to do with differences in male and female brains, or the way in which men and women are injured when their heads hit something.

Whatever the case, "you cannot treat women like you treat men," said neuropsychologist Dave Ellemberg, PhD, an associate professor who studies brain injuries at the University of Montreal. "But in the field of the management of brain injuries, everyone is managed the same. The data mainly comes from men, and the management programs are all based on evidence that comes from them."

At issue are concussions, also known as mild traumatic brain injuries. According to the Brain Injury Association of America, "mild" refers to the initial blunt trauma itself, not its consequences, which can be severe.

Concussions have gotten tremendous attention in recent years in the world of sports, and some research has shown that female athletes suffer concussions at a higher rate than male athletes playing similar sports, the researchers noted.

Study Details

The recent study, which was led by Dr. Chi-Jen Chen and conducted by scientists at Taipei Medical University Shuang-Ho Hospital in New Taipei City, involved using functional magnetic resonance imaging (fMRI) scans to study the brains of 30 men and 30 women.

Half of each group had suffered mild traumatic brain injuries from playing sports, car crashes, falls or assault. Their brains were scanned a month after their injuries and again after another six weeks had passed. The other halves of both groups had not suffered brain injuries.

While other studies have found differences in how the brains of males and females react to brain injuries, the new research is unique because it used brain scans, said Dr. Ellemberg, who was not involved with the study.

In the first round of scans, the Taiwanese researchers found that the sections of the

Hidden Bone Loss Danger

Low bone density is known to boost fracture risk, but a new study shows that it also impairs balance and hearing. Participants age 65 and older with low bone density were almost four times more likely (and those 40 and older twice as likely) to fail a balance test than those with normal density.

Explanation: Bone loss affects the entire body, including bones in the skull that house the organs for balance and hearing.

Angelico Mendy, MD, MPH, researcher in epidemiology, The University of Iowa College of Public Health, Iowa City.

brain devoted to "working memory" were more active in brain-injured men and less active in brain-injured women, compared to their uninjured peers.

Expert Response

"Working memory is short-term memory," explained Steven Broglio, PhD, a brain researcher and director of the NeuroSport Research Laboratory at the University of Michigan in Ann Arbor. "For example, remembering the price of something when you take it off the shelf and to the register at a store."

The working memory in the brain-injured men, at least when viewed via brain scans, seemed to have bounced back to normal when they returned six weeks after their first scan. But the brains of the injured women were still affected.

"We know women have higher brain injury rates and longer recoveries, but we aren't entirely sure why," said Dr. Broglio, who was not involved with the study. One theory is that women have weaker muscles in the neck that are a factor in how head injuries affect them. Another theory suggests that women are more likely to report brain injuries and to tell doctors about ongoing symptoms, he said.

The study likely won't affect treatment of concussions, said Dr. Broglio. It's still crucial to treat injuries based on individual symptoms, he said, and there's inconclusive research about the value of using brain scans as a tool for concussion patients.

Dr. Ellemberg said that physical and mental rest are more important for women and they must take the time they need away from athletics and mentally taxing activities for a full recovery.

The study appears online in the journal *Radiology*.

Visit the US Centers for Disease Control and Prevention at *www.cdc.gov/Traumatic BrainInjury/* for more on brain injuries.

Menopausal Drug for Bone Care

A new drug for menopausal hot flashes may also prevent osteoporosis, we hear from Michelle Warren, MD.

Recent finding: Women taking the drug Duavee had 74% fewer moderate-to-severe hot flashes, compared with just 47% in women taking a placebo. It also significantly increased bone mineral density in the hip and spine. The drug is not recommended for use by women who have a history of blood clots, bleeding disorders, liver problems or breast or uterine cancer.

Michelle Warren, MD, founder and medical director of the Center for Menopause, Hormonal Disorders & Women's Health, Columbia University Medical Center, New York City.

Protect Your Bones from Osteoporosis with Resveratrol

Marie Juul Ornstrup, MD, PhD candidate, department of endocrinology and metabolism, Aarhus University Hospital, Aarhus, Denmark. Her study was published in *Journal of Clinical Endocrinology and Metabolism*.

S trong bones and teeth are not just kid stuff—we especially need ways to promote them as we age because age-related bone loss is no joke. Forget the mere scraped knee if you slip and fall—one false step could mean a broken hip. But a popular supplement, often taken for cardiovascular vigor, can help build strong bones in adults, possibly protecting against osteoporosis.

The supplement is resveratrol, an antioxidant and anti-inflammatory compound famously found in red wine, red grape juice, grapes (it's in the skins) and cacao, peanuts and blueberries.

Because resveratrol has such strong anti-inflammatory properties, Danish researchers reasoned that it might help put the brakes on the inflammation that causes bone weakening. They decided to investigate this in people who have metabolic syndrome, a combination of high blood pressure, high cholesterol and high blood sugar, because their condition puts them at risk for bone weakening. But you don't have to have metabolic syndrome to suffer from systemic inflammation and bone loss...so, anyone who wants to maintain strong bones, pay attention.

The researchers recruited 66 middle-aged men with metabolic syndrome but not osteoporosis and started tracking the effect of resveratrol on bone-forming enzymes and bone density in the men's lower spines. They did this by dividing the participants into three groups. One group received 1,000 milligrams (mg) per day of a natural formulation of resveratrol called transresveratrol (as a 500-mg pill taken twice a day), another group received 150 mg (as a 75-mg pill taken twice a day), and the third group received placebo pills.

The results: It didn't take long for the resveratrol to make its mark. After only four months, the men who took the higher daily dosage of resveratrol had a 16% increase in a bone-forming enzyme called bone alkaline phosphatase, commonly found in children who are going through growth spurts. They also had 3% more bone density than they had at the start of the study. Meanwhile no changes were seen in the placebo group, and minimal changes were seen in the low-dose resveratrol group.

Does this mean that resveratrol can be a natural substitute for osteoporosis drugs, such as Forteo and Fosamax? Probably not—studies show that these drugs have a stronger effect on bone mass than the 3% improvement seen in this study of resveratrol. But who knows? Additional studies of the supplement that look at the impact of different doses over longer time periods may provide more promising information about resveratrol and bone health. In the meantime, resveratrol supplementation might be a smart way to support your body's bone-building potential to protect against bone loss.

Get It Right

If you are interested in taking a resveratrol supplement, check labels to make sure you are purchasing transresveratrol, since a synthetic formulation of resveratrol may not deliver the same health benefit as transresveratrol.

Drug-Free Bone Builders

Ray Hinish, PharmD, CN, certified nutritionist and author of *The Osteoporosis Diet: The Natural Approach to Osteoporosis Treatment.* He is a certified personal trainer and host of the weekly radio show *Wake Up Healthy.* ExpertNutrition.com

Bone is constantly breaking down and rebuilding, a process called remodeling. If you have osteoporosis or osteopenia (an earlier stage of bone thinning), the rate of breakdown exceeds that of reconstruction.

Result: Porous bones that are brittle and prone to fractures.

A broken bone means pain, tests, repeated doctor visits and maybe even surgery—and that could be just the beginning.

About half of women with osteoporosis (and one in eight men) eventually will have a bone fracture, and many will have more than one.

Drugs Are Not the Solution

The main class of drugs for treating osteoporosis, the bisphosphonates, have been linked to rare but serious side effects, including severe bone, muscle and joint pain and possibly an increased risk for esophageal cancer (due to inflammation of the esophagus). Other rare side effects include atypical femoral fracture, in which the thighbone cracks, and osteonecrosis of the jaw, in which a section of the jawbone dies and deteriorates.

The risks might be justified if the drugs worked—but often they don't. One study published in *The Journal of the American Medical Association* found that 99.8% of patients who took *alendronate* (Fosamax) did not suffer a subsequent fracture. That sounds impressive, but it turns out that people in the study who took placebos had nearly the same result.

It's estimated that 81 women would have to take alendronate to prevent just one fracture. Put another way, 80 out of 81 patients who take the drug won't benefit at all. Here are effective, safer treatments…

Calcium-Plus

Everyone knows that calcium is important for strong bones. But calcium alone isn't enough. Bones are made up of a variety of minerals. You need all of them to increase—or just maintain—bone strength. *Examples…*

•**Magnesium.** Up to 80% of Americans don't get enough magnesium. There is some evidence that people who are low in magnesium are more likely to develop osteoporosis.

My advice: Eat magnesium-rich foods, including dark leafy greens, nuts, fish and whole grains. Because most people don't get enough magnesium from food, I also recommend a daily supplement that contains 500 milligrams (mg).

•**Phosphorus.** It's the second-most-abundant mineral in the body after calcium, and 80% to 90% is found in the bones and teeth.

My advice: Eat phosphorus-rich foods, which include meats, fish, nuts, beans and dairy. Aim for 700 mg of phosphorous a day.

Examples: Salmon (three ounces) has 315 mg…beef (three ounces), 243 mg…yogurt (one cup), 386 mg.

•**Calcium.** You can't have strong bones without calcium—but despite what you've heard, you do not have to consume dairy to get sufficient calcium. Leafy green vegetables—such as kale, spinach and collard greens—are rich in calcium. A four-ounce serving of steamed collard greens or kale has about the same amount of calcium as one cup of milk.

My advice: Since many people don't get enough calcium from their diets, a supplement is helpful. Take 600 mg to 800 mg daily. I recommend any calcium supplement other than calcium carbonate, which is poorly absorbed. Combined with the calcium that you get from foods, it will get you into the recommended daily range of 1,200 mg to 1,500 mg.

Some studies have shown a link between calcium supplements and heart attacks, but a recent study by researchers at Brigham and Women's Hospital found no correlation between calcium supplementation and coronary artery disease, and previous research failed to show a link when calcium was taken with other supplements such as vitamin D and magnesium.

Vitamin D

Vitamin D increases the body's ability to absorb calcium from foods and supplements. It also appears to inhibit both the production and activity of osteoclasts, cells that break down bone.

One study found that people who took a daily vitamin-D supplement had a 23% decrease in nonvertebral fractures and a 26% decrease in hip fractures.

Vitamin D is called the "sunshine vitamin" because it is produced in the skin when you're exposed to sun. But most people don't get enough sun to produce adequate amounts.

My advice: Take 2,000 international units (IU) to 4,000 IU of vitamin D daily. And take it with meals for up to 50% better absorption. I recommend the natural D-3 form. It raises blood levels 1.7 times more than the synthetic D-2 form.

Leafy Greens

Leafy greens are not only high in calcium, they are rich in vitamin K. Vitamin K works with vitamin D to increase the activity of bone-building osteoblasts.

The Harvard Nurses' Health Study found that women who ate a daily serving of leafy green vegetables, such as spinach, dark green lettuce or kale, were 50% less likely to suffer a fracture than those who had only one serving a week.

My advice: Eat a salad every day. Make side dishes that include spinach, kale or beet greens. Other green vegetables, such as broccoli, cabbage, asparagus and Brussels sprouts, also are high in vitamin K.

One Part Protein to Four Parts Vegetables

This ratio seems to be ideal for bone health. You need protein to decrease calcium loss from the body and to increase levels of bone growth factors. But too much protein (particularly from animal sources) increases acidity, which depletes bone minerals.

It's a delicate balancing act. The Framingham Osteoporosis Study found that people who ate the least protein were more likely to have a bone fracture than those who ate the most. But a Harvard study found that people who ate the most protein (from animal sources) had a higher risk for forearm fractures. (Those who got their protein from soy or other nonmeat sources didn't have the same risk.)

My advice: For every serving of a meat-based protein, consume three to four servings of vegetables to alkalinize your body. An alkaline (low-acid) environment helps prevent bone loss.

Exercise with Weights

You need to stress the bones to promote new growth. Lifting weights is the best way to do this, particularly when it's combined with aerobic workouts. A University of Washington study found that women who did both during a 50-to-60-minute session, three times a week, gained 5.2% in spinal mineral density in just nine months.

Don't make it easy. If you can lift a weight more than 10 times, you're not stressing the bones enough. Pick a weight that you can lift only between six and 10 times. You want the last few lifts to be a struggle. When that gets too easy, move up to a heavier weight.

Walking is another good way to build bone. One study found that people who were sedentary lost an average of 7% of bone mass in the spine, while those in a walking program gained 0.5%.

My advice: Wear a weighted vest when you walk. You can build more bone by adding to your body weight. You can buy weighted vests at sporting-goods stores and discount stores such as Target and Walmart. Most are adjustable—you can start with five pounds and work your way up to about 10% of your body weight.

Keep Your Hips Forever!

Mitchell Yass, DPT, physical therapist and founder/owner of PT2 Physical Therapy and Personal Training in Farmingdale, New York. He is the author of *Overpower Pain: The Strength-Training Program That Stops Pain Without Drugs or Surgery.* MitchellYass.com

If you're tired of hobbling around on an aching hip, surgery to replace that failing joint might sound pretty good.

Every year, more than 330,000 Americans get this operation. For those who have severe joint damage (for example, bone-on-bone damage that prevents full range of motion), hip replacement can be an excellent choice.

Here's the rub: Many people who receive a hip replacement aren't in this category. They undergo hip replacement but don't realize that the cause of their pain could be in hip muscles, not joints.

Identify the Problem

If you complain about persistent groin pain (one of the most common symptoms of hip dysfunction), your doctor will probably order an imaging test (such as an X-ray and/or MRI scan).

What you need to know: Even though imaging tests can give doctors a great deal of information about the condition of a joint, they aren't as conclusive as you might think. For example, an X-ray can show a decrease in cartilage and less space between the thighbone and hip socket, but doctors differ in deciding at what point surgery becomes necessary. Virtually everyone who's age 50 or older will show some degree of joint damage just from normal wear and tear. A decrease in range of motion at the hip joint is key to the need for surgery.

Does a diagnosis of arthritis at the hip joint mean that you need surgery? Not necessarily. Most hip and groin pain is caused by muscle weakness or a muscle imbalance. People who correctly exercise these muscles can often eliminate—or at least greatly reduce—their discomfort. Strengthening these muscles also can help ease pain in those who have already had hip replacements...and improve balance.

The Best Workouts

The following exercises are ideal for hip or groin pain. After getting your doctor's OK, start by trying to repeat each one 10 times. Take a one-minute break, then repeat two more sets. The whole routine, which should be done two or three times a week, takes about 20 minutes.

•**Hamstring curl.** The hamstrings (in the back of the thigh) play a key role in the functioning of the hip joints. However, the hamstrings are weak in most people—mainly because these muscles aren't used much in normal daily movements.

How this exercise helps: It strengthens hamstrings and helps prevent the opposing muscles (the quadriceps, in the front of the thigh) from shortening and causing muscle strain and/or spasms.

How to do it: Attach one end of a piece of elastic exercise tubing (available in sporting-goods stores and online) to your left ankle. Stand on the other end with your right foot. Leaving more slack will reduce resistance...taking up the slack will increase it.

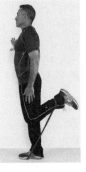

With your feet a few inches apart and knees slightly bent, raise your left foot and curl it backward toward your buttocks as far as you comfortably can. Then return to the starting position. If you feel unsteady, put one hand (on the side opposite the leg you're working) on a wall. Switch legs and repeat.

•**Hip abduction.** This is great for hip or groin pain because the abductor muscles (on the outer thighs) tend to be much weaker than the opposing adductor muscles.

How this exercise helps: Weakness in the abductors can allow the pelvis to drop on one side, which can cause groin muscles to tighten and become painful.

How to do it: Lie on the side that's not painful (or less painful) on a mat or a carpeted floor. Your painful side will be on top. Place

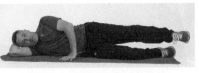

your arm under your head, and bend your other leg's knee for better support and balance.

Slowly raise your affected leg, keeping it in line with your torso. Keep the knee straight, and don't roll forward or backward. Raise your leg only to hip height (a few inches). Then slowly lower your leg back to the starting position. After performing a set, roll over

and repeat the exercise with the other leg, only after pain has eased in the affected leg. Otherwise, focus only on strengthening the painful side.

•**Hip flexor stretch.** This exercise is vital. Most of us spend a lot of time sitting, causing these muscles to shorten and tighten.

How this exercise helps: It stretches tight hip flexors, which can stress the low back.

How to do it: Kneel on your right knee on a mat or a carpeted area. (If you need more padding, you can put a folded towel under the knee.) Place your left foot flat on the floor in front of you, with the knee bent. Rest your left hand on your left thigh and your right hand on your right hip. Keeping your back straight and abdominal mus-

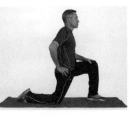

cles tight, lean forward so that more of your weight is on the front leg. You'll feel a stretch in your right upper thigh. Hold for 20 to 30 seconds. Switch sides.

•**Quad stretch.** Overly tight quad muscles can pull the pelvis downward—a common cause of low-back and hip pain.

How this exercise helps: Stretching the quads helps distribute weight evenly through the pelvis.

How to do it: Stand near a wall for support. Rest your right hand on the wall, then reach back with your left hand to grip your left foot/ankle. Pull your heel upward toward your buttocks—and eventually behind the hip. Keep pulling, gently, until you feel a stretch in the front of your thigh. Tighten your

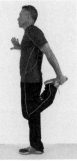

abdominal muscles. Hold for about 20 to 30 seconds. Repeat on the other side.

If your pain doesn't improve after a month of performing these exercises, consult your doctor.

Hip Replacements Fail Most Often in Women

Although the risk of total hip-replacement failure is low, women are 29% more likely than men to need repeat surgery within three years.

Reasons for the failures: Women need prosthetic hips with a smaller-sized femoral head—the rounded ball end of the femur (thighbone)—but a smaller femoral head is more likely to dislocate. Because of differences in anatomy, women's prosthetic hips also are implanted at an angle that is different from men's.

If you need a hip replacement: Ask your surgeon what type of implant you are going to receive. Failure is less common with metal-on-polyethylene or ceramic-on-polyethylene implants than with metal-on-metal implants.

Study of 35,000 people by researchers at Icahn School of Medicine at Mount Sinai, New York City, published in *The Journal of the American Medical Association.*

Don't Rush to Have Surgery for a Torn Meniscus

People who had meniscal tears repaired surgically had almost exactly the same improvements in their knees as people who had a sham procedure. Both groups had chronic meniscal tears and did not have arthritis. Meniscal repair still may be needed for an acute tear, such as a sports injury…and for unstable tears that cause locking of the knee.

David T. Felson, MD, MPH, professor of medicine and epidemiology and chief of the Multidisciplinary Clinical Research Center Grant, Boston University School of Medicine.

The Painkiller Trap

Jane Ballantyne, MD, professor in the department of anesthesiology and pain medicine at the University of Washington School of Medicine in Seattle, where she serves as director of the UW Pain Fellowship. She is coauthor of *Expert Decision Making on Opioid Treatments.*

If you have ever suffered from severe pain, you probably know that a strong pain pill can seem like the holy grail. In fact, with chronic pain affecting about one-third of Americans—or roughly 100 million people—it's perhaps no surprise that the most commonly prescribed medication in the US is a painkiller, *hydrocodone* (Vicodin).

Frightening trend: Hydrocodone and the other prescription opioid painkillers (also known as narcotics) have now overtaken heroin and cocaine as the leading cause of fatal overdoses, according to the Centers for Disease Control and Prevention.

Why the Shift?

Until recently, prescription opioids were used to treat only acute (severe, short-lived) pain, such as pain after surgery or an injury or pain related to cancer.

Now: As doctors have stepped up their efforts to better control pain in all patients, opioids are much more widely prescribed. These powerful medications are now being used to treat chronic painful conditions such as low-back pain, chronic headaches and fibromyalgia.

What pain sufferers need to know…

Dangers of Opioids

Each day, an estimated 4.3 million Americans take hydrocodone or other widely used opioids, such as *oxycodone* (OxyContin), *hydromorphone* (Dilaudid), codeine and morphine. For some patients, opioids are prescribed as an alternative to nonsteroidal anti-inflammatory drugs (NSAIDs), which are notorious for causing gastrointestinal bleeding and other side effects, including increased risk for heart attack and kidney disease.

Opioids work by mimicking natural pain-relieving chemicals in the body and attaching to receptors that block the transmission of pain messages to and within the brain. These drugs can be highly effective pain relievers, especially for arthritis patients who can't tolerate NSAIDs.

But opioids also have potentially serious side effects, especially when they're used long term (usually defined as more than 90 days). While the effectiveness of the medications often decreases over time (because the patient builds up a tolerance to the drug), the risk for side effects—including constipation, drowsiness or even addiction—increases due to the higher and more toxic doses used to overcome tolerance.

Continuous use of these pain medications also can have far-reaching health effects that can include a heightened risk for falls and fractures…slowed breathing…concentration problems…and vision impairment. And these drugs can compromise the immune system, resulting in susceptibility to infection.

Men who take opioids long term are five times more likely to have low testosterone levels, which can curb libido and result in erectile dysfunction. Even at low doses, such as 20 mg of morphine, opioids can diminish alertness and have been shown to increase risk for car accidents by 21%.

Best Nondrug Alternatives

If your doctor suggests taking an opioid for back pain, chronic headaches or migraines, or fibromyalgia, ask him/her about trying the following nondrug treatments first. Opioids should be considered only as a last resort.

•**Back pain.** For long-term low-back pain, exercises that strengthen the abdomen and back (or "core") muscles are the most effective treatment. If the pain is so severe that you can't exercise, over-the-counter painkillers sometimes can alleviate the pain enough to start an effective exercise regimen.

Bonus: Exercise can ease depression, which is common in back pain sufferers.

Yoga may also be effective because it stretches the muscles and ligaments in addition to reducing mental stress.

Other possible options: If the approaches described above don't provide adequate relief, you may be a candidate for steroid injections into the spine or joints…a spinal fusion…or disk-replacement surgery. In general, these treatments have less risk for adverse effects than long-term use of opioids.

•**Chronic headaches or migraines.** With chronic headaches or migraines, opioids can worsen pain by causing "rebound" headaches that occur when the drug is overused. Try lifestyle changes, such as daily meditation, and the sparing use of mild painkillers, such as NSAIDs. Supplements, including magnesium and feverfew, also have been shown to relieve headache pain.

•**Fibromyalgia.** With this condition, which has no known cure, opioids have been found to intensify existing pain.

Much better: A review of 46 studies has found aerobic exercise, such as brisk walking or pool aerobics (done two to three times a week for an hour), may reduce system-wide inflammation, making it an effective treatment for fibromyalgia.

If you're in too much pain to do aerobic exercise, a mild painkiller or a nondrug approach, such as massage, may allow you to start.

Cognitive behavioral therapy is another good choice. With this treatment, a therapist

Sudden Noises May Lead to Knee Injuries

Startling noises, such as honking horns and sirens, can disrupt circuits in the brain that control the muscles and ligaments that stabilize the knee, causing people to fall.

Study of 36 people in their early 20s by researchers at University of Delaware, Newark, published in *Scandinavian Journal of Medicine & Science in Sports.*

can help you reframe negative thoughts that may be fueling fibromyalgia pain.

Additional nondrug approaches that may help all of these conditions: acupuncture, relaxation exercises and heating pads.

What's Your Risk for Addiction?

Some people who take opioids are more likely to become addicted than others. *Risk factors include…*

•**Depression, anxiety or some other psychiatric condition (current or in the past).**

•**Substance abuse.** This includes alcohol or other drugs (current or in the past).

•**Poor coping skills.** Those with "catastrophizing" personalities—they tend to imagine the worst possible outcomes in trying situations—are more likely to develop chronic pain and drug dependence.

Before using an opioid, discuss your potential for addiction with your physician. You want a doctor who understands the risks and benefits of the drug…who is aware of your potential for dependence and addiction…and who will take you off the drug if he/she notices problematic behavior. See your doctor often—at least monthly when you first start taking the drug.

Eczema Increases Risk For Broken Bones

Eczema increases risk for broken bones and other bone/joint injuries by 44%.

Possible reasons: People with the chronic skin condition may fall more often because they use sedating antihistamines during the day.

Also: Chronic inflammation—or oral steroids used to relieve symptoms—may have weakened their bones.

Self-defense: Take sedating antihistamines only at night. Avoid using prednisone and other oral steroids.

Jonathan Silverberg, MD, PhD, MPH, director of Northwestern Medicine Eczema Center, at Northwestern University's Feinberg School of Medicine, Chicago. He is senior author of a study published in *JAMA Dermatology.*

Is Your Back Still Hurting Months After a Fall?

David G. Borenstein, MD, clinical professor of medicine at The George Washington University Medical Center, Washington, DC, and the author of *Heal Your Back. ARAPC.com*

The coccyx is essentially the tail of the spine and is protected by the buttocks. Unless you fell on your coccyx, you probably have strained the muscles and connective tissue over the sacrum, the part of the spine between the hips. These muscle strains usually improve within three months after an injury.

A physical therapist can be helpful in devising an exercise program that can improve range of motion and decrease pain. An over-the-counter pain reliever can also be helpful. Less pain makes it easier to do physical therapy exercises.

Massage can help ease pain as well. Some people like massage with ice in the affected area, while others prefer the application of wet heat.

If these therapies don't resolve your pain, see your doctor again.

When Is It Time for a Scooter?

Gregory Thielman, MSPT, EdD, associate professor of physical therapy, University of the Sciences, Philadelphia.

If you, or your loved one's health is declining, you may be thinking about getting an electric scooter. Would your condition become worse if you don't walk as much?

Texting Is as Dangerous as Drunk Driving

Both of these behaviors led to the same degree of slowed braking time and increased speeding in a recent study.

Study by several Australian universities, published in *Traffic Injury Prevention*.

There is no easy answer, but your top priorities should be your (or your loved one's) safety and independence. You need to maintain mobility as much as possible while still conserving energy for those activities that are important to you.

If what you're using now, likely a rolling walker, leaves you vulnerable to falls, then a scooter is the way to go. But before you order that scooter, you may want to consider another alternative—a rollator (a four-wheeled walker with a seat and brakes). The seat allows one to take breaks while walking, and the hand-braking system allows for greater control.

If you participate in activities that require some endurance, such as visiting parks or shopping, a scooter is especially useful. Scooters are more mobile than a power wheelchair, and they are now made light enough to be taken apart and placed in the trunk of a car.

One Drink Too Many...

Even small amounts of alcohol may be too much if you're driving. Adults over age 55 who drank roughly the equivalent of one glass of wine had worse driving skills—such as more difficulty controlling the wheel—in a simulated test than sober peers and younger drivers who drank the same amounts of alcohol.

Reason: Alcohol is more potent in older adults.

Sara Jo Nixon, PhD, chief, division of addiction research, University of Florida College of Medicine, Gainesville.

A Mystery Car Crash Solved

Richard O'Brien, MD, associate professor of emergency medicine at The Commonwealth Medical College of Pennsylvania in Scranton. He is also a spokesperson for the American College of Emergency Physicians, *ACEP.org*, and a recipient of the group's Communications Lifetime Achievement Award.

It was a sunny day when a healthy 39-year-old woman named Margrette was driving on a familiar road near her home. Temporarily "blinded" by the bright sun, she drove her car a few feet off the road and hit a utility pole. Fortunately, she was traveling only about 25 mph and was wearing her seat belt, and the air bags in her car worked. Even though she didn't think she was injured, Margrette called an ambulance just to get "checked over" in the hospital.

The emergency technician filled me in on the details of the accident and explained that Margrette's vital signs had been stable during the ride to the hospital. As I was about to begin her exam, I happened to notice that she had trouble reading a form she had been asked to sign. Everything checked out fine during Margrette's exam, except for one unusual finding. When I used a penlight to peer into her eyes, I saw an obvious cataract in each of them. Wanting to confirm this discovery, I looked again—this time using a slit lamp (a type of microscope for the eye) and could see that the natural lens in both eyes had clouded dramatically—a surprising discovery in someone not yet 40. I then asked Margrette to read a handheld eye chart, and she had only 20/200 vision in each eye—generally considered a sign of severe visual impairment.

Being blinded by bright light and having difficulty reading black print on white paper are common symptoms of cataracts, so Margrette's momentary inability to see the road while driving into the sun and her trouble signing an unfamiliar form were beginning to make sense. If she had been driving at night, the oncoming headlights would most likely have affected her vision, too. Any sort of light can appear to a person with cataracts as though it has a bright "halo" around it—an extremely disconcerting sight.

As I probed further into Margrette's background, even more pieces of her story fell into place. She confessed that she had not had her eyes examined since she was a teenager, even though she had begun having trouble reading around age 30. At first, drugstore reading glasses helped, but after just a few years, she found that reading glasses were useless. Frighteningly, she described her vision as "looking through a window smeared with cooking oil." Her impairment went undetected, in part, because her state of residence does not require eye exams to renew driver's licenses for people of her age. I was relieved when Margrette had cataract surgery shortly thereafter, and she was again reading 20/20 in time for her 40th birthday.

Why did Margrette get cataracts at such an early age? She explained that she had lived in Florida from birth until age 33 and hardly ever wore a wide-brimmed hat or sunglasses to protect her eyes. She also used oral and nasal steroids for asthma and environmental allergies. Excessive sun exposure and regular use of oral steroids have clearly been shown to cause premature cataracts. The evidence linking nasal steroids to cataracts is mixed, but Margrette said that she often used large doses, likely increasing her risk for this eye disease.

Lesson Learned: Subtle changes in vision can occur slowly over a period of several years. That's why a professional eye exam every two years is critical to diagnose any eye disease early—before it becomes a serious problem. Cataracts are the world's leading cause of blindness.

Fast Music = More Driving Errors for Teens

Teen risk for traffic violations increases when they listen to fast music. When teenagers were allowed to drive while listening to music with fast-paced vocals, about 98% of them made driving errors, such as speeding. When they listened to a softer, easy-listening background, driver errors declined by 20%.

Study of 85 teens by researchers at Ben-Gurion University of the Negev, Beer-Sheva, Israel, published in *Accident Analysis & Prevention.*

Make Your Bathroom Safer

Highly glazed ceramic floor tile can be slippery. Consider replacing it with slip-resistant tiles or tiles with a surface that mimics natural stone. Also, opt for smaller tiles because smaller tiles mean more grout, and grout is less slippery.

Alternative: Rubber or vinyl flooring.

Also: Install screw-mounted grab bars—suction cups can come away from the wall. Attach to the wall studs, not just drywall. And it's best if the bars run horizontally, not vertically or at an angle, as your hand could slip.

Sheila Barton, LCSW, social worker at Mount Sinai School of Medicine, New York City, writing in *Focus on Healthy Aging.*

If Trauma Makes You Faint...

When people experience a sudden, painful injury, often the heart rate can slow and blood pressure drops. Blood flow to the brain is reduced, resulting in light-headedness or fainting.

If you feel faint: Lie down. Lying down puts the brain at the same level as the heart and restores full circulation. If you can't lie down, sit down. The light-headedness should disappear within a few minutes.

Don't follow the old advice of putting your head between your knees. If you're in a chair, you might fall flat on your head out of the chair. Also, with your head between your knees, you potentially are crimping off your airway a bit and making it more difficult to breathe.

Richard O'Brien, MD, associate professor of emergency medicine, The Commonwealth Medical College of Pennsylvania, Scranton, and spokesperson for the American College of Emergency Physicians. *ACEP.org*

Do You Walk Wrong? 7 Mistakes That Can Sabotage Your Walking Workout

Robert Sweetgall, president of Creative Walking, a Kirkwood, Missouri, company that designs walking and fitness programs for schools, corporations and other clients. Sweetgall is coauthor, with Barry Franklin, PhD, of *One Heart, Two Feet: Enhancing Heart Health One Step at a Time. CreativeWalking.com*

We all know that walking is very good for us. Studies have shown that walking promotes heart health, strengthens bones, spurs weight loss, boosts mood and even cuts risk for cancer and Alzheimer's.

But what most people don't realize is that they could significantly improve the health benefits of their walks by tweaking their walking techniques and using the right equipment.

Here are common walking mistakes—and what you should be doing instead…

Mistake #1: Tilting forward. Some walkers tilt their upper bodies forward, as though they're walking into the wind. They think that this position increases speed. It does not—and it greatly increases pressure on the lower back while straining the shins.

Better: Walk with your head high and still, shoulders relaxed and chest slightly out. In this position, you can rotate your eyes downward to survey the path and look ahead to view the scenery around you.

Mistake #2: Swinging the arms inefficiently. Many walkers waste energy by swinging their arms side to side or pumping their arms up and down. These exaggerated movements add little to cardiovascular fitness and make walking less efficient because arm energy is directed upward or sideways rather than straight ahead.

Better: For maximum efficiency, pump your arms straight ahead on a horizontal plane, like you're reeling in a string through your midsection. This motion improves balance, posture and walking speed.

Mistake #3: Using hand and/or ankle weights. While some people like to walk with weights to boost the intensity of a walking workout, the risk for injury far outweighs the benefits of using weights. The repetitive stress of swinging weights can cause microtears in the soft tissues of the arms and legs.

Better: To increase exertion, walk uphill or on an inclined treadmill.

Another good option: Try Nordic walking for a total-body workout. With this type of walking, you use specially designed walking poles (one in each hand) to help propel your body forward.

Compared with regular walking, Nordic walking can increase your energy expenditure by 20%, according to a study from The Cooper Institute. It works the abdominal, arm and back muscles and reduces stress on the feet, ankles, knees and hips while improving endurance.

Mistake #4: Not doing a warm-up. You're inviting muscle soreness and potential injury if you hit your top speed at the start.

Better: Be sure to warm up. Start slowly, accelerating over the first five to 10 minutes… and end slowly, decelerating over the last five minutes. A slow start allows your muscles to warm up and become flexible, while enabling your cardiorespiratory system to get used to higher workloads. Finish up at a slow pace to eliminate the buildup of lactic acid, which can lead to muscle soreness.

Mistake #5: Doing the same walk every day. It's best to alter your routine for maximum health benefits and to maintain motivation.

Better: Do shorter, faster-paced walks some days (cardiovascular conditioning) and longer, moderate-paced walks on other days (calorie burning). Also try walks on steeper terrains and walks that alternate faster intervals with slower intervals.

Mistake #6: Not keeping a walking log or journal. Every day, indicate how far and fast you walked and any other observations you wish to record in a notebook or on your computer. Keeping a journal helps foster a sense of accomplishment and self-esteem and is the single most effective method for ensuring that you'll stick to a walking program.

Mistake #7: Choosing cushy shoes. A study in *The American Journal of Sports Medicine* found that, on average, expensive, high-tech footwear caused twice the injuries as shoes costing half as much.

Some high-priced, cushiony shoes can make you feel as if you're walking on a foam mattress, but they have an inherent "wobble" that can cause your foot to move side to side, leading to potential foot, ankle, knee and hip injuries.

Better: Thin-soled shoes with minimal support. They force the muscles in the legs and feet to work harder, which improves strength and balance and helps prevent injuries.

When transitioning to thinner-soled shoes, make the switch gradually, breaking them in on shorter walks. They can feel awkward at first, so give your feet time to adjust.

Of course the right shoe is a very individual choice, but I like Karhu shoes, which promote forward momentum.

Cost: About $55 to $140, depending on the model. Other people like the so-called "barefoot" shoes, such as Vibram FiveFingers.

Helpful: Avoid cotton socks, which can lose their support and shape after a few washings. Try socks made from blends that include acrylic fibers, Coolmax and/or spandex/elastic. Soft wool socks also can work.

Tip: Powder your feet with cornstarch before a long walk to reduce friction, heat buildup and blisters.

Take the Longevity Test

The more steps it takes you to walk the same distance each year, the weaker your core muscles are becoming.

Self-test: Each year on your birthday, go to a track and walk one lap, recording the number of steps on your pedometer. Aim to complete the lap in about the same number of steps each year. If it takes you more steps each year, you are regressing toward the "senior shuffle" and compromising your core-muscle strength and overall vitality.

What to do: In addition to walking regularly, start a core-muscle strengthening regimen and a stretching program to tone your hip and leg muscles.

Helmets Save Lives

Helmets do save skiers' and snowboarders' lives. Helmets do not, as previously thought, give athletes a false sense of security and encourage risky behavior. Skiers and snowboarders who wear helmets have significantly lower risk for head injuries than those who don't wear helmets. About 600,000 injuries from skiing and snowboarding are reported annually...up to 20% of those are head injuries.

Study by researchers at Johns Hopkins University School of Medicine, Baltimore, published in *The Journal of Trauma and Acute Care Surgery.*

Chapter 7

BEST WAYS TO CONTROL— EVEN CURE—DIABETES

How America's Top Diabetes Doctor Avoids Diabetes

You might think that a diabetes researcher would never develop the disease that he has dedicated his life to studying. But I can't count on it.

My family's story: My father was diagnosed with diabetes at age 72 and was promptly placed on three medications to control his insulin levels. What he did next made all the difference: Even though he began taking diabetes medication, he simultaneously went into action—walking an hour a day and going on the diet described below. A year and a half later, he no longer needed the prescriptions. He still had diabetes, but diet and exercise kept it under control.

As a diabetes researcher and physician whose own diabetes risk is increased by his family history, I've got a lot at stake in finding the absolute best ways to avoid and fight this disease.

Here are the steps I take to prevent diabetes—all of which can benefit you whether you want to avoid this disease or have already been diagnosed with it and are trying to control or even reverse it...

Step 1: Follow a rural Asian diet (RAD). This diet includes the most healthful foods of a traditional Asian diet—it consists of 70% complex carbohydrates...15% fat...15% protein...and 15 g of fiber for every 1,000 calories. Don't worry too much about all these numbers—the diet is actually pretty simple to follow once you get the hang of it.

You might be surprised by "70% complex carbohydrates," since most doctors recommend lower daily intakes of carbohydrates. The difference is, I'm recommending high amounts of complex, unrefined (not processed) carbohydrates. This type of carb is highly desirable because it's found in foods—such as whole grains, legumes, vegetables and fruits—that are chock-full of fiber. If your goal is to reduce diabetes risk, fiber is the holy grail.

Why I do it: The RAD diet has been proven in research to promote weight loss...

George L. King, MD, chief scientific officer at the Boston-based Joslin Diabetes Center, one of the country's leading diabetes clinical care and research centers. He is also a professor of medicine at Harvard Medical School and the author, with Royce Flippin, of *The Diabetes Reset: Avoid It, Control It, Even Reverse It—A Doctor's Scientific Program.*

improve insulin sensitivity (a key factor in the development and treatment of diabetes) and glucose control…and decrease total cholesterol and LDL "bad" cholesterol levels.

To keep it simple, I advise patients to follow a 2-1-1 formula when creating meals—two portions of nonstarchy veggies (such as spinach, carrots or asparagus)…one portion of whole grains (such as brown rice or quinoa), legumes (such as lentils or chickpeas) or starchy veggies (such as sweet potatoes or winter squash)…and one portion of protein (such as salmon, lean beef, tofu or eggs). Have a piece of fruit (such as an apple or a pear) on the side. Portion size is also important. Portions fill a nine-inch-diameter plate, which is smaller than a typical 12-inch American dinner plate.

Helpful: I take my time when eating—I chew each bite at least 10 times before swallowing. Eating too quickly can cause glucose levels to peak higher than usual after a meal.

Step 2: Fill up on dark green vegetables. I include dark, leafy greens in my diet every day. These leafy greens are one of the two portions of nonstarchy veggies in the 2-1-1 formula.

Why I do it: Dark green vegetables contain antioxidants and compounds that help your body fight insulin resistance (a main driver of diabetes).

My secret "power veggie": A Chinese vegetable called bitter melon. It is a good source of fiber and has been shown to lower blood sugar. True to its name, bitter melon tastes a little bitter but is delicious when used in soups and stir-fries. It is available at Asian groceries. Eat bitter melon as one of the two portions of nonstarchy veggies in the 2-1-1 formula.

Step 3: Adopt an every-other-day workout routine. I try to not be sedentary and to walk as much as I can (by using a pedometer, I can tell whether I've reached my daily goal of 10,000 steps).

While this daily practice helps, it's not enough to significantly affect my diabetes risk. For that, I have an every-other-day workout routine that consists of 30 minutes of jogging on the treadmill (fast enough so that I'm breathing hard but can still carry on a conversation)…followed by 30 minutes of strength training (using handheld weights, resistance bands or weight machines).

Why I do it: Working out temporarily reduces your insulin resistance and activates enzymes and proteins that help your muscles use glucose instead of allowing the body to accumulate fat—a beneficial effect that lasts for 48 hours (the reason for my every-other-day routine). Strength training is crucial—your muscles are what really kick your body's glucose-burning into high gear. A weekly game of tennis helps shake up my routine.

Step 4: Keep the temperature chilly. At the courts where I play tennis, the temperature is naturally cool, but I wear a very thin T-shirt that leaves my neck exposed. This helps activate the "brown fat" in my body. Most people have this special type of body fat—mainly around the neck, collarbone and shoulders.

Why I do it: Brown fat burns calories at high rates when triggered by the cold. To help burn brown fat, exercise in temperatures of 64°F or lower…set your home's thermostat in the mid-60s…and dress as lightly as possible in cool weather. Walking for 50 or 60 minutes a day in cool weather also helps.

Step 5: Get the "sleep cure." I make a point to sleep at least six hours a night during the week and seven hours nightly on weekends.

Why I do it: Lack of sleep has been proven to dramatically harm the body's ability to properly metabolize glucose—a problem that sets the stage for diabetes. Research shows that seven to eight hours a night are ideal. However, because of my work schedule, I'm not always able to get that much sleep on weekdays. That's why I sleep a bit longer on weekends.

Research now shows that the body has some capacity to "catch up" on lost sleep and reverse some—but not all-—of the damage that occurs to one's insulin sensitivity when you're sleep deprived.

Big Breakfasts May Be Better for People with Diabetes

People with type 2 diabetes who ate a large breakfast that included protein and fat for three months had lower blood glucose levels and lower blood pressure than people who ate smaller breakfasts. Nearly one-third of the big-breakfast eaters were able to reduce the amount of diabetes medication they took. And big-breakfast eaters reported themselves less hungry later in the day.

Caution: The calorie, protein and fat contents of the large breakfasts (which were about one-third of the subjects' daily calories) were carefully arranged and monitored. Talk to your doctor before making any changes in your diet.

Study by researchers at Hebrew University of Jerusalem, presented at the annual meeting of the European Association for the Study of Diabetes in Barcelona.

The Secret Invasion That Causes Diabetes

George L. King, MD, research director and chief scientific officer of Harvard's Joslin Diabetes Center, where he heads the vascular cell biology research section, and professor of medicine at Harvard School of Public Health in Boston. Dr. King is coauthor, with Royce Flippin, of *The Diabetes Reset: Avoid It, Control It, Even Reverse It—A Doctor's Scientific Program.*

It's easy to get the impression that diabetes is all about blood sugar. Most people with diabetes check their glucose levels at least once a day. Even people without diabetes are advised to have glucose tests every few years—just to make sure that the disease isn't creeping up on them.

But glucose is only part of the picture. Scientists now know that chronic inflammation increases the risk that you'll develop diabetes. If you already have insulin resistance (a precursor to diabetes) or full-blown diabetes,

Hidden Epidemic

Diabetes now affects nearly 10% of US adults. The percentage has doubled since 1988 and totals 21 million people. Obesity rates track closely with the increase in diabetes.

Study by researchers at The Johns Hopkins Bloomberg School of Public Health, Baltimore, published in *Annals of Internal Medicine.*

inflammation will make your glucose levels harder to manage.

A common mistake: Unfortunately, many doctors still don't test for inflammation even though it accompanies all of the main diabetes risk factors, including smoking, obesity and high-fat/sugar diets. *What you need to know about this important aspect of diabetes care...*

Silent Damage

You hear a lot about inflammation, but what exactly is it—and when is it a problem? Normal inflammation is protective. It comes on suddenly and lasts for just a few days or weeks—usually in response to an injury or infection. Inflammation kills or encapsulates microbes...assists in the formation of protective scar tissue...and helps regenerate damaged tissues.

But chronic inflammation—caused, for example, by infection or injuries that lead to continuously elevated levels of toxins—does not turn itself off. It persists for years or even decades, particularly in those who are obese, eat poor diets, don't get enough sleep or have chronic diseases, including seemingly minor conditions such as gum disease.

The diabetes link: Persistently high levels of inflammatory molecules interfere with the ability of insulin to regulate glucose—one cause of high blood sugar. Inflammation also appears to damage beta cells, the insulin-producing cells in the pancreas.

Studies have shown that when inflammation is aggressively lowered—with salsalate (an anti-inflammatory drug), for example—glucose levels can drop significantly. Inflammation is typically identified with a blood test that measures a marker known as CRP, or C-reactive protein (see next page).

How to Fight Inflammation

Even though salsalate reduces inflammation, when taken in high doses, it causes too many side effects, such as stomach bleeding and ringing in the ears, to be used long term. *Safer ways to reduce inflammation and keep it down…*

•**Breathe clean air.** Smoke and smog threaten more than just your lungs. Recent research has shown that areas with the highest levels of airborne particulates that are small enough to penetrate deeply into the lungs have more than 20% higher rates of type 2 diabetes than areas with the lowest levels of these particulates.

Air pollution (including cigarette smoke) increases inflammation in fatty tissues and in the vascular system. In animal studies, exposure to air pollution increases both insulin resistance and the risk for full-fledged diabetes.

My advice: Most people—and especially those who live in polluted areas—could benefit from using an indoor HEPA filter or an electrostatic air filter.

Products such as the Honeywell Long-Life Pure HEPA QuietCare Air Purifier (available at Amazon.com for about $90) will trap nearly 100% of harmful airborne particulates from indoor air.

If you live in a large metropolitan area, avoid outdoor exercise during high-traffic times of day.

•**Take care of your gums.** Even people who take good care of their teeth often neglect their gums. It's estimated that almost half of American adults have some degree of periodontal (gum) disease.

Why it matters: The immune system can't always eliminate infections that occur in gum pockets, the areas between the teeth and gums. A persistent gum infection causes equally persistent inflammation that contributes to other illnesses. For example, research

shows that people with gum disease were twice as likely to develop diabetes as those without it.

My advice: After every meal (or at least twice a day), floss and brush, in that order. And clean your gums—gently use a soft brush. Twice a day, also use an antiseptic mouthwash (such as Listerine).

It's particularly important to follow these steps before you go to bed to remove bacteria that otherwise will remain undisturbed until morning.

•**Get more exercise.** It's among the best ways to control chronic inflammation because it burns fat. When you have less fat, you'll also produce fewer inflammation-promoting cytokines.

Data from the Nurses' Health Study and the Health Professionals Follow-Up Study found that walking briskly for a half hour daily reduced the risk of developing diabetes by nearly one-third.

My advice: Take 10,000 steps per day. To do this, walk whenever possible for daily activities, such as shopping, and even walk inside your home if you don't want to go out. Wear a pedometer to make sure you reach your daily goal.

•**Enjoy cocoa.** Cocoa contains a type of antioxidant known as flavanols, which have anti-inflammatory properties. Known primarily for their cardiovascular benefits, flavanols are now being found to help regulate insulin levels.

My advice: For inflammation-fighting effects, have one square of dark chocolate (with at least 70% cocoa) daily.

•**Try rose hip tea.** Rose hips are among the richest sources of vitamin C, with five times as much per cup than what is found in one orange. A type of rose hip known as rosa canina is particularly potent because it may contain an additional anti-inflammatory compound known as glycoside of mono and diglycerol (GOPO). It inhibits the production of a number of inflammatory molecules, including chemokines and interleukins.

My advice: Drink several cups of tangy rose hip tea a day. It's available both in bags and as a loose-leaf tea. If you're not a tea drinker, you can take rose hip supplements. Follow the directions on the label.

• **Season with turmeric.** This spice contains curcumin, one of the most potent anti-inflammatory agents. It inhibits the action of eicosanoids, "signaling molecules" that are involved in the inflammatory response.

My advice: Eat more turmeric—it's a standard spice in curries and yellow (not Dijon) mustard. You will want something more potent if you already have diabetes and/or elevated CRP. I often recommend Curamin, a potent form of curcumin that's combined with boswellia, another anti-inflammatory herb.

Important: Be sure to talk to your doctor before trying rose hip or turmeric supplements if you take medication or have a chronic health condition.

Check Your CRP Level

An inexpensive and accurate blood test that is often used to estimate heart attack risk is also recommended for people who have diabetes or are at increased risk for it. The blood test measures C-reactive protein (CRP), a marker for inflammation, which can lead to heart disease and impair the body's ability to regulate glucose.

Doctors may recommend the test for patients beginning in their 30s. It's wise to get it earlier if you have diabetes risk factors, such as obesity or a family history.

A high-sensitivity CRP (hsCRP) test typically costs about $20 and is usually covered by insurance. A reading of less than 1 mg/L is ideal. Levels above 3 mg/L indicate a high risk for insulin resistance and diabetes as well as for heart attack.

If the first test shows that your CRP level is elevated, you'll want to do everything you can to lower it—for example, through exercise, a healthful diet and weight loss. Repeat the test every four to six months to see how well your lifestyle improvements are working.

Diabetes May Be Bigger Threat to the Female Heart

Rachel Huxley, D.Phil, director, Queensland Clinical Trials and Biostatistics Centre, The University of Queensland, Australia.

Mary Ann Bauman, MD, medical director for Women's Health and Community Relations, Integris Health, Oklahoma City, Oklahoma.

Tara Narula, MD, associate director, Cardiac Care Unit, Lenox Hill Hospital, New York City.

Diabetes appears to pose a greater risk to heart health for women than men, a recent analysis of current research contends.

"The risk of coronary heart disease conferred by diabetes is between 40% to 50% greater for women than for men," said study co-author Rachel Huxley, director of the Queensland Clinical Trials and Biostatistics Centre at the University of Queensland in Australia.

The results support findings from an earlier analysis that found that women with diabetes have a nearly 50 percent increased risk of death from heart disease compared to men with diabetes, the study authors said.

This difference could stem from the fact that men develop full-blown type 2 diabetes earlier than women and at a lower weight, Huxley said. Because of this, men receive aggressive treatment sooner both for their diabetes and potential heart health risks, such as high blood pressure or elevated cholesterol levels.

Meanwhile, women may have to deteriorate further than men before full-blown type 2 diabetes develops, so they're at a worse starting point even before treatment begins. The study authors cited data that show the body mass index (BMI) of women at the time of their diabetes diagnosis tends to be nearly two units higher than it is in men. BMI is a score that measures if a person is considered overweight in relation to their height.

The study seems to suggest that, "it is not so much that women are not being treated, it is more that they are further along when they are diagnosed," said Mary Ann Bauman, MD, medical director for Women's Health and Community Relations at Integris Health in Oklahoma City, and a spokeswoman for the American Heart Association.

Research Details

The study authors reviewed health data on more than 850,000 people gathered from 64 different studies conducted between 1966 and 2013. The most recent report was released online in the journal *Diabetologia*.

Although the studies didn't identify what type of diabetes the study volunteers had, type 2 diabetes is by far the most common type of diabetes, according to the American Diabetes Association.

Nearly 30,000 people in the studies had some form of heart disease, the study authors noted. When the researchers looked at the risk by gender, they discovered that diabetic women were nearly three times more likely to develop heart disease than women without diabetes. For men with diabetes, the risk of heart disease was slightly more than twice as likely compared to men without diabetes.

Although the study found an association between women with diabetes and heart disease, it doesn't prove a cause-and-effect relationship between diabetes, gender and heart disease.

Implications

The study findings do strongly suggest that doctors need to consider gender when treating chronic disease, said Tara Narula, MD, associate director of the Cardiac Care Unit at Lenox Hill Hospital in New York City.

"The days of lumping men and women together are coming to an end," Dr. Narula said. "We need to see women as unique entities regarding their risk factors and, if we recognize there's this gender differential, we need to be more aggressive in screening and treating women for diabetes or heart disease."

Women likely need to receive more aggressive treatment while in prediabetes, rather than waiting for full-blown diabetes to develop, according to both Drs. Narula and Bauman. In pre-diabetes, people have started to build up resistance to insulin but do not have the high blood sugar levels needed for a diagnosis of diabetes.

It may be that spending a longer period of time in pre-diabetes takes a toll on the blood vessels of the heart, causing them to harden and narrow, they said.

"If that turns out to be true, then we might need to look more in the pre-diabetic phase, to maybe be more aggressive than we already are," Dr. Bauman said. "We can keep these things from happening. Heart disease is largely preventable."

The study authors recommend increased screening for pre-diabetes in women, as well as more stringent follow-up of women at high risk of diabetes.

For more about women and diabetes, visit the U.S. Department of Health and Human Services' Office on Women's Health at *http://www.womenshealth.gov/*.

The Shocking Diabetes Trigger That Can Strike Anyone

Hyla Cass, MD, a board-certified psychiatrist and nationally recognized expert on integrative medicine based in Los Angeles. She is the author of 10 books, including 8 Weeks to Vibrant Health *and* The Addicted Brain and How to Break Free. *CassMD.com*

Everyone knows about high blood sugar and the devastating effects it can have on one's health and longevity. But low blood sugar (hypoglycemia) can be just as dangerous—and it does not get nearly the attention that it should.

Simply put, hypoglycemia occurs when the body does not have enough glucose to use as fuel. It most commonly affects people with type 2 diabetes who take medication that sometimes works too well, resulting in low blood sugar.

Who gets overlooked: In other people, hypoglycemia can be a precursor to diabetes that is often downplayed by doctors and/or missed by tests. Having low blood sugar might even make you think that you are far from having diabetes…when, in fact, the opposite is true.

Hypoglycemia can also be an underlying cause of anxiety that gets mistakenly treated with psychiatric drugs rather than the simple steps (see next page) that can stabilize blood sugar levels. That's why anyone who seems to be suffering from an anxiety disorder needs to be seen by a doctor who takes a complete medical history and orders blood tests. When a patient comes to me complaining of anxiety, hypoglycemia is one of the first things I test for.

What's the link between hypoglycemia and anxiety? A sudden drop in blood sugar deprives the brain of oxygen. This, in turn, causes the adrenal glands to release adrenaline, the "emergency" hormone, which may lead to agitation, or anxiety, as the body's fight-or-flight mechanism kicks in.

The Dangers of Hypoglycemia

Hypoglycemia has sometimes been called carbohydrate intolerance, because the body's insulin-releasing mechanism is impaired in a manner similar to what occurs in diabetics. In people without diabetes, hypoglycemia is usually the result of eating too many simple carbohydrates (such as sugar and white flour). The pancreas then overreacts and releases too much insulin, thereby excessively lowering blood sugar.

The good news is that hypoglycemia—if it's identified—is not that difficult to control through diet and the use of specific supplements. Hypoglycemia should be considered a warning sign that you must adjust your carbohydrate intake or risk developing type 2 diabetes.

Caution: An episode of hypoglycemia in a person who already has diabetes can be life-threatening and requires prompt care, including the immediate intake of sugar—a glass of orange juice or even a sugar cube can be used.

Common symptoms of hypoglycemia include: Fatigue, dizziness, shakiness and faintness…irritability and depression…weakness or cramps in the feet and legs…numbness or tingling in the hands, feet or face…ringing in the ears…swollen feet or legs…tightness in the chest…heart palpitations…nightmares and panic attacks…"drenching" night sweats (not menopausal or perimenopausal hot flashes)…constant hunger…headaches and migraines…impaired memory and concentration…blurred vision…nasal congestion…abdominal cramps, loose stools and diarrhea.

A Tricky Diagnosis

Under-the-radar hypoglycemia (known as "subclinical hypoglycemia") is difficult to diagnose because symptoms may be subtle and irregular, and test results can be within normal ranges. Technically, if your blood sugar drops below 70 mg/dL, you are considered hypoglycemic. But people without diabetes do not check their blood sugar levels on their own, so it is important to be aware of hypoglycemia symptoms.

If you suspect that you may have hypoglycemia, talk to your physician. Ideally, you should arrange to have your blood glucose levels tested when you are experiencing symptoms. You will then be asked to eat food so that your blood glucose can be tested again. If this approach is impractical for you, however, talk to your doctor about other testing methods.

The Right Treatment

If you have been diagnosed with diabetes, hypoglycemia may indicate that your diabetes medication dose needs to be adjusted. The sugar treatment described earlier can work in an emergency but is not recommended as a long-term treatment for hypoglycemia. Left untreated, hypoglycemia in a person with diabetes can lead to loss of consciousness and even death.

In addition to getting their medication adjusted, people with diabetes—and those who are at risk for it due to hypoglycemia—can benefit from the following…

•A high-protein diet and healthful fats. To keep your blood sugar levels stabilized, consume slowly absorbed, unrefined carbohydrates, such as brown rice, quinoa, oatmeal and sweet potatoes. Also, get moderate amounts of healthful fats, such as those found in avocado, olive oil and fatty fish, including salmon…and protein, such as fish, meat, chicken, soy and eggs.

Recommended protein intake: 10% to 35% of daily calories. If you have kidney disease, get your doctor's advice on protein intake.

•Eat several small meals daily. Start with breakfast to give your body fuel for the day (if you don't, stored blood sugar will be released into your bloodstream) and then have a small "meal" every three to four waking hours.

•Avoid tobacco and limit your use of alcohol and caffeine. They cause an excessive release of neurotransmitters that, in turn, trigger the pancreas to deliver insulin inappropriately.

The supplements below also help stabilize blood sugar levels (and can be used in addition to a daily multivitamin)…*

•Chromium and vitamin B-6. Chromium helps release accumulated sugars in the liver, which can lead to a dangerous condition called fatty liver. Vitamin B-6 supports chromium's function and helps stabilize glucose levels.

Typical daily dose: 200 micrograms (mcg) of chromium with 100 mg of vitamin B-6.

•Glutamine. As the most common amino acid found in muscle tissue, glutamine plays a vital role in controlling blood sugar. Glutamine is easily converted to glucose when blood sugar is low.

*Consult your doctor before trying any supplements, especially if you take prescription medication and/or have a chronic medical condition, including diabetes.

Typical daily dose: Up to four 500-mg capsules daily…or add glutamine powder to a protein drink or a smoothie that does not contain added sugar—these drinks are good options for your morning routine. Glutamine is best taken 30 minutes before a meal to cut your appetite by balancing your blood sugar.

PTSD May Raise Women's Risk for Diabetes

Alexander Neumeister, MD, director, Molecular Imaging Program for Anxiety and Mood Disorders, New York University School of Medicine.
Karestan Koenen, PhD, director, Psychiatric-Neurological Epidemiology Cluster, and professor, epidemiology, Columbia University Mailman School of Public Health, New York City.
JAMA Psychiatry.

Women with post-traumatic stress disorder seem more likely than others to develop type 2 diabetes, with severe PTSD almost doubling the risk, a recent study suggests.

The research "brings to attention an unrecognized problem," said Alexander Neumeister, MD, director of the molecular imaging program for anxiety and mood disorders at New York University School of Medicine. It's crucial to treat both PTSD and diabetes when they're interconnected in women, he said. Otherwise, "you can try to treat diabetes as much as you want, but you'll never be fully successful," he added.

PTSD is an anxiety disorder that develops after living through or witnessing a dangerous event. People with the disorder may feel intense stress, suffer from flashbacks or experience a "fight or flight" response when there's no apparent danger.

It's estimated that one in 10 U.S. women will develop PTSD in their lifetime, with potentially severe effects, according to the study.

"In the past few years, there has been an increasing attention to PTSD as not only a mental disorder but one that also has very profound effects on brain and body function," said Dr. Neumeister, who wasn't involved in the new study. Among other things, PTSD sufferers gain more weight and have an increased risk of cardiac disease compared to other people, he said.

Study Details

The new study followed 49,739 female nurses from 1989 to 2008—aged 24 to 42 at the beginning—and tracked weight, smoking, exposure to trauma, PTSD symptoms and type 2 diabetes.

People with type 2 diabetes have higher than normal blood sugar levels. Untreated, the disease can cause serious problems such as blindness or kidney damage.

Over the course of the study, more than 3,000 of the nurses, or 6%, developed type 2 diabetes, which is linked to being overweight and sedentary. Those with the most PTSD symptoms were almost twice as likely to develop diabetes as those without PTSD, said study co-author Karestan Koenen, PhD, professor of epidemiology at Columbia University Mailman School of Public Health in New York City.

The study doesn't prove that PTSD directly causes diabetes, although Dr. Koenen said the study's design allows the researchers to "know that PTSD came before type 2 diabetes."

Since PTSD disrupts various systems in the body, such as those that manage stress hormones, "it may be that something about PTSD changes women's biology and increases risk" of diabetes, she said.

Obesity Not the Only Cause of Diabetes

Use of antidepressants and higher body weight accounted for almost half the increased risk, Dr. Koenen said. "The antidepressant finding was surprising because as far as we know, no one has shown it before," she said. "Much more research needs to be done to determine what the finding means."

Obesity explains some, but not all, of the relationship, she said.

Dr. Neumeister said there could be a connection from PTSD to overeating to diabetes, but he believes the situation is more complex than it sounds.

"Many PTSD patients are on the overweight end of the spectrum, and that's true for both men and women," he said. "We don't understand this link." Some factor, perhaps genetic, could make people more prone to both conditions, he said.

What About Men?

"Our findings are consistent with findings for male veterans," Dr. Koenen said. "Studies need to be done in men in the general population, but based on these data we would expect findings to be similar."

For now, Dr. Neumeister said doctors should pay more attention to the possible

4 Foods That Fight Diabetes

•**Reduce risk for type 2 diabetes with blueberries, grapes and apples.**
People who ate at least three servings of these fruits per week were up to 26% less likely to develop type 2 diabetes than people who ate less of these fruits, according to a recent study. Eat the whole fruit, not just the juice. Fruit juice increases risk for diabetes.

Study of 187,382 health professionals by researchers from the US, UK and Singapore, published in *BMJ.*

•**Yogurt may protect against diabetes.**
People who ate at least four-and-a-half servings of low-fat yogurt weekly—one serving equals 4.4 ounces—had 28% lower risk for diabetes than people who did not eat yogurt. The calcium, magnesium and vitamin D in fortified, fermented dairy products such as yogurt may have a protective effect.

Nita Forouhi, PhD, group leader, nutritional epidemiology program, University of Cambridge, UK, and leader of a study of 4,255 people, published in *Diabetologia.*

causes of diabetes. "Physicians in general don't ask enough questions, but when they do, they forget to ask questions about psychological factors that potentially contribute to medical problems."

The study appears in a January 2015 issue of *JAMA Psychiatry*.

For more about PTSD, see the US Department of Veteran Affairs at *http://www.ptsd.va.gov*.

Fake Sugar Is Not the Way to Go

Artificial sweeteners may increase diabetes risk in some people.

Recent finding: Studies in mice and people show that some users of artificial sweeteners have different gut bacteria from those of non-users—and have higher glucose intolerance, which puts them at increased risk for diabetes.

Eran Segal, PhD, professor in the department of computer science and applied mathematics, Weizmann Institute of Science, Rehovot, Israel. He is coauthor of a study published in *Nature*.

Pencil Test for Diabetes

David L. Katz, MD, MPH, internist and preventive medicine specialist and clinical instructor at the Yale School of Medicine in New Haven, Connecticut. Dr. Katz is the author of *Disease-Proof: The Remarkable Truth About What Makes Us Well*.

This test* checks the nerve function in your feet—if abnormal, this could indicate diabetes, certain types of infections or autoimmune disease.

The prop you'll need: A pencil that is freshly sharpened at one end with a flat eraser on the other end…and a friend to help.

*This self-test is not a substitute for a thorough physical exam from your doctor. Use it only as a way to identify potential problem areas to discuss with your physician.

What to do: Sit down so that all sides of your bare feet are accessible. Close your eyes, and keep them closed throughout the test.

Have your friend lightly touch your foot with either the sharp end or the eraser end of the pencil. With each touch, say which end of the pencil you think was used.

Ask your friend to repeat the test in at least three different locations on the tops and bottoms of both feet (12 locations total). Have your friend keep track of your right and wrong answers.

Watch out: Most people can easily tell the difference between "sharp" and "dull" sensations on their sensitive feet. If you give the wrong answer for more than two or three locations on your feet, have your doctor repeat the test to determine whether you have nerve damage (neuropathy).

Beware: Neuropathy is a common sign of diabetes…certain autoimmune disorders, including lupus and Sjögren's syndrome…infection, such as Lyme disease, shingles or hepatitis C…or excessive exposure to toxins, such as pesticides or heavy metals (mercury or lead).

Fight Diabetes Naturally—3 Proven Nondrug Remedies

Bill Gottlieb, CHC, a health coach certified by the American Association of Drugless Practitioners. Based in northern California, he is author of *Defeat High Blood Sugar—Naturally! Super-Supplements and Super-Foods Selected by America's Best Alternative Doctors. BillGottliebHealth.com*

Scientific research and the experience of doctors and other health professionals show that supplements and superfoods can be even more effective than drugs when it comes to preventing and treating diabetes. I reviewed thousands of scientific studies and talked to more than 60 health professionals about these glucose-controlling natural remedies. One is magnesium. Studies show that magnesium significantly reduces the risk for diabetes. (Note: High doses of magnesium can cause diarrhea.)

Here are three more standout natural remedies…

Caution: If you are taking insulin or other medications to control diabetes, talk to your doctor before taking any supplement or changing your diet.

Gymnema

Gymnema has been the standard antidiabetes recommendation for the past 2,000 years from practitioners of Ayurveda, the ancient system of natural healing from India. Derived from a vinelike plant found in the tropical forests of southern and central India, the herb also is called gurmar, or "sugar destroyer"—if you chew on the leaf of the plant, you temporarily will lose your ability to taste sweets.

Modern science has figured out the molecular interactions underlying this strange phenomenon. The gymnemic acids in the herb have a structure similar to glucose molecules, filling up glucose receptor sites on the taste buds. They also fill up sugar receptors in the intestine, blocking the absorption of glucose. And gymnemic acids stimulate (and even may regenerate) the cells of the pancreas that manufacture insulin, the hormone that ushers glucose out of the bloodstream and into cells.

Standout research: Studies published in *Journal of Ethnopharmacology* showed that three months of using a unique gymnema extract, formulated over several decades by two Indian scientists, reduced fasting blood glucose (a blood sample is taken after an overnight fast) by 23% in people with type 2 diabetes (defined as fasting blood sugar levels of 126 mg/dL or higher). People with prediabetes (defined as those with blood sugar levels of 100 mg/dL to 125 mg/dL) had a 30% reduction.

Important: The newest (and more powerful) version of this extract is called ProBeta, which is available at *PharmaTerra.com*. A na-

turopathic physician who uses ProBeta with his patients told me that the supplement can lower fasting glucose in the 200s down to the 120s or 130s after five to six months of use.

Typical daily dose: ProBeta—two capsules, two to three times a day. Other types of gymnema—400 milligrams (mg), three times a day.

Apple Cider Vinegar

Numerous studies have proved that apple cider vinegar works to control type 2 diabetes. Several of the studies were conducted by Carol Johnston, PhD, RD, a professor of nutrition at Arizona State University.

Standout scientific research: Dr. Johnston's studies showed that an intake of apple cider vinegar with a meal lowered insulin resistance (the inability of cells to use insulin) by an average of 64% in people with prediabetes and type 2 diabetes…improved insulin sensitivity (the ability of cells to use insulin) by up to 34%…and lowered postmeal spikes in blood sugar by an average of 20%. Research conducted in Greece, Sweden, Japan and the Middle East has confirmed many of Dr. Johnston's findings.

How it works: The acetic acid in vinegar—the compound that gives vinegar its tart flavor and pungent odor—blunts the activity of disaccharidase enzymes that help break down the type of carbohydrates found in starchy foods such as potatoes, rice, bread and pasta. As a result, those foods are digested and absorbed more slowly, lowering blood glucose and insulin levels.

Suggested daily intake: Two tablespoons right before or early in the meal. (More is not more effective.)

If you're using vinegar in a salad dressing, the ideal ratio for blood sugar control is two tablespoons of vinegar to one tablespoon of oil. Eat the salad early in the meal so that it disrupts the carb-digesting enzymes before they get a chance to work. Or dip premeal whole-grain bread in a vinaigrette dressing.

Soy Foods

A new 10-year study published in *Journal of the American Society of Nephrology* found that the mortality rate for people with diabetes and kidney disease was more than 31%. Statistically, that makes kidney disease the number-one risk factor for death in people with diabetes.

Fortunately, researchers have found that there is a simple way to counter kidney disease in diabetes—eat more soy foods.

Standout scientific research: Dozens of scientific studies show that soy is a nutritional ally for diabetes patients with kidney disease. But the best and most recent of these studies, published in *Diabetes Care*, shows that eating lots of soy can help reverse signs of kidney disease, reduce risk factors for heart disease—and reduce blood sugar, too.

The study involved 41 diabetes patients with kidney disease, divided into two groups. One group ate a diet with protein from 70% animal and 30% vegetable sources. The other group ate a diet with protein from 35% animal sources, 35% textured soy protein and 30% vegetable proteins. After four years, those eating the soy-rich diet had lower levels of several biomarkers for kidney disease. (In another, smaller experiment, the same researchers found that soy improved biomarkers for kidney disease in just seven weeks.) In fact, the health of the participants' kidneys actually improved, a finding that surprised the researchers, since diabetic nephropathy (diabetes-caused kidney disease) is considered to be a progressive, irreversible disease.

Those eating soy also had lower fasting blood sugar, lower LDL cholesterol, lower total cholesterol, lower triglycerides and lower C-reactive protein, a biomarker for chronic inflammation.

How it works: Substituting soy for animal protein may ease stress on the delicate filters of the kidneys. Soy itself also stops the overproduction of cells in the kidney that clog the filters…boosts the production of nitric oxide, which improves blood flow in the kidneys…and normalizes the movement of minerals within the kidneys, thus improving filtration.

Suggested daily intake: The diabetes patients in the study ate 16 grams of soy protein daily. Examples: Four ounces of tofu provide 13 grams of soy protein…one soy burger, 13 grams…one-quarter cup of soy nuts, 11 grams…one-half cup of shelled edamame (edible soybeans in the pod), 11 grams…one cup of soy milk, 6 grams.

What's Wrong with Diabetes Drugs?

Doctors typically try to control high blood sugar with a glucose-lowering medication such as *metformin* (Glucophage), a drug most experts consider safe. But other diabetes drugs may not be safe.

Example #1: Recent studies show that *sitagliptin* (Januvia) and *exenatide* (Byetta) double the risk for hospitalization for pancreatitis (inflamed pancreas) and triple the risk for pancreatic cancer.

Example #2: *Pioglitazone* (Actos) can triple the risk for eye problems and vision loss, double the risk for bone fractures in women and double the risk for bladder cancer.

Better Glucose-Meter Accuracy

Glucose meters that check blood sugar should be tested for accuracy every time users open a new pack of test strips, get a new meter or suspect a malfunction. A new survey found that only 23% of patients with diabetes who use glucose meters said they followed these manufacturer recommendations.

Here's how to test a glucose meter: Use one drop of the control-solution liquid on the test strip (just like you would check your own blood sugar) to test the accuracy of both the meter and packages of test strips.

Katherine O'Neal, PharmD, assistant professor, The University of Oklahoma College of Pharmacy, Tulsa.

Acid-Producing Diet Increases Diabetes Risk

Study titled "Dietary acid load and risk of type 2 diabetes: the E3N-EPIC cohort study," published in *Diabetologia*.

When you sit down to a meal, you may think about how many calories it has…the amount of fat or carbs you're consuming…and which vitamins and minerals you're getting. You probably don't think about the meal's acid load. You should. Why? Because once they're inside you, certain foods lead to the production of a lot of acid—and that acid may increase your risk of developing diabetes, a new study shows.

Shocker: Foods that you'd generally think of as acidic (oranges, tomatoes, lemons, etc.) are not the ones to worry about. Instead, the acid producers include some foods you probably consider healthful. *Here's what to watch out for…*

Acid Scoring

To understand the new study, let's review a little chemistry. Remember that pH, ranging from zero to 14, is a measure of the acidity or alkalinity of a substance, which has to do with the concentration of hydrogen ions. A pH of 7.0 is neutral…numbers below 7.0 are more acid…numbers above 7.0 are more alkaline. The normal healthy pH range for human blood and tissues is slightly more alkaline than acid, with a pH of about 7.35 to 7.45.

Severe pH imbalances are known to be life-threatening, and moderate imbalances can compromise bone health and lead to kidney stones. Researchers decided to investigate how pH affects diabetes risk. They drew on data from more than 66,000 women who did not have diabetes at the start of the study. In 1993, these women completed questionnaires about how often and in what quantities they consumed 208 different foods. The researchers then did a nutritional analysis, calculating each woman's dietary acid load

based on the potential renal acid load (PRAL) scores of the foods she ate. The PRAL score takes into account the intestinal absorption rates of protein, phosphorus, potassium, calcium and magnesium, all of which contribute to maintaining the acid-alkaline balance. Negative PRAL scores reflect alkaline-forming potential, while positive PRAL scores reflect acid-forming potential.

Based on their PRAL scores, participants were divided into four equal-sized groups. The lowest-scoring group had the most alkaline-forming diet…the highest-scoring group had the most acid-forming diet. Then, for the next 14 years, the researchers kept track of who developed diabetes—as almost 3,500 of the women did.

What the researchers found: Women with the lowest PRAL scores were the least likely to develop diabetes. Compared to that group, women with the highest scores (representing a high acid load) were 56% more likely to develop diabetes. This held even after researchers adjusted for other diabetes risk factors, such as body mass index (BMI), physical activity, smoking, high blood pressure, high cholesterol and family history of diabetes. Surprisingly, the association between a high acid load and diabetes risk was even more pronounced among women of normal weight (with a BMI of 25 or less) than among overweight women.

Which Foods Are Acid-Forming?

In this study, the high-risk high-PRAL diets were characterized by higher consumption of fat and protein (mainly from animal protein—meat, poultry, fish) and also by consumption of bread and soft drinks, especially artificially sweetened drinks. In contrast, women who followed a low-risk low-PRAL diet tended to consume more fruits, vegetables, dairy products and coffee. PRAL examples: A three-ounce chicken breast without the skin has a PRAL score of 9.43…whereas an orange scores -4.24 and a cup of broccoli scores -5.6.

What might be the metabolic mechanism behind these findings? Our lungs and kidneys are responsible for maintaining a healthy pH by eliminating excess amounts of acid or alkaline from the body. The lungs take care of carbon dioxide and the kidneys take care of all other acids. But when the kidneys aren't able to keep up with the task, a condition called metabolic acidosis arises. According to the study researchers, a diet that creates a high acid load may contribute to chronic metabolic acidosis, which in turn leads to insulin resistance and metabolic syndrome—which are risk factors for diabetes. Additional evidence: Animal studies have shown that metabolic acidosis decreases the ability of insulin to bind to insulin receptors...and human studies have shown that some markers of metabolic acidosis are associated with insulin resistance.

Bottom line: The study doesn't mean that you should shy away from fish, which has been shown to have cardiovascular health benefits. But it does give you one more excellent reason to make sure that your diet includes plenty of fruits and vegetables and a moderate amount of dairy.

Don't Be One of the Millions of Americans Overtreated for Diabetes

Kasia Joanna Lipska, MD, MHS, assistant professor of medicine (endocrinology), department of internal medicine, Yale School of Medicine, New Haven, Connecticut. Her study was published in *JAMA Internal Medicine*.

Bringing blood sugar down with diabetes drugs might be too simple an approach and, worse, ineffective and even harmful for some of us, especially those of us who are 65 or older. What's more, the reason why so many Americans have diabetes might not be because their blood sugar levels are dangerously high but because the system that defines what constitutes diabetes is rigged. And even doctors might not realize it!

Here's how to really protect your health and protect yourself from overtreatment when a doctor tells you that your blood sugar is high...

Follow the Money

Diabetes management has become big business, amassing billions of dollars in annual sales. In 2014, sales of diabetes drugs alone reached $23 billion. For this we can thank, in part, the changing definition of what exactly diabetes is. Since 1997, the American Diabetes Association and other professional endocrinology groups have twice lowered blood sugar thresholds for type 2 diabetes and prediabetes. Each time they did this, millions more Americans were suddenly considered, by definition, diabetic or prediabetic.

But the doctors making these blood sugar threshold changes have strong incentives to do so that have nothing to do with your well-being, according to a recent exposé published by the medical news outlet *MedPage Today* and the *Milwaukee Journal Sentinel*. Many of these doctors receive speaking and consulting fees from diabetes-drug manufacturers. In one analysis, the authors of the exposé found that 13 of 19 members of a committee responsible for diabetes guidelines accumulated a combined sum of more than $2 million in speaking and consulting fees from companies that make diabetes drugs. Whether doctors responsible for diabetes guidelines are intentionally and systematically basing their decisions on their bank account balances isn't known, but the findings do reveal an obvious and material conflict of interest.

Effectiveness of Therapies Questioned

The authors of the exposé also pointed out that although they reduce blood sugar, none of the 30 diabetes drugs approved since 2004 has been definitively proven to reduce the risk of heart attack and stroke, blindness or any other diabetes-related complication. "In order to approve a new diabetes drug, the FDA requires evidence that the drug effectively reduces hemoglobin A1C levels—a measure of blood glucose—and that it doesn't result in an unacceptable increase in heart disease risk. The evidence that the drug reduces the risk of complications of diabetes, such as heart attacks and stroke, is not required," explained endocrinologist Kasia Lipska, MD, assistant professor of medicine at Yale School of Medicine. She is the leader of a recent, related study that showed that mature adults are being treated too aggressively for diabetes, sometimes with dangerous consequences. The study population of nearly 1,300 adults, selected from the National Health and Nutrition Examination Survey database, represents a cross section of senior Americans with diabetes.

Similar to a recent study showing that tight blood pressure control may not be beneficial in older adults, prior studies suggest that tight blood sugar control in people 65 and older who have serious health problems actually may do more harm than good. Tight blood sugar control is defined by the American Diabetes Association as a hemoglobin A1C level of less than 7%.

Dangerous Side Effects

When it comes to drug treatment for diabetes, most doctors will turn to the older drug metformin first, said Dr. Lipska. It has been used in the United States since 1994 and has had a good safety record here and in Europe, where it has been used much longer. It is considered safe and effective. In addition, it does not cause low blood sugar reactions or weight gain. However, after metformin, there is no clear "winner" among the diabetes drugs, and the choice of drug depends on a number of trade-offs and risks, particularly for older adults, she said. Insulin and sulfonylurea drugs such as *glipizide* (Glucotrol), *glyburide* (Micronase) and *glimepiride* (Amaryl) have been associated with dangerously low blood sugar (hypoglycemia), and other drugs, such as *pioglitazone* (Actos), with risk of fluid retention and fractures. Some drugs, such as *saxagliptin* (Onglyza), may be associated with heart failure, while, for very new drugs, such as *canagliflozin* (Invokana), the risks are not yet known.

Although the American Diabetes Association and other professional groups have been lowering the threshold for what constitutes "diabetes" (and, thereby, driving the market for diabetes drugs, at least according to the Medpage exposé), the American Diabetes Association and the American Geriatrics Society discourage tight blood sugar control in older adults. They acknowledge that older adults whose blood sugar is too aggressively controlled are more vulnerable to the dangerous side effects mentioned above, said Dr. Lipska. She added that one treatment standard does not fit all in older adults, because their health and treatment preferences vary greatly. Tight control may be safe and appropriate for one person and not another.

Avoid Overtreatment

Diabetes in older people should be generally managed through lifestyle modification first, including exercise, according to Dr. Lipska. Nevertheless, medications are often required to bring down blood sugar levels, she said. "For many older people with serious health problems or a history of hypoglycemia, tight blood sugar control may not be worth the risks involved. But for some relatively healthy people, tight blood sugar control may make sense. Treatment should be individualized, which requires a careful case-by-case approach," she said. Unfortunately, this is not always the case in practice. Her study found absolutely no difference in how people were treated based on their health. In other words, patients in poor health and at risk for hypoglycemia tended to be treated as aggressively as far healthier patients. What's more, 55% of older adults with diabetes who achieved tight blood sugar control were taking insulin or sulfonylureas—drugs that can lead to hypoglycemia—regardless of whether they were healthy, had complex health issues and/or were in poor health.

To avoid overtreatment for diabetes, Dr. Lipska recommends that you make the necessary lifestyle changes and work together with doctors and other health-care providers on a personalized approach to your specific health needs and safety. You need to be engaged and part of the plan. The plan should involve much more than simply prescribing a diabetes drug if your blood sugar is above the recommended threshold.

For Some, Insulin Might Not Be the Way to Go

Some diabetics may be better off not starting insulin. For adults over age 50 who have type 2 diabetes but a low risk for complications because their glucose levels are under control (A1C level of 8% to 8.5%), the side effects of taking a daily insulin shot or other diabetes medications may do more harm than good, a recent study reports. Common side effects such as low blood sugar may be worse than the small benefit of the medication. Diet and exercise may be better for these patients.

Caution: Do not stop taking insulin or other diabetes drugs without first consulting your doctor.

Sandeep Vijan, MD, professor of internal medicine, University of Michigan Medical School, Ann Arbor.

Diabetes Drug Danger

Steven E. Nissen, MD, chairman of the department of cardiovascular medicine at Cleveland Clinic Foundation and professor of medicine at the Cleveland Clinic Lerner College of Medicine at Case Western Reserve University. *ClevelandClinic.org*

The Food and Drug Administration (FDA) recently lifted its restrictions on the type 2 diabetes treatment Avandia. But it would be a mistake to assume that the drug is safe—it is not.

Avandia (*rosiglitazone*) was originally approved as a treatment for type 2 diabetes in 1999 after small-scale, short-term studies suggested that it lowered blood glucose concentrations. It became the world's top-selling antidiabetes drug—until further studies found that it significantly increased users' risk for heart attacks and related cardiovascular events.

Avandia was banned by European regulators and restricted to use as a drug of last resort in the US in 2010. The maker of the drug (Glaxo-SmithKline) initially concealed Avandia's dangers but eventually pled guilty to criminal misconduct and paid a $3 billion fine.

Now the FDA has removed the restrictions on Avandia—though the evidence continues to strongly suggest that the drug increases users' risk for heart attack. The FDA pointed to a trial that failed to confirm Avandia's cardiovascular dangers when it announced that it was lifting the restrictions. But reviewers have found major flaws in the methodology of that trial, calling its results into question. Better studies by independent researchers (including myself), by the FDA itself and even by GlaxoSmithKline continue to strongly suggest that the drug does, in fact, increase the odds of heart attack.

New Weekly Diabetes Drug

A weekly injectable drug for type 2 diabetes is now available. Recently approved by the FDA, *dulaglutide* (Trulicity) is a once-a-week injectable, single-dose pen that has been shown to safely improve blood sugar levels in six separate trials of more than 3,300 people with type 2 diabetes. The medication, which requires no mixing (as do competing drugs), can be used alone or in combination with other diabetes medication, including metformin and mealtime insulin. Potential side effects include nausea, diarrhea and abdominal pain. People at risk for thyroid or endocrine gland tumors should not take dulaglutide.

Ralph A. DeFronzo, MD, deputy director, Texas Diabetes Institute, San Antonio.

A Promising Treatment for Type I Diabetes

There's a new drug for type 1 diabetes. According to a recent study, people with type 1 diabetes were given an Alpha1-Antitrypsin (AAT) infusion once a week for eight weeks. AAT is made from an anti-inflammatory blood protein.

Breakthrough: Half of those who received AAT produced more of their own insulin for more than two years. AAT is expected to be FDA-approved for diabetes within two years. Until then, doctors can prescribe it "off-label."

Eli C. Lewis, PhD, director of the Clinical Islet Laboratory, Ben-Gurion University of the Negev, Beer-Sheva, Israel. His study was published in *The Journal of Clinical Endocrinology & Metabolism.*

How to Beat the 3 Big Mistakes That Worsen Diabetes

Osama Hamdy, MD, PhD, medical director of the Joslin Diabetes Center's Obesity Clinical Program and an assistant professor of medicine at Harvard Medical School, both in Boston. He also is coauthor of *The Diabetes Breakthrough.*

Despite what you may have heard, type 2 diabetes doesn't have to be a lifelong condition. It can be controlled and even reversed in the early stages or stopped from progressing in the later stages—with none of the dire consequences of out-of-control blood sugar.

Sounds great, right? What person with diabetes wouldn't want to do everything possible to help prevent serious complications such as coronary heart disease, kidney disease, blindness or even amputation?

The problem is, even people who are following all the doctor's orders may still be sabotaging their efforts with seemingly minor missteps that can have big consequences. Among the most common mistakes that harm people with diabetes are oversights in the way they eat and exercise. *For example...*

Mistake #1: Skimping on protein. The majority of people with type 2 diabetes are overweight or obese. These individuals know

Diabetes Drug Can Affect Your Thyroid

Your diabetes drug may affect thyroid levels. People taking metformin for type 2 diabetes while being treated for hypothyroidism (underactive thyroid) were 55% more likely to have low thyroid-stimulating hormone (TSH) levels than those taking sulfonylurea diabetes drugs. Low TSH is associated with hyperthyroidism (overactive thyroid).

Implication: Hypothyroidism patients on metformin may need to have their TSH levels monitored and thyroid medication adapted.

Laurent Azoulay, PhD, assistant professor of cancer epidemiology, McGill University, Montreal, Quebec, Canada.

that they need to lose weight but sometimes fail despite their best efforts.

Here's what often happens: We have had it drummed into our heads that the best way to lose weight is to go on a low-fat diet. However, these diets tend to be low in protein—and you need more protein, not less, if you have type 2 diabetes and are cutting calories to lose weight.

What's so special about protein? You need protein to maintain muscle mass. The average adult starts losing lean muscle mass every year after about age 40. If you have diabetes, you'll probably lose more muscle mass than someone without it. And the loss will be even greater if your diabetes is not well controlled.

Muscle is important because it burns more calories than other tissues in your body. Also, people with a higher and more active muscle mass find it easier to maintain healthy blood-glucose levels, since active muscle doesn't require insulin to clear high glucose from the blood.

My advice: Protein should provide 20% to 30% of total daily calories. If you're on an 1,800-calorie diet (a reasonable amount for an average man who wants to lose weight), that's about 90 g to 135 g of protein a day.

If you're on a 1,200- to 1,500-calorie diet (a sensible amount for an average woman who is dieting), that's about 60 g to 113 g of protein a day.

Examples: Good protein sources include fish, skinless poultry, nonfat or low-fat dairy, legumes and nuts and seeds. A three-ounce chicken breast has about 30 g of protein…a three-ounce piece of haddock, 17 g …one-half cup of low-fat cottage cheese, 14 g…and one-quarter cup of whole almonds, 7 g of protein.

Note: If you have kidney problems, you may need to limit your protein intake. Check with your doctor.

Mistake #2: Not doing resistance training. It's widely known that aerobic exercise is good for weight loss and blood sugar control. What usually gets short shrift is resistance training, such as lifting weights and using stretch bands.

When you build muscle, you use more glucose, which helps reduce glucose levels in the blood. If you take insulin for your diabetes, toned muscles will also make your body more sensitive to it.

An added benefit: People who do resistance training can often reduce their doses of insulin or other medications within a few months.

My advice: Do a combination of resistance, aerobic and flexibility exercises. Start with 20 minutes total, four days a week—splitting the time equally among the three types of exercise. Try to work up to 60 minutes total, six days a week. An exercise physiologist or personal trainer certified in resistance training can help choose the best workout for you.

Mistake #3: Ignoring hunger cues. Many individuals are so conditioned to eat at certain times that they virtually ignore their body's hunger signals. Learning how to read these cues can be one of the best ways to achieve (and maintain) a healthy body weight.

The key is to recognize that there are different levels of hunger. It's easy to overeat when you do not acknowledge the difference between feeling satisfied and stuffing yourself.

My advice: Imagine a five-point hunger scale: 1 means you're feeling starved…2 is hungry…3 is comfortable…4 is full…and 5 is stuffed. Before you start eating, rate your hunger between 1 and 5. Halfway through the meal, rate it again.

Here's the secret: Stop eating when you rate your hunger somewhere between "comfortable" and "full." If you give your hunger a ranking of 4 and you still want to eat, get away from the table and do something else!

Note: It can take up to 20 minutes for the "satiety signal" to kick in, so eat slowly. If you eat too quickly, you may miss the signal and overeat.

After just a few weeks of eating this way, it usually becomes second nature.

If You Take Diabetes Meds…

Sometimes, diet and exercise aren't enough to tame out-of-control blood sugar. *Traps to avoid…*

•**Drug-induced weight gain.** Ironically, the drugs that are used to treat diabetes also can cause weight gain as a side effect. If you start taking insulin, you can expect to gain about 10 pounds within six months—with oral drugs, such as *glipizide* (Glucotrol), you'll probably gain from four to seven pounds.

My advice: Ask your doctor if you can switch to one of the newer, "weight-friendly" medications.

Examples: A form of insulin called Levemir causes less weight gain than Lantus,

"Bionic" Pancreas Passes Muster

In recent testing, an external device effectively monitored blood sugar levels and administered medication as needed in people with type 1 diabetes. More tests are planned, and the device should become available by 2017.

American Diabetes Association.

Humulin N or Novolin N. Newer oral drugs called DPP-4 inhibitors, such as Januvia, Onglyza and Nesina, don't have weight gain as a side effect.

Important: The newer drugs are more expensive and may not be covered by insurance. But if they don't cause you to gain weight, you might get by with a lower dose—and reduced cost.

•**Erratic testing.** You should test your blood sugar levels at least four to six times a day, particularly when you're making lifestyle changes that could affect the frequency and doses of medication. Your doctor has probably advised you to test before and after exercise—and before meals.

My advice: Be sure to also test after meals. This will help determine the effects of different types and amounts of foods.

Statins Help with Diabetes Complications

According to recent research, statins, in addition to lowering risk for heart attack and stroke, also lowered risk for diabetes complications. People with diabetes taking statins were 34% less likely to be diagnosed with diabetes-related nerve damage (neuropathy)…40% less likely to develop diabetes-related damage to the retina…and 12% less likely to develop gangrene than diabetics not taking statins.

Børge G. Nordestgaard, MD, DMSc, chief physician at Copenhagen University Hospital, Herlev, Denmark, and leader of a study of 60,000 people, published in *The Lancet Diabetes Endocrinology.*

New Insulin Gets FDA Nod

The new diabetes drug Afrezza is a fast-acting inhalable insulin that comes in a small inhaler that looks like a whistle. No needles are required.

How it works: At the beginning of each meal, the user inhales powder from the device. People with chronic obstructive pulmonary disease (COPD) or other lung conditions should not use Afrezza.

Osama Hamdy, MD, PhD, medical director, Obesity Clinical Program, Joslin Diabetes Center, Boston.

If You Have Diabetes… How to Fast Safely for a Medical Test

Paula Vetter, RN, MSN, diabetes educator, holistic family nurse practitioner, personal wellness coach and former critical care nursing instructor at the Cleveland Clinic. Based in Paso Robles, California, she currently is writing a self-help guide for people with type 2 diabetes. *CrazyDiabetesMyths.com*

Recently, an employee at *Bottom Line Health* was scheduled for a colonoscopy, the screening test for colon cancer. The medical test turned into medical mayhem.

The day before the test, the woman followed her doctor's orders to start ingesting a "clear liquid" diet, which includes soft drinks, Jell-O and other clear beverages and foods. But when she drank the "prep"—the bowel-cleaning solution that is consumed the evening before a colonoscopy (and sometimes also the morning of)—she vomited. Over and over. As a result, her colon wasn't sufficiently emptied to conduct the test, which had to be postponed.

What Went Wrong?

The woman has diabetes—and her glucose (blood sugar) levels had become unstable, triggering nausea and vomiting. Yet not one medical professional—not a doctor, not a nurse, not a medical technician—had warned her that people with diabetes need to take special precautions with food and diabetes medicine whenever they have any medical test that involves an extended period of little or no eating. Unfortunately, this lack of diabetes-customized instruction about medical tests is very common. *What you need to know...*

Do It Early

If you're undergoing a test that requires only overnight fasting, which includes many types of CT scans, MRIs and X-rays, make sure that the test is scheduled for early in the morning—no later than 9 a.m. That way, you will be able to eat after the test by 10 a.m. or 11 a.m., which will help to stabilize your blood sugar as much as possible

Don't expect your blood sugar levels to be perfect after the test. The important thing is to keep them from getting too high or too low.

The Right Clear Liquids

Conventional dietitians and doctors specify clear liquids and foods that reflect the conventional American diet, such as regular soda, sports drinks, Popsicles, Kool-Aid and Jell-O (no red or purple). But the pH of these products is highly acidic. And that could contribute to diabetic ketoacidosis, a potentially life-threatening condition where the body burns fat instead of glucose for fuel, producing ketones, substances toxic to the liver and brain.

When my clients with diabetes are on a clear-liquid diet before a test, I recommend that they consume liquids with essential nutrients and a more balanced pH, such as apple juice, white grape juice and clear, fat-free broth (vegetable, chicken or beef). A typical "dinner" could include up to three-quarters cup of juice (to limit sugar) and any amount of broth. A bedtime "snack" could include one-half cup of juice and any amount of broth. Plenty of good pure water between "meals" also is important to stay well-hydrated.

Check Blood Sugar Often

Many people with diabetes check their blood sugar a few times a day—typically right before a meal and again one to two hours afterward. But if you're on a clear-liquid diet or fasting before a medical test, you

should check your glucose level every two to three hours. If it's too low, correct it with a fast-acting carbohydrate, such as four ounces of 100% fruit juice or a glucose gel (a squeezable, over-the-counter product).

Important: Take fruit juice or a glucose gel with you to the test—if the test is delayed for any reason, you can ingest the carb and keep your blood sugar on track.

Stop Taking Metformin

Your doctor likely will recommend that you stop taking the diabetes medication metformin 24 hours before the test. *Metformin* (Glucophage) also can contribute to acidosis and typically is stopped 24 hours before and up to 72 hours after any test that requires a contrast agent (an injected dye often used in an X-ray, CT scan or MRI that helps create the image). Talk to your doctor about when to stop taking your medication and when to resume or about the possible need for an alternative diabetes drug during this period.

An unexpected threat: Metformin is a component of many multi-ingredient diabetes drugs—so you may not realize you're taking it and therefore may need to discontinue it. Drugs that include metformin are Actoplus Met and Actoplus Met XR...Avandamet...Glucovance...Janumet and Janumet XR...Jentadueto...Kazano...Kombiglyze XR...Metaglip...and PrandiMet. New drugs are being developed constantly, so check with your pharmacist to see if yours contains metformin.

Also important: Many X-rays, CT scans and MRIs utilize an injected dye or a contrast agent that can damage the kidneys in people with diabetes (contrast-induced nephropathy). Before restarting metformin, have a kidney function test (such as BUN, which requires a blood sample, and creatinine clearance, which requires a urine sample and a blood sample) that confirms that your kidneys are working normally. These tests are recommended 24 to 48 hours after your procedure is completed and usually are covered by insurance.

Plant-Based Diet Eases Diabetic Nerve Pain

In a 20-week study of people with diabetic neuropathy (which often leads to pain and numbness in the legs and feet), half ate a low-fat vegan diet and took a vitamin B-12 supplement (diabetes patients are often deficient in B-12), and the other half took only the supplement.

Result: The group eating the plant-based diet had significantly greater pain relief and lost more weight than the other group.

Anne Bunner, PhD, associate director of clinical research, Physicians Committee for Responsible Medicine, Washington, DC.

Decrease Insulin

Insulin is the hormone used by the body to regulate blood sugar—and many people with advanced diabetes give themselves shots of short- and/or long-acting insulin to keep glucose levels steady. But if you're consuming only clear liquids or fasting before a medical test, you likely will need to take less insulin.

Excellent guidelines for insulin use before a medical procedure have been created by the University of Michigan Comprehensive Diabetes Center. *In general, it recommends…*

•**Take one-half of your usual dose of long-acting insulin the evening before the procedure.**

•**Take one-half of your usual dose of long-acting insulin the morning of the test and no short-acting insulin the morning of the test.**

You can find the complete guidelines in downloadable PDF form at *Med.UMich.edu/ 1libr/MEND/Diabetes-OutpatientProcedure. pdf.* Print them out, and discuss them with your doctor.

Reduce Anxiety

Anxiety triggers the release of the stress hormone cortisol, which in turn sparks the production of glucose. *To keep blood sugar balanced before a test, use these two methods to keep anxiety in check…*

•**Get all your questions answered.** Fear of the unknown is the greatest stress. Before your procedure, create a list of questions to ask your doctor or nurse practitioner. Examples: What is going to happen during the procedure? What is it going to feel like? What are the potential side effects from the test, and how can I best avoid them? When will I be informed of the test results? How will the test results affect future decision-making about my health?

•**Breathe deeply.** Deep breathing is the easiest and simplest way to reduce anxiety. My recommendation, based on the approach of Andrew Weil, MD…

Repeat this breathing exercise three times, and do it three times a day every day: Inhale for a count of four…hold for a count of seven…exhale for a count of eight. (Don't worry if you can't do the entire count—shorter counts also work.) Do this exercise when you get up in the morning, at midday and at bedtime. You can do it more often, but most people find three times simple and easy to integrate into their routines.

Also, you can use this breathing technique in any situation that you find anxiety-producing, such as before and during the test itself. Breathe deeply three times every 10 or 15 minutes, and be sure to keep the 4:7:8 ratio—inhale for four, hold for seven, exhale for eight.

First Treatment Approved for Diabetic Retinopathy

The FDA recently approved injections of the drug Lucentis—also used to treat macular degeneration in older adults—for diabetic retinopathy in patients with macular edema (swelling that occurs when fluid builds up in the eye). Diabetic retinopathy, which causes bleeding and/or abnormal blood-vessel growth in the retina, is the leading cause of blindness in Americans with diabetes.

Deeba Husain, MD, retina specialist and associate professor of ophthalmology at Harvard Medical School, Boston.

New Eye Implant for Diabetes Patients

Anyone with type 1 or type 2 diabetes is at risk for vision loss caused by diabetic macular edema (DME), which affects up to 28% of diabetics. Once the Iluvien implant is in place, it slowly delivers a submicrogram dose of the corticosteroid fluocinolone acetonide for 36 months—which helps to control inflammation in the eye. Possible side effects include cataracts and increased intraocular pressure.

Joel Zonszein, MD, professor of clinical medicine at Albert Einstein College of Medicine and director of the Clinical Diabetes Center at Montefiore Medical Center, the Bronx, New York.

Are Two Large Meals Good for Diabetes?

A recent, highly publicized Czech study suggested that eating only breakfast and lunch is better for controlling blood sugar, weight and other factors than six smaller meals a day. But the study was very small and went against years of diabetes research.

Best for people with diabetes: Patients who use insulin before meals to adjust blood sugar levels must wait at least five or six hours after a meal before adjusting blood sugar levels again and eating another meal. Patients who do not adjust blood sugar levels before meals may be able to control sugar levels with smaller, frequent meals.

Richard K. Bernstein, MD, diabetes specialist in private practice in Mamaroneck, New York, and author of several books on diabetes, including *Dr. Bernstein's Diabetes Solution: A Complete Guide to Achieving Normal Blood Sugars*. His free monthly teleseminars are available at *AskDrBernstein.net*.

Chapter 8

FIGHT INFLUENZA AND PNEUMONIA

Boost Your Ability to Fight the Flu

With the outbreak of the H1N1 virus (commonly known as the swine flu) in 2009, most people relied solely on public health authorities for advice on the best ways to avoid infection.

While such recommendations can be helpful, there almost always are additional steps you can take to stay healthy when a highly contagious disease threatens large numbers of people.

Overlooked infection-fighting strategy: By enhancing your body's natural infection-fighting mechanisms (immunity), you often can avoid illness—even if you are exposed to infectious organisms that are making other people sick.

How Infections Begin

Bacteria and viruses are the main causes of potentially deadly infections. Whether bacterial or viral, these infections pass from person to person in much the same way—from people touching contaminated surfaces, through hand-to-hand contact or via coughs and/or sneezes. Hand-washing is the most widely recommended infection-control measure.

With the flu, antiviral medications can help prevent infection or at least lessen the severity of the infection, depending on the strain that has caused the illness. The antivirals *oseltamivir* (Tamiflu) and *zanamivir* (Relenza) have been shown in laboratory tests to shorten the duration of H1N1 symptoms by one to two days (when taken within 48 hours of the onset of symptoms).

As we all know, antibiotics are prescribed for bacterial infections—and should not be taken unnecessarily.

Reason: Antibiotics kill not only dangerous bacteria, but also friendly immune-boosting bacteria that help ward off dangerous bugs. Antibiotics are not effective against viral infections.

Robert Rountree, MD, physician in private practice and owner of Boulder Wellcare in Boulder, Colorado. He is co-author of numerous books, including *Immunotics: A Revolutionary Way to Fight Infection, Beat Chronic Illness and Stay Well* and *Clinical Natural Medical Handbook.* He also is medical editor of the journal *Alternative and Complementary Therapies* and a member of the advisory board for the Alternative Medicine Foundation, a nonprofit educational organization based in Washington, DC.

Simple Lifestyle Strategies

Our lifestyles play a critical role in whether our immune systems are able to fight off illness. Recommendations for reducing your infection risk...

•**Eat immune-boosting foods.** Blueberries and other berries (the darker, the better), purple grape juice and pomegranate juice are rich sources of plant-based compounds (phytochemicals) that boost the immune system.

Cruciferous vegetables contain sulforaphane, a compound with immunity-enhancing properties that help fight off infection.

Good sources of sulforaphane: Broccoli (especially BroccoSprouts, high-potency broccoli sprouts available at supermarkets and health-food stores)...cabbage...cauliflower...and Brussels sprouts. Aim to eat at least one serving of immune-boosting foods with every meal.

•**Get eight hours of sleep a night.** Lack of sleep has been shown to weaken the immune system—especially the activity of natural killer cells, a type of white blood cell thats key to preventing infection.

Supplements to Consider

Most health-conscious adults take a multivitamin to ensure that they are getting enough key nutrients. In addition, certain individual supplements (which can be taken indefinitely with your doctors approval) have important infection-fighting properties. *For example...*

•**Vitamin D.** Scientists have found that vitamin D helps protect against viral infections and stimulates the body to produce natural antibiotics.

Important: Studies now suggest that at least half of the people in northern latitudes (in the US, generally north of Atlanta) are vitamin D–deficient in the fall and winter, when the suns angle is too low to stimulate the body's natural production of vitamin D.

Advice: Take a daily supplement of 2,000 international units (IU) of vitamin D-3 (the most readily absorbed form). It's best to take this vitamin with food high in fat, such as milk or cheese, which also improves absorption.

After two to four months, ask your doctor to order a 25-hydroxy vitamin D blood test to see if the supplement is doing its job (a healthy blood level is 40 ng/mL to 50 ng/mL). If not, you may want to increase your daily dose of vitamin D-3.

•**Probiotics.** These "good bacteria" work in the gut to prime the immune system.

Advice: Look for a product that contains lactobacillus, acidophilus or bifidus and provides a total daily dose of 10 billion to 30 billion organisms (sometimes expressed as CFUs, or colony-forming units). Refrigerated probiotic supplements, which are sold in the supplement section of most health-food stores, are best—refrigeration helps preserve potency of the probiotics.

Also helpful: Certain products, such as the yogurt Activia and the drinks DanActive and Yakult, contain high amounts of probiotics.

•**Sulforaphane.** This antimicrobial compound found in cruciferous vegetables is believed to boost the immune system by replenishing nutrients in the dendritic cells in the membranes of the mouth, nose, bladder and gut. These cells bolster the body's first line of defense against invading microorganisms.

Animal studies also have shown that sulforaphane is very effective at ridding the body of toxins in our environment that dampen the immune response. Such toxins could include arsenic, *polychlorinated biphenyls* (PCBs) and bisphenol A (BPA), the chemical used in certain plastic water and beverage bottles and the lining of many food cans.

In addition to BroccoSprouts (described earlier), scientists at Johns Hopkins have now developed a tea called Brassica Tea—both products provide concentrated doses of sulforaphane. To learn more, visit the product website, *www.brassica.com* or call 410-732-1200.

Is It a Cold, Flu, Allergies...or Something Else?

Murray Grossan, MD, an otolaryngologist and head and neck surgeon with the Tower Ear, Nose and Throat Clinic at Cedars-Sinai Medical Center in Los Angeles and the founder of the Web-based Grossan Sinus & Health Institute. He is the author of *Free Yourself from Sinus and Allergy Problems Permanently. Grossan Institute.com*

Sniffling, sneezing and wiping your eyes? You might assume you have a cold...but not so fast. These symptoms also can come from the flu or allergies...from something that's similar to an allergy...and even from something else entirely—sinusitis!

Telling these five conditions apart can be tricky—even for doctors and for people who may have developed allergies later in life. *But knowing the difference is the key to getting the most effective treatment...*

Colds

Colds are caused by more than 100 different viruses. Your symptoms will depend on the specific virus you are infected with.

Telltale signs: In addition to common cold symptoms, such as sneezing, a sore throat, congestion and/or a cough, you may also have a low-grade fever, mild body aches and aching, swollen sinuses. Symptoms usually last a week or two.

My favorite cold remedies: Get into bed and rest. Also, have chicken soup and de-caffeinated green tea with lemon and honey. Chicken soup and green tea have anti-inflammatory properties that help fight infection. If you can, watch a funny movie. Research shows that laughing promotes healing. If you need help sleeping, try 25 mg to 50 mg of *diphenhydramine* (Benadryl).

For an immune-boosting herbal cough syrup: Mix one-half teaspoon each of cayenne pepper and freshly grated gingerroot... two tablespoons each of honey and apple cider vinegar...and four tablespoons of water. Take one teaspoon every few waking hours.

The Flu

The flu will make you feel awful.

Telltale signs: Symptoms can be the same as a cold, but you'll have significant body aches and probably a fever. Also, the flu comes on more suddenly than a cold.

My advice: Get a flu shot. If you still come down with the flu, stay home for at least 24 hours after any fever is gone so you won't spread the virus. Adults over age 65 and those with any chronic health problem should take an antiviral drug, such as *oseltamivir* (Tamiflu), to avoid flu complications, including pneumonia. Antivirals work best if taken within 48 hours of starting to feel sick.

Allergies

Allergic rhinitis (nasal allergy) is caused by a hypersensitive immune system that identifies an innocuous substance as harmful, then attacks it, causing symptoms.

Telltale signs: Nasal allergies can cause symptoms that are nearly indistinguishable from a cold—congestion, sneezing, red and runny eyes, scratchy throat, etc.—but allergies do not cause the mild fever or achiness of a cold. With seasonal allergies, you get symptoms from exposure to pollen (trees in spring, grass in summer and weeds in fall). Allergies to pet dander, dust, etc., tend to occur year-round.

Helpful: Use a diary to track your symptoms and the times they occur. It will help you distinguish allergies from other conditions.

My advice: Prescription nasal sprays, like *fluticasone propionate* (Flonase) or *azelastine* (Astelin), work for most people with less risk for side effects than antihistamine pills. Also, avoid spicy foods, which can worsen nasal allergies.

Nonallergic Rhinitis (Vasomotor Rhinitis)

This condition causes virtually the same symptoms as allergies, but it's not a true allergy that involves the immune system. Rather, it's triggered by specific irritants, such as certain odors, smoke and exhaust—or even changes in the weather.

Telltale signs: With nonallergic rhinitis, standard allergy medications fail to relieve symptoms, and allergy tests are negative. Post-nasal drip, an irritating flow of mucus down the back of the throat, tends to be worse with nonallergic rhinitis than with seasonal allergies.

My advice: Avoid irritants that you're sensitive to…and consider using the prescription drug *ipratropium bromide* (Atrovent), available as a nasal spray. It helps relax and open nasal passages. This drug can cause side effects, including dizziness, so use it only when needed and at the lowest dose possible.

Sinusitis

Sinusitis is tough to diagnose because it often occurs in conjunction with colds and allergies.

Reason: The excess mucus from congestion provides an optimal breeding ground for bacteria and viruses.

Telltale signs: Congestion with tenderness and a feeling of pressure around the eyes, cheeks or forehead. Also, when you blow your nose, the mucus will usually have a yellow or greenish color. Fever may be present as well. Symptoms can last for several weeks (acute) or even longer (chronic).

My advice: The prescription nasal sprays mentioned under "Allergies" help open the airways. *Acetaminophen* (Tylenol) or *naproxen* (Aleve) work for sinus pain. Bromelain (from pineapple) and papain (from papaya) also help reduce pain. Antibiotics are not always needed for acute sinusitis—a virus is sometimes the cause.

More from Dr. Grossan…

Natural Remedies for All Sinus Problems!

Nasal cilia (tiny, hairlike strands) help clear mucus from the nasal cavity. Slow-moving cilia can lead to nasal and sinus irritation and congestion. *To stimulate cilia…*

• **Hum.** It may sound far-fetched, but the vibrations from humming break up and thin accumulated mucus. Patients of mine who hum for a few minutes several times a day tend to get fewer sinus infections.

• **Keep the nose moist by using a preservative-free saline nasal spray such as Simply Saline,** available in drugstores. Avoid daily irrigation with a neti pot—the neti pot can easily get contaminated with bacteria, and irrigation can wash away protective elements in the nose.

• **Stay warm and drink hot tea.** Cold temperatures can slow the movement of nasal cilia, so wear a jacket, hat and scarf to keep warm. Additionally, avoid cold beverages and drink hot green or black tea—both contain L-theanine, an amino acid that increases ciliary activity. The excess fluid also will help thin and clear mucus, speeding recovery.

Beating the Flu Just Became Easier

William Schaffner, MD, professor of preventive medicine and infectious disease specialist, Vanderbilt University School of Medicine, Nashville. Dr. Schaffner is an associate editor of *The Journal of Infectious Diseases*.

Mention the subject of flu vaccination in a group discussion and at least one person will swear that he or she caught the flu from a flu shot. Sorry—that's not possible. But it is possible—and even expected—that some people will catch the flu despite getting vaccinated because their immune systems need more protection than what a regular flu vaccine can provide, and they may be exposed to a strain not covered by the vaccine. People age 65 and older are particularly vulnerable.

"Older people—those 65 and older—don't respond as strongly as younger people to any vaccine, including the flu vaccine, because their immune systems simply have become weaker from aging," said William Schaffner, MD, a professor of preventive medicine and infectious disease specialist at Vanderbilt University School of Medicine. But good news—getting stronger immunity to avoid the flu just became easier for older adults thanks to a new high-dose vaccine that packs more immune-producing antigens into the shot than standard-dose vaccines. The high-dose trivalent vaccine, which protects against three flu strains, became available a few years ago, and research is now showing that it really does deliver in terms of better protection against the flu for older adults.

More Vaccine, Better Protection

A two-year research study to track the effectiveness of the new high-dose flu vaccine involved 32,000 men and women age 65 and older. The study participants were randomly assigned to receive either the standard-dose trivalent vaccine or the high-dose trivalent vaccine.

After vaccination, the participants (who didn't know which vaccine they had received) were instructed to report any illness to the research team. Participants also received weekly or twice weekly phone calls from the researchers from the time they were vaccinated until the end of flu season in April. If a participant came down with flu-like symptoms, the research team took a cell swab from inside the nose to see whether the influenza virus was the cause.

At the study's end, researchers found that the high-dose vaccine was 24% more effective than the standard vaccine in preventing flu in these older adults. This means that among older people who get vaccinated, the new vaccine can keep an additional one-quarter of them from getting the flu. That's a lot of people!

Surprising Benefits of the Flu Vaccine

A review of six studies of more than 6,700 adults found that the flu vaccine lowered risk for heart attack, stroke, heart failure or death from any cardiac cause by 36%.

Theory: The vaccine may reduce flu-related inflammation that can make plaque in the arteries unstable and trigger a heart attack or other cardiac event. Violent coughing, elevated heart rate, pneumonia and other flu symptoms also may stress the heart.

Jacob A. Udell, MD, MPH, cardiologist, Women's College Hospital, University of Toronto, Canada.

"The extra protection did come with some extra 'ouch,' though," said Dr. Schaffner. There were slightly more sore arms and short-term fevers after the high-dose vaccine, as the higher dose kicks the immune system in the shorts more briskly!

Something to Consider

Among flu vaccines available in 2013 was a newly developed type with quadrivalent (four-strain) protection, though it was in scant supply. In 2014, more standard-dose vaccines offered quadrivalent protection. The high-dose vaccine, though, offered only trivalent protection because the manufacturer was unable to squeeze all the antigen needed for a high-dose quadrivalent vaccine into a syringe that won't terrify people with its size.

If you are 65 or older, you may be wondering whether you should get the standard-dose quadrivalent vaccine (for protection from four strains) or the high-dose trivalent vaccine (for extra-strong protection against three strains). Dr. Schaffner recommends the latter. "If you have a choice between the quadrivalent vaccine or the high-dose vaccine, opt for the high-dose vaccine. Although the quadrivalent vaccine has broader protection against flu strains, the high-dose vaccine has been proven, in the two-year study described, to provide more optimal protection against the flu in older people. The same kind of documented proof isn't yet available for the quadrivalent vaccine," he said.

If you are concerned about allergic reactions to the flu vaccine, development of a serious neurologic disorder called Guillain-Barré syndrome or the presence of a mercury-based preservative in some vaccines, put your mind at ease by reading the following article for important myth-busting information.

"Let's acknowledge that the flu vaccine is good but it's not perfect," said Dr. Schaffner. "It's the best protection we currently have." In 2013, the vaccine prevented between 50% and 60% of potential flu illnesses. The extra protection provided by the high-dose vaccine for people 65 and older boosts that number to 62% to 74%, and that's a very significant bonus. It may mean the difference between life and death for you or a loved one.

The Truth About Flu Shots

Fiona Havers, MD, medical epidemiologist at the influenza division, National Center for Immunization and Respiratory Diseases, Centers for Disease Control and Prevention in Atlanta, Georgia.

What's your take on flu shots? Are you dutiful about it, or do you take your chances and tough it out? Is it all about you, or do you consider the impact of viral illnesses and vaccination on the world at large? Are you afraid that you'll have a serious adverse reaction to the vaccine? Here, Fiona Havers, MD, a medical epidemiologist at the National Center for Immunization and Respiratory Diseases at the Centers for Disease Control and Prevention (CDC) in Atlanta fleshes out these concerns about the flu and the vaccine to see who should and who shouldn't get vaccinated…

Myth-Busting the Flu Vaccine

Commonly held misconceptions, according to research from the CDC, are that the vaccine is not safe, has dangerous side effects and gives you the flu. Other people believe that the vaccine doesn't work or that an annual flu shot is just not necessary.

The truth is, serious allergic reactions to flu vaccine can occur—but the truth also is that these reactions are extremely rare. What causes these rare reactions is not always known. The cause can be an allergic reaction to a preservative added to the vaccine to extend its shelf life, an antibiotic added to inhibit bacterial contamination or the material (eggs for most flu vaccines) that the virus for the vaccine is grown in. To help prevent severe allergic reactions, doctors are trained to examine and question patients to decide whether they may react badly to the vaccine and to have antidotes on hand should a bad reaction occur.

Another truth: Despite what many people think, an association between an uncommon neurologic disease called Guillain-Barré syndrome and currently available flu vaccines is unlikely. In Guillain-Barré syndrome, the immune system attacks the neuromuscular system, causing muscle weakness. The syndrome tends to develop after a person has had a respiratory infection or the flu. Most people recover, but some can have permanent nerve damage or even die, usually from breathing difficulties.

Although a bona-fide association was seen between Guillain-Barré syndrome and the swine flu vaccine of 1976, scientists are now questioning whether a link exists beyond that one year's vaccine. The latest research shows that a person is 17 times more likely to acquire Guillain-Barré syndrome after having the flu than after getting the flu vaccine.

As for whether the flu vaccine can give you the flu, the evidence strongly says no. Although it's true that people who get vaccinated can still get the flu—no one ever claimed that the vaccine is 100% effective—it isn't the vaccine that makes these people sick. Their immune systems might not be strong enough (even after vaccination) to fight off a flu virus they become exposed to—in which case they come down with a milder version of the flu than they would otherwise. Or else they may become infected with a flu strain that differs from that in the vaccine they received. With the introduction of a quadrivalent vaccine (which protects against four different flu strains) and a new high-dose trivalent vaccine (which packs stronger protection against three different flu strains), getting the flu after vaccination is becoming less and less likely.

Yes, you might have a sore arm after getting the flu shot, but what is that compared with days or weeks of being sick and possibly being hospitalized if you catch the flu?

As for fears about mercury-laced vaccines, most currently available vaccines either do not contain the mercury-containing preservative thimerosal or are available in two versions—one with and one without thimerosal.

The amount of thimerosal used in vaccines has been proved to be safe in people of all ages—including people with thimerosal allergies, who are simply more likely to have a sore arm after vaccination. Despite what many people think (and despite many heartbreaking personal anecdotes from parents whose children are autistic), there is no scientific evidence of a correlation between thimerosal in vaccines and autism or any health problem besides injection-site soreness. In any case, thimerosal-free vaccines have been made available to ease public concerns. You can request one from your doctor.

Because a shot in the arm might be traumatic, a nasal-spray vaccine, called FluMist, is also available, but it's not for everyone. You have to be healthy, not pregnant, have no respiratory problems (or allergies) and be between two and 49 years old. It's particularly effective in children and is mainly being made for them. Eligibility is limited because FluMist is the last-standing activated flu vaccine out there. Activated vaccines are made from live virus strains and are associated with more side effects—both mild (sore arms and mild, short-term flu-like symptoms) and severe (allergy-associated anaphylaxis, with estimated incidence of one in 500,000 vaccinations)—than inactivated vaccines.

Flu Vaccine Precautions

The CDC recommend that virtually everyone older than six months get the flu vaccine. Still, if you've had a bad allergic response to the flu vaccine in the past, discuss with your doctor whether any of the current vaccines would be safe for you—or if you need to avoid the vaccine altogether.

Also, because nearly all flu vaccines contain a small amount of egg as an ingredient, people with egg allergies need to proceed with caution when it comes to flu vaccines. They can't just walk into a local pharmacy for any free flu shot—but they may be able to be safely vaccinated depending on the severity of the allergy. Vaccination is, therefore, something that a person with an egg allergy needs to carefully discuss with his or her physician.

There is good news for some people with egg allergies, though. An egg-free vaccine called Flublok was recently approved by the FDA for people with egg allergies who are between the ages of 18 and 49. If you have an egg allergy, this is the vaccine to ask your doctor about. If it is right for you, the doctor may have it on hand or may have to order it for you.

Finally, if you come down with bronchitis or a "stomach flu" (which is usually not caused by the seasonal flu but another cause) just when you've decided to run out to get your flu shot, you should postpone getting vaccinated until you feel better. Mild head cold or sore throat is not a deterrent to vaccination.

Many different types of flu vaccines are now available. You can view a list of those approved for this year's flu season at the CDC website, *www.cdc.gov/*. The list includes information on precautions and whether and how much mercury and egg are in each vaccine.

If you are on the fence about getting a flu shot because of safety concerns about mercury content in a vaccine, an egg allergy or other personal medical condition or anything else, print out the CDC list and talk to your doctor about which flu vaccine is best for you.

Natural Flu Prevention: The 4-Point Plan

Leo Galland, MD, director of the Foundation for Integrated Medicine in New York City. He has held faculty positions at Rockefeller University, Albert Einstein College of Medicine of Yeshiva University and Stony Brook University. He specializes in the medicinal use of supplements and is the developer of the website *PillAdvised.com*, which discusses how to avoid dangerous interactions when combining medications with supplements.

When autumn's around the corner, most of us would rather think about the season's multihued foliage than the onset of influenza. But think about the flu we must...because this is when we need to begin preparing our bodies to fight it off, says Leo Galland, MD, founder and director of the Foundation for Integrated Medicine in New York City and creator of *www.PillAdvised.com*. Dr. Galland urges his patients to amp up their immune power starting early September.

Preseason Flu Fighters

There are easy ways to fortify your immune system before the various strains of flu start gathering strength. If you do this, you can greatly increase your ability to fight them off, said Dr. Galland. All of the following products are widely available in health-food stores, Whole Foods and the like...

• **N-acetyl-cysteine (NAC).** A metabolite of the amino acid cysteine, NAC not only helps the body fight flu, research shows that it also dramatically reduces symptoms in those who do fall prey. Italian researchers designed a study to weigh NAC's effectiveness at reducing flu symptoms in older people (65 and older). One group began taking NAC supplements three months before the start of flu season and continued throughout the winter months, while the other took no special precautions. The group taking NAC had symptoms that were, on average, 75% reduced compared with those who did not take NAC.

Other reasons NAC is helpful: It's an antioxidant and a precursor to glutathione, said to be the master antioxidant of all. Dr. Galland typically prescribes 1,500 mg of NAC daily, best taken between meals.

Caution: Pregnant or nursing women should not take NAC—and, if you take nitroglycerin, you may find that NAC magnifies its effects and also increases side effects, including headache. Check with your doctor.

• **Zinc and selenium.** These two minerals are immune system strengtheners and boost the protective antibody response to the flu vaccine. This is especially helpful for older adults, who are most likely to have low blood levels of zinc and/or selenium. Zinc and selenium supplements won't help you immediately, as it takes several months for your body to build up effective stores—so begin taking them early September, suggests Dr. Galland, who typically prescribes about 25 mg of zinc daily (with food to prevent nausea) and 100 mcg of selenium.

• **Vitamin D.** Most people don't connect the multipurpose vitamin D with flu resistance, but there is growing evidence that people with healthy vitamin D levels get fewer colds and cases of flu. In fact, some experts speculate that the relative lack of sunshine in

---

Flu-Fighting Electrolyte Punch

Store-bought electrolyte drinks, such as Gatorade and Pedialyte, are full of artificial flavors. To fight dehydration, try this homemade recipe—blend in a blender two cups of filtered water...one-half cup of fresh orange juice...one-half cup of fresh lemon juice...one-eighth teaspoon of sea salt...and two to four tablespoons of organic raw honey.

Mark Stengler, NMD, naturopathic medical doctor and founder of Stengler Center for Integrative Medicine, Encinitas, California. He has served on a medical advisory committee for the Yale University Complementary Medicine Outcomes Research Project and has been an associate clinical professor at the National College of Naturopathic Medicine in Portland, Oregon. He is coauthor of *The Natural Physician's Healing Therapies*. MyBottomLine.com

winter and our bodies' resulting diminished levels of vitamin D contribute to the season's numerous respiratory ailments. So, as the sun's path sinks low in the sky—which is starting right about now—begin to buttress your vitamin D levels by taking 1,000 IU to 2,000 IU of vitamin D-3 (avoid D-2) daily.

Caution: Consult your doctor first if you take *digoxin* (Digitek) for congestive heart failure.

• **Black elderberry.** In the herbal category, Dr. Galland suggests purchasing black elderberry capsules or syrup to have at the ready if and when you begin feeling poorly. These contain flavonoids, including anthocyanins, that can bolster immunity and keep viruses from effectively implanting in mucous membranes.

Dr. Galland says it's not known for sure whether black elderberry helps prevent flu, but it will help reduce symptoms if you do get sick. He usually tells patients to take 750-mg supplements twice daily with food. If you use the syrup, check the label for dosage.

Tried and True Flu Fighters

Dr. Galland also recommends these time-tested, scientifically proven flu-fighting strategies…

• **Frequent hand washing**—one of the most effective ways we know to prevent flu. Carry and use portable hand sanitizer when you're out in communal facilities that might lack easy restroom access (such as public transportation, houses of worship, supermarkets or parks).

• **Regular exercise, but not too much**—a moderate amount of exercise, 30 minutes a day, boosts immunity, while high-intensity exercise (90 minutes a day or more) actually suppresses it.

• **A good night's rest**—research shows that about seven hours of sleep each night increases immunity.

• **Reduced sugar, alcohol and fat in your diet**—all are believed to have negative effects on immunity.

Whether or not you should be vaccinated with the flu shot is a topic to discuss with your doctor, but in the meantime, you can get started on Dr. Galland's four flu-fighting strategies as described above.

All Pregnant Women Need the Flu Shot

Laura Riley, MD, chair, Immunization Expert Work Group, American College of Obstetricians and Gynecologists, Washington, DC.

American College of Obstetricians and Gynecologists, news release.

A group representing U.S. obstetricians is calling for all pregnant women to get a flu shot.

According to the American College of Obstetricians and Gynecologists (ACOG), several studies released in recent years have upheld the safety and effectiveness of flu vaccination during pregnancy.

"The flu virus is highly infectious and can be particularly dangerous to pregnant women, as it can cause pneumonia, premature labor, and other complications," said Laura Riley, MD, chair of the college's Immunization Expert Work Group.

When to Get the Flu Shot

"Vaccination every year, early in the season and regardless of the stage of pregnancy, is the best line of defense," Dr. Riley advised.

The best time to get vaccinated is early in the flu season, regardless of the stage of pregnancy, the guidelines state. However, pregnant women can get a flu shot at any time during flu season, which typically lasts from October to May.

Get the Inactived Vaccine

All women who are or become pregnant during the flu season should get the inactivated flu vaccine, which is also safe for women who have just given birth and those who are breast-feeding. However, pregnant women should not be given the live attenuated version of the flu vaccine (the nasal mist), according to the guidelines.

The guidelines appeared in the journal *Obstetrics & Gynecology*.

Flu Shot Protects Baby Too

Flu shots not only protect pregnant women, but their infants as well. Babies can't be given flu vaccine until they are 6 months old, but receive flu antibodies from their vaccinated mother while in the womb. This provides them with protection until they can be vaccinated directly.

Before the 2009 H1N1 swine flu pandemic, flu vaccination rates for pregnant women were only 15%. That rose to 50% in the 2009-2010 flu season and has been around that mark every flu season since. However, vaccination rates could and should be even higher, according to ACOG.

For more information about pregnancy and the flu vaccination, visit the Web site of the U.S. Centers for Disease Control and Prevention, *cdc.gov*. Search "pregnancy and flu."

Why Pregnant Women Get Sicker From Flu

Catherine Blish, MD, PhD, assistant professor of medicine—infectious diseases, Stanford University School of Medicine, California.

Alexander Kay, MD, instructor in pediatric infectious diseases, Stanford University School of Medicine, California.

Stanford University School of Medicine, Lucile Packard Children's Hospital, Stanford, news release.

Pregnant women appear to have an unusually strong immune response to the flu, according to a new study.

And this strong immune response may help explain why pregnant women get sicker from the flu than other healthy adults.

The reason: Many symptoms of flu are the result of the immune system responding to the virus, the researchers said.

This finding was unexpected because it's generally believed that pregnancy weakens the immune system to keep it from attacking the growing fetus, according to researchers from the Stanford University School of Medicine and Lucile Packard Children's Hospital, Stanford.

"We were surprised by the overall finding," said the study's senior author, Catherine Blish, MD, PhD, assistant professor of medicine—infectious diseases, at Stanford University School of Medicine. "We now understand that severe influenza in pregnancy is a hyperinflammatory disease rather than a state of immunodeficiency."

The Study

In conducting the study, the researchers examined the reactions of immune cells taken from 21 pregnant women and 29 healthy women who weren't pregnant. The cells were taken from samples of the women's blood before and seven days after they received a flu shot. The researchers also tested cells taken from pregnant women six weeks after their baby was born.

In a lab, the women's cells were exposed to two flu viruses: the H1N1 strain that caused the 2009 pandemic and a strain of the seasonal flu, known as H3N2.

The researchers found pregnancy heightened the immune response of two different types of white blood cells (natural killer and T cells) to both strains of the flu. These cells produced more cytokines and chemokines, which are molecules that help attract other immune cells to an infection site, the study authors explained.

The study was published in the *Proceedings of the National Academy of Sciences*.

Implications

"If the chemokine levels are too high, that can bring in too many immune cells," Dr. Blish explained. "That's a bad thing in a lung where you need air space." Getting the flu while pregnant increases women's risk for pneumonia and death, she said.

Although pregnant women with the flu are usually treated with drugs to slow the

Fist Bump for Fewer Germs

To cut down on the spread of germs, greet friends with a fist bump.

Why: In a study, researchers wearing gloves dipped in bacteria transferred 10 times more germs while shaking hands than when they used the knuckle greeting. Other microorganisms, such as cold and flu viruses, are also spread this way.

Reason: A handshake lasts longer than a fist bump, and more surface area of the hand is touched.

David Whitworth, PhD, senior lecturer, Institute of Biological, Environmental and Rural Sciences, Aberystwyth University, Wales, UK.

replication of the virus inside their bodies, the study's authors suggested their findings could lead to improved treatments for these women.

"If our finding ends up bearing out in future studies, it opens the possibility that we can develop new immune-modulating treatment approaches in the setting of severe influenza, especially in pregnant women," concluded the study's lead author, Alexander Kay, MD, instructor in pediatric infectious diseases at Stanford University School of Medicine.

Although the study revealed that pregnant women's immune cells have a greater response to the flu, it remains unclear if these immune cells would have a similar response to other viruses.

"I suspect this is peculiar to influenza for a variety of reasons. I wonder if this is an inflammatory pathway that is normally activated later in pregnancy to prepare the body for birth, but that flu happens to overlap with the pathway and aberrantly activates it too early," Dr. Blish suggested.

Important

The study's authors said they hoped their findings would remind women about the importance of getting an annual flu shot. "Flu vaccination is very important to avoid this in-

flammatory response we're seeing," Dr. Kay pointed out. "But only 50% of pregnant women are currently vaccinated for influenza."

The U.S. Centers for Disease Control and Prevention provides more information on the flu in pregnant women, at *cdc.gov*. Search "pregnancy and flu."

Should You Take an Antiviral for the Flu?

Fiona Havers, MD, medical epidemiologist at the influenza division, National Center for Immunization and Respiratory Diseases, Centers for Disease Control and Prevention in Atlanta, Georgia. Her study appeared in *Clinical Infectious Diseases*.

O ops—score one for people who don't think very highly of flu vaccinations. Every year, the World Health Organization and the FDA try to predict which three or four strains of flu virus will be most prevalent in the next flu season, and vaccines are made to target those strains. But in the 2014-2015 flu season, one of the strains mutated, which meant that if you had been vaccinated against the flu, you were not as well-protected against it as you thought. The flu vaccine can help protect you against the flu and, overall, it significantly reduces the number of people who land in the hospital or die during annual flu outbreaks, but it isn't a guarantee of protection.

What is your best line of defense if you get the flu, particularly if you have a health condition that puts you at risk for a severe infection or complications?

The good news first: There are two readily available prescription antiviral drugs that can help tamp down flu symptoms and shorten the time you spend being sick. They are *oseltamivir* (Tamiflu) and *zanamivir* (Relenza).

Now for the bad news: Too many doctors are failing to prescribe these antiviral medications to those who can really benefit from them. In fact, the CDC reported that, in seasons past, many doctors were not properly treating patients with serious flu symptoms. The CDC caught them red-handed in a study that looked at prescribing practices during the 2012 to 2013 flu season. The study, headed by Fiona Havers, MD, a medical epidemiologist at the CDC's National Center for Immunization and Respiratory Diseases in Atlanta, looked at prescriptions of 6,766 patients given a diagnosis of "acute respiratory illness"—that is, a serious lung infection that can land you in the hospital. Although many of the patients could have benefited from an antiviral because they probably had the flu, only 8% were given a prescription for one. When the study's researchers looked at patients who were at high risk for deadly flu complications because they were very young or old or had more than one chronic illness, they discovered that only 19% of them were given a prescription for an antiviral.

And—you aren't going to like this—when researchers looked at patients whose lab tests positively confirmed that they had the flu, they saw that an antiviral was prescribed to only 15% of these people…and instead of an antiviral, patients were often prescribed an antibiotic.

It means that doctors are missing opportunities to improve health care for high-risk patients who have the flu and could benefit from antiviral treatment, said Dr. Havers… while giving them antibiotics, which are generally useless for the flu!

Antiviral drugs can lessen symptoms and shorten the time you are sick by up to two days, she said. More importantly, these drugs can prevent serious complications, such as pneumonia. For some people, namely those with medical conditions such as heart and lung diseases, treatment with an antiviral drug can mean the difference between having a mild illness and a very serious one that could result in a hospital stay. The CDC recommends prompt treatment with antivirals primarily for these high-risk people.

What to Do If You Get the Flu

If you feel flu symptoms coming on, time is of the essence. If you are in the high-risk category (if you have heart or lung disease or another chronic illness), get to your doctor for antiviral treatment as soon as possible, Dr. Havers said. If you are not in the high-risk zone and want to lessen the impact of flu symptoms, you can still be prescribed an antiviral, although there is disagreement among medical researchers about whether antivirals really make that big a difference in lessening flu symptoms in otherwise healthy people.

If you do have an interest in taking an antiviral for the flu, you will need to get to your doctor for a prescription within 48 hours of feeling sick. That is when an antiviral will be most effective, said Dr. Havers. The usual length of treatment is five days. Flu antivirals can have side effects, including nausea, vomiting, diarrhea and headache. The gastrointestinal effects can be reduced if the antiviral is taken with food, said Dr. Havers.

Whereas Tamiflu is approved for people as young as two weeks old, Relenza is recommended for treatment of adults and for children who are seven years or older. It is given via an inhaler, though, and should not be used by people who have breathing problems, such as asthma.

The CDC has issued an alert to doctors that they should get on the ball and prescribe these antivirals to those who need them to dampen the effects of a mutated flu virus. If you visit your doctor with flu symptoms and he or she wants to hand you a prescription for an antibiotic, be sure to thoroughly question the doctor about why.

Tenacious Flu Virus

Flu virus can survive on your fingers for up to 30 minutes. Even though most flu germs are transmitted through airborne droplets when people sneeze, cough or talk, they also are transmitted if your fingers come in contact with the virus and you touch your eyes, nose or mouth.

Self-defense: Wash your hands often with soap and water or use a hand sanitizer, and avoid touching your face.

Study by researchers at University Hospitals of Geneva, Kantonales Laboratorium, Basel, and Federal Office of Public Health, Bern, Switzerland, published in *Clinical Microbiology and Infection*.

Don't Catch Pneumonia from Your Dentures

Study titled "Denture wearing during sleep doubles the risk of pneumonia in the very elderly," published in *Journal of Dental Research*.

Could you be giving yourself pneumonia because of some innocent thing that you do each and every night? A new study from Japan says that's exactly what may be happening to denture wearers around the globe. *Here's what everyone who wears dentures needs to know...*

What Not to Wear to Bed

The Japanese study included 524 men and women who ranged in age from 85 to 102. At the beginning of the study, each participant had a dental exam and a face-to-face interview to answer questions about his or her general and oral health. The participants who wore dentures were also asked questions such as how and how often they cleaned their dentures. And they were asked if they wore their dentures to bed.

Over the course of the next three years, 20 of the participants died of pneumonia. Another 28 were hospitalized with pneumonia but eventually recovered. When the researchers analyzed the data, they found that factors associated with increased risk of pneumonia included difficulty swallowing, cognitive impairment and whether the person had ever had a stroke or a serious or chronic respiratory disease...and whether he or she wore dentures to bed.

Sleeping with dentures was the only risk factor directly related to behavior. In fact, people who wore dentures to bed had double the risk of pneumonia of those who removed their dentures at night.

People who slept wearing dentures also tended to clean their dentures less frequently. As you can guess, bacteria can easily congregate on dentures. When it does, a bacterial film forms—similar to the layer of soap scum that accumulates in a bathtub that doesn't get cleaned. Eventually, the bacteria find their way from a person's mouth to the throat. From there, the organisms can be inhaled (aspirated) into the lungs—and this is what the researchers think is happening among people who sleep wearing dentures.

A Variety of Flu Vaccines

In the US, flu vaccines are available from six different manufacturers. These vaccines all have specific indications for who can get them. For example, there is a high-dose flu vaccine that is designed specifically for people who are age 65 and older. Older people's immune responses to vaccination tend to be weaker than those of younger people. The high-dose flu vaccine contains four times the amount of antigen (the part of the vaccine that prompts the body to make an antibody response) contained in regular flu shots. The additional antigen is intended to create a stronger immune response (more antibody) in the person getting the vaccine.

Even though older adults may benefit from the high-dose vaccine, the type of flu vaccine that's used is less important than simply getting vaccinated—with your doctor's OK, of course. A nasal flu vaccine is also available but not recommended for adults over age 49.

Benjamin N. Haynes, senior press officer, infectious disease team, Centers for Disease Control and Prevention, Atlanta.

Pneumonia Increases Heart Disease Risk That Can Last for Years

Pneumonia increases heart disease risk, including stroke and heart attack. That risk rises fourfold in the first month after pneumonia and stays elevated—one-and-half-times higher than normal—for several additional years in older adults. Researchers are currently looking into the possibility that aspirin or statins may lower risk by reducing persistent inflammation in the bloodstream.

Sachin Yende, MD, vice president of critical care at VA Pittsburgh and program director of the clinical epidemiology program, CRISMA Center, University of Pittsburgh. He led a study of data on almost 22,000 patients, published in *Journal of the American Medical Association*.

Good Denture Hygeine and Sleep

But is the problem wearing dentures to sleep or wearing dirty dentures to sleep? Some American dentists think that sleeptime denture-wearing helps prevent sleep apnea because it helps keep the airways open. Rather than dentures, though, the American Academy of Dental Sleep Medicine recommends that people with sleep apnea be fitted for an oral appliance specifically made to be worn at night and designed to prevent sleep apnea. You can find dentists certified in dental sleep medicine in your area through the Academy.

If you wear dentures (full or partial) or know someone who does and are concerned about health risks of sleeping with dentures—or health risks of sleeping without them—talk to your dentist. Most importantly, especially if you choose not to remove them while sleeping, make sure to keep them clean, as suggested in the Japanese study, by washing them daily in peroxide-based cleaner, such as Polident.

Seniors Should Get Two Pneumonia Shots

Seniors should get two different pneumonia vaccines for optimal protection. People age 65 and older who have never been immunized against pneumonia should get the newly recommended Prevnar 13 shot first, followed by a Pneumovax 23 shot six to 12 months later. Seniors who have already received Pneumovax 23—which has been recommended for several years—should ask their doctors about Prevnar 13.

For more information on pneumococcal vaccine, visit the U.S. Centers for Disease Control and Prevention at *www.cdc.go*v

E. Neil Schachter, MD, professor of medicine and medical director of the respiratory-care department, Icahn School of Medicine at Mount Sinai, New York City, and author of *The Good Doctor's Guide to Colds & Flu*.

Bird Flu Alert

As of June 2015, 10% of the US poultry supply (encompassing 16 states) has been affected by avian flu strains, according to the Centers for Disease Control and Prevention. Should you be concerned about eating poultry or eggs?

No. You cannot get avian flu from eating poultry or eggs. Bird flu is transferred through respiratory secretions or bird droppings, so to contract the virus, you typically need to have come in close contact with live poultry infected with avian flu.

William Schaffner, MD, professor of preventive medicine, department of health policy, and professor of medicine, Division of Infectious Diseases at Vanderbilt University School of Medicine, Nashville.

Recover Fast from Stomach "Flu"

Jamison Starbuck, ND, naturopathic physician in family practice and a guest lecturer at the University of Montana, both in Missoula. She is past president of the American Association of Naturopathic Physicians and a contributing editor to *The Alternative Advisor: The Complete Guide to Natural Therapies and Alternative Treatments.*

Though commonly known as the "stomach flu," this short-lived gastrointestinal (GI) bug is technically gastroenteritis, a medical term meaning inflammation of the stomach and intestines. It can be caused by bacteria, parasites or a virus—which are spread by human contact as well as contaminated food or water. One of its most common causes, norovirus, is often spread when you use a doorknob, for example, that has been touched by someone with the virus on his/her hands, and you then put your fingers (or food you touch) in your mouth. The symptoms of gastroenteritis are well known—nausea, diarrhea, loss of appetite, sometimes vomiting and a mild (99-degree) fever. *How to reduce the severity and duration of your misery…**

• **Stick to clear fluids.** At the first sign of gastroenteritis (typically diarrhea), have only chicken, beef or vegetable broth, herbal tea, diluted fruit juice, ginger ale, club soda and water. Consume these liquids cold, hot or at room temperature—whatever feels most soothing. Avoiding solid foods will reduce both diarrhea and nausea and give your GI tract time to recuperate. When nausea and diarrhea are gone, ease back into eating solid foods with rice, steamed veggies and/or three ounces of chicken or fish.

• **Take a good probiotic.** I recommend a powdered formula containing 3 billion colony forming units (CFUs) of Lactobacillus acidophilus and Bifidobacterium, taken three times a day. If your probiotic comes in a capsule, open it and dissolve the powder it contains directly in your mouth or in only two ounces of water to avoid the vomiting that can accompany gastroenteritis.

• **Consider chamomile.** Lots of herbal teas—such as cinnamon, ginger, chamomile, lemon balm, peppermint and spearmint—soothe nausea and diarrhea. However, I prefer chamomile because it also kills microorganisms, decreases inflammation and reduces intestinal gas. For gastroenteritis, I suggest drinking 32 to 48 ounces of chamomile tea daily. People who are allergic to plants in the daisy family—daisy, ragweed, marigold, chrysanthemum—should avoid chamomile.

• **Use natural antiseptics.** Two natural antiseptics can speed your body's process of shedding an unwanted stomach bug. Oregon graperoot is an antimicrobial, and activated charcoal binds to microorganisms so they can be eliminated via the stool. Use these medicines separately, or the charcoal will also sweep the Oregon graperoot out of your body.

My advice: Take one-eighth teaspoon of Oregon graperoot tincture in four ounces water, followed two hours later by two charcoal capsules, opened and mixed with four ounces of water. Do this until you get four doses of each medicine in 24 hours. Consult a pediatrician before giving Oregon graperoot and/or activated charcoal to children.

*If you are frail, elderly or have a compromised immune system…or if vomiting or diarrhea lasts more than 48 hours, see your physician.

Chapter 9

REMEDIES FOR KIDNEY, BLADDER AND LIVER DISEASE

Protect Your Kidneys Before It's Too Late

Imagine this: You've just had a routine checkup, and your doctor gives you some surprising news. Your blood and urine tests show that you've got chronic kidney disease (CKD). How could that be? You feel fine.

What most people don't realize: Kidney disease can be "silent" and often sneaks up on you. Nine out of 10 people who already have early-stage CKD don't realize it, and as a result, they aren't taking the necessary steps to protect their kidneys.

Are You At Risk?

Our kidneys naturally lose some function as we age. If you are 60 or older, there's a one-in-four chance that you already have CKD—though you may not know it.

You're also at increased risk for this disease if you have high blood pressure, diabetes or a family history of CKD (in a first-degree relative such as a parent or sibling).

With the right tests (see list at the end of this article), it's relatively easy to find out if you have CKD. But once your kidneys are damaged, you won't be able to reverse the damage. The goal is to not develop the disease or slow its progression.

Protect Your Kidneys

Whether you're trying to avoid CKD or prevent it from worsening, the best way to protect your kidney function is to control your blood sugar (crucial if you have diabetes), blood pressure and cholesterol levels, and to avoid smoking.

Other promising new approaches…

• **Watch out for sleep apnea.** Researchers have found that sleep apnea is associated with increased protein levels in the urine (an indicator of CKD). For this reason, sleep apnea is now considered an independent risk factor for CKD—and it may cause the disease to progress in people who already have it.

My advice: If you have sleep apnea, be sure to get your kidney function tested. Similarly, if you know you have CKD, you may also have sleep apnea, especially if you snore or sleep restlessly. Get tested.

Mildred Lam, MD, professor of medicine at Case Western Reserve University School of Medicine and a nephrologist at MetroHealth Medical Center, both in Cleveland. Dr. Lam's clinical interests include acute and chronic kidney disease, hypertension and dialysis.

If you're diagnosed with sleep apnea, be vigilant about wearing your continuous positive airway pressure (CPAP) mask—the preferred treatment for this condition—while sleeping. Getting the proper amount of oxygen at night will help maintain your kidney function.

• **Keep an eye on your diet.** At one time, salt was the only potential dietary danger for anyone concerned about kidney health. People with CKD, especially those who also have high blood pressure, are still urged to follow a "no-salt-added" diet—that is, avoiding salty foods, such as canned soups, chips and lunch meats, and not adding salt to food when cooking or eating.

Other dietary advice…

• **Eat more vegetable protein (instead of animal protein).** Eating large amounts of any kind of protein can tax the kidneys. But when you do eat protein, vegetable protein—found in such foods as soybeans, legumes, nuts and quinoa—is healthier because it generally contains fewer calories, less saturated fat, less sodium and less acid than meat protein.

• **Avoid soft drinks.** High amounts of sugar (glucose) in your blood—a given with sugary soft drinks—will stress your kidneys. According to a recent Japanese study, consuming at least two soft drinks per day may increase protein levels in the urine and, in turn, one's risk for CKD. If you're at increased risk or already have CKD, it's safest to drink water and avoid sugary soft drinks, especially if you have diabetes.

• **Use caution with painkillers.** Long-term use (more than 10 consecutive days) of nonsteroidal anti-inflammatory drugs (NSAIDs), such as *ibuprofen* (Motrin) or *naproxen* (Aleve), can harm the kidneys. If you're a frequent NSAID user, be sure that your doctor tests your kidney function routinely.

If you know that you have CKD, take an NSAID only if pain is severe and for no more than three to five consecutive days…or talk to your doctor about pain relievers that may be safer to take such as *acetaminophen* (Tylenol). Additionally, recent research has found that when an NSAID is combined with blood pressure drugs—an ACE inhibitor or angiotensin receptor blocker (ARB) and a diuretic ("water pill")—it may create a "triple threat" that can cause acute kidney injury, further damaging the kidneys.

My advice: People who are concerned about their kidney health or who already have CKD should always ask a doctor before taking any new drug—even if it's over-the-counter.

Also: Many supplements (such as potassium) and herbs (including periwinkle and aloe) can cause harm in people with kidney disease. Before taking any dietary supplement, consult your doctor—especially if you have CKD.

The Tests You Need

If you are over age 40, you should have annual urine and blood tests to monitor your kidneys. People with diabetes or other chronic conditions should start sooner, and may need to be tested more often. *What needs to be checked…*

• **Albumin.** If this protein appears in your urine, it can be a sign of early kidney disease. Urine microalbumin/creatinine ratio (a very sensitive indicator of early kidney damage) should be less than 30 mg/g. Urine protein/creatinine ratio should be less than 150 mg/g.

• **Creatinine.** If your blood level of creatinine (a waste product filtered by the kidneys) is higher than 1.2 for women or 1.4 for men, you may have chronic kidney disease (CKD).

Your doctor may refer you to a nephrologist (kidney specialist) for more blood and urine tests and a renal ultrasound to check for kidney scarring or other conditions, such as kidney stones or a tumor.

• **Estimated glomerular filtration rate (eGFR). Your creatinine result can also be calculated in a formula that includes your age,** weight, race and sex to determine your eGFR, which indicates how well your kidneys are filtering blood and getting rid of waste. A normal reading for eGFR ranges from 90 ml/min to 130 ml/min, with no protein in the urine. A reading of 60 to 89 may indicate a mild decrease in kidney function. Many people are diagnosed with CKD at stage 3 (an eGFR of 30 to 59), which is considered "moderate."

A Recent Blood Test Shows High Creatinine... What to Do

Joseph Kellerstein, ND, naturopathic physician in private practice in Toronto and Oshawa, Ontario, Canada. *DrJoeND.com*

A high creatinine level (over 1.1 mg/dL for women) means that your kidneys aren't functioning as well as they should. You need an evaluation from a kidney specialist (nephrologist).

Meanwhile, because creatinine is a substance that is formed when food is metabolized, eating certain foods and avoiding others may lower creatinine levels and reduce stress on the kidneys—improving kidney function. For example, to reduce creatinine, minimize your intake of animal proteins (meat, poultry and fish) and eat lots of vegetables.

Drinking a cup or two of nettle leaf tea each day also can help flush creatinine from the body, but check first with your doctor if you take medication or have a chronic condition. Chitosan supplements (avoid these if you're allergic to shellfish) also can reduce creatinine levels. Follow label instructions. But make sure you see a nephrologist!

Revisit Metformin

For diabetes patients with kidney disease, the benefits of metformin may outweigh the risks. The drug metformin is very effective for type 2 diabetes, but an FDA label dating to 1994 restricts its use in patients with kidney problems. Recent evidence now shows that metformin is safe for patients with mild-to-moderate kidney disease.

Remedies for Kidney, Bladder and Liver Disease

James H. Flory, MD, MSCE, fellow in endocrinology at Weill Cornell Medical College, New York City.

A Walk Does Wonders for Chronic Kidney Disease

Che-Yi Chou, MD, PhD, Kidney Institute, division of nephrology, department of internal medicine, both at China Medical University Hospital, Taiwan. Dr. Chou's study appeared in the *Clinical Journal of the American Society of Nephrology*.

I f you have chronic kidney disease (CKD), there is a stone simple way that you might save yourself from needing dialysis or a kidney transplant. CKD, a condition in which the kidneys struggle to filter waste from the blood, is a silent health threat that you can be completely unaware of until serious damage is done. One in three adults with diabetes and one in five with high blood pressure has CKD, and like so many illnesses, incidence increases after age 50. If left unchecked, end-stage renal disease—kidney failure—occurs. That's when you'll need to be hooked up to a dialysis machine to filter your blood or will require a kidney transplant to stay alive.

Although there is no cure once CKD sets in, it can often be kept from advancing, and now doctors have confirmed that a certain simple exercise can not only help you avoid dialysis or transplantation but also add years to your life. And that exercise is...walking! *Here's what to do...*

A Proven Benefit

We all know that exercise improves cardiovascular fitness, and researchers had already confirmed that it improves fitness in people with CKD. But could walking actually help with the disease itself—and in a significant way? That question had never been tested by research...so a group of Taiwanese researchers decided to find out.

The study started out with 6,363 patients whose average age was 70. All had moderate to severe CKD, and 53% had CKD severe enough to need dialysis or a kidney transplant. The researchers recorded and monitored exercise activity and a range of other health and medical measurements in the group and identified 1,341 people who walked as their favorite form of exercise. These patients were compared with patients who did not walk nor exercise in any other way.

The results: Walkers were 33% less likely to die of kidney disease and 21% less likely to need dialysis or a kidney transplant than nonwalkers/nonexercisers. And the more a person walked, the more likely he or she was not on dialysis or in need of a kidney transplant and still alive when the study ended. So, for example, someone who walked once or twice a week for an average 30 minutes to an hour had a 17% lower risk of death and a 19% lower risk of needing dialysis or a kidney transplant compared with someone who didn't walk or exercise. And someone who walked for an average 30 minutes to an hour seven or more times a week had a 59% lower risk of death and a 44% lower risk of needing dialysis or a kidney transplant.

Now, when researchers see this kind of dramatic result, they always should explore whether there was some reason other than the activity that was studied (in this case, walking) that could explain things. These are called confounding factors—for example, could it be that walkers walked because they were healthier, as opposed to being healthier because they walked? But no confounding factors were found. The average age, average body size and degree of kidney disease was the same in the two groups, as was the prevalence of diabetes-associated coronary artery disease, cigarette smoking and use of medications for CKD.

The bottom line for people with CKD... walk! Walk everywhere! Walk often! Even a 30-minute walk once or twice a week can help. The more you walk, the greater the benefit.

Are You At Risk?

If you have diabetes or high blood pressure, your doctor should give you a simple blood test to see whether CKD is developing. Otherwise, here are telltale signs to keep an eye out for—these may signal that you should be evaluated for CKD...

- **Unexplained fatigue**
- **Trouble concentrating**
- **Poor appetite**
- **Trouble sleeping**
- **Nighttime muscle cramps**
- **Swollen feet and ankles**
- **Eye puffiness, especially in the morning**
- **Dry, itchy skin**
- **Frequent urination, especially at night**

Be sure to tell your doctor what medications you're on when you are examined for CKD. Because the kidneys also filter medications out of your body, meds can build up to toxic levels in your system if the kidneys aren't doing their job. If you have CKD, your doctor may take you off some medications and lower the dose of others.

While there's no cure for CKD once it sets in, it need not advance to severe and deadly stages that require dialysis or a kidney transplant. Besides exercising and keeping the underlying cause (whether it be diabetes, high blood pressure or something else) in check, mild CKD is managed by diet. *To do it right...*

- **Make walking a priority.**
- **Work with your doctor to manage the underlying cause,** and work with a dietitian to manage your nutrition requirements. A dietitian will plan a regimen that controls the amount of protein, salt, potassium and phosphorus you consume, all of which can build up to toxic levels in people with CKD. A dietitian will also balance your CKD diet needs with those related to glucose control or whatever condition may be associated with your CKD.

Older Women Have Less Access to Kidney Transplants

Despite comparable risks and survival rates, women over age 55 are 15% less likely to be referred to a waiting list for a kidney transplant than men of the same age...the disparity rises to 59% in women over 75.

Best: If you are approaching kidney failure, insist that your doctor refer you for a transplant.

Dorry Segev, MD, PhD, director of clinical research, transplant surgery, Johns Hopkins Medicine, Baltimore, and lead author of a study of 563,197 patients, published in *Journal of the American Society of Nephrology.*

This Urine Test Could Save Your Life

David L. Katz, MD, MPH, internist and preventive medicine specialist. He is cofounder and director of the Yale-Griffin Prevention Research Center in Derby, Connecticut, and clinical instructor at the Yale School of Medicine in New Haven, Connecticut. Dr. Katz is also president of the American College of Lifestyle Medicine and the author of *Disease-Proof: The Remarkable Truth About What Makes Us Well.*

Why this test? It helps evaluate the functioning of your kidneys.*

The prop you'll need: A clear plastic cup or clean, disposable clear jar.

What to do: In the middle of the day (urine will be too concentrated if you do this first thing in the morning), urinate into the cup or jar until you have caught at least an inch of urine. Throughout the day, note how often you urinate (about once every three waking hours is typical).

Watch out: The urine should be a pale, straw color—not deep yellow, brown or pinkish. Urine that's discolored could indi-

*This self-test is not a substitute for a thorough physical exam from your doctor. Use this only as a way to identify potential problem areas to discuss with your physician.

Blood Pressure Alert

According to recent research, one in 12 adults age 65 and older who began taking thiazide diuretics for high blood pressure had adverse effects, such as low levels of sodium and/or potassium and decreased kidney function.

Upshot: Older adults need to be monitored with a metabolic blood test within a month of starting thiazide diuretics. In some cases, a potassium supplement may be prescribed.

Anil N. Makam, MD, assistant professor of medicine, The University of Texas Southwestern Medical Center, Dallas.

cate dehydration, abnormal kidney function or another health problem.

Next, smell the urine. It should have nothing more than a very faint urine odor (unless you recently ate asparagus).

Beware: While dark-colored or smelly urine could simply mean that you are dehydrated, there are too many other potentially serious causes to ignore the signs.

Some of the disorders that can affect urine include...

• **Kidney or bladder infection, which can cause discolored urine and frequent urination.**

• **Kidney disease, which can cause smelly, discolored urine.** Interestingly, both too frequent urination and infrequent urination are signs of kidney disease.

• **Diabetes or enlarged prostate, which can cause frequent urination.**

Poor Kidney Function Linked to Cancer

A large-scale study involving nearly 1.2 million adults found that even mild kidney disease can increase kidney cancer risk by up to 39%. The worse the kidney function, the higher the risk.

Possible explanation: Kidney dysfunction can lead to chronic inflammation and oxidative stress, which may trigger cancer.

Alan Go, MD, director, Comprehensive Clinical Research Unit, Kaiser Permanente Northern California, Oakland.

Kidney-Donation Caution

Dorry Segev, MD, PhD, associate professor of surgery, The Johns Hopkins University School of Medicine, Baltimore.

A recent study of more than 1,000 kidney donors found that 7% had difficulties obtaining health insurance, and 25% reported problems getting life insurance. New guidelines under the Affordable Care Act should make getting health insurance easier for organ donors, since insurers are not supposed to deny coverage or charge higher rates, but unfortunately it still seems to be happening in some cases.

The insurance company could have rejected your wife's claim because it misinterpreted blood work in her medical record—for example, her serum creatinine (a measure of

---

Exercise Reduces Risk for Kidney Stones

According to a recent finding, active postmenopausal women were 16% to 31% less likely than sedentary women to develop kidney stones over an eight-year period. Maximum effects were found at the equivalent of three hours a week of moderate-paced walking, one hour of moderate-paced jogging or four hours of light gardening.

Study of 84,225 women led by researchers at University of Washington School of Medicine, Seattle, published in *Journal of the American Society of Nephrology*.

---

kidney function). Call the insurance company and clarify that your wife donated a kidney after passing a detailed health screening and that the creatinine level in her record is only a reflection of the fact that she has one kidney, not that she has kidney disease. If the insurer still refuses to cover her or tries to charge her a higher premium, ask her transplant center to call on her behalf.

Surprising Ways to Avoid Kidney Stones

Mathew D. Sorensen, MD, assistant professor of urology at the University of Washington School of Medicine in Seattle and director of the Comprehensive Metabolic Stone Clinic at the Puget Sound VA. His specialties include the treatment and prevention of kidney stones.

Plenty of people who develop kidney stones are shocked when this common condition occurs. How do these extremely painful stones take hold—and what can be done to prevent them?

Before you tell yourself that kidney stones are something that you'd never suffer, consider this—one of every 10 people is destined to develop at least one of these excruciating stones in his/her life. Each year, more than 1 million people see their doctors because of kidney stones. Already had a kidney stone? You're not off the hook—about half of kidney stone sufferers will develop another stone in five to seven years. *How to stay in the stone-free zone...*

How Stones Form

The good news is that kidney stones can usually be prevented by making the right changes to your diet and lifestyle. The problem is that many of the prevention strategies are counterintuitive...and involve some surprising approaches, such as cutting back on foods that are widely considered to be healthful.

The majority of kidney stones are made of calcium and oxalate. During normal digestion, oxalate (found in many healthful foods, such as spinach and beets) combines with calcium (another generally healthful nutrient) and makes its way through the digestive system before being excreted.

If there is excess oxalate, however, it gets absorbed into the bloodstream and carried to the kidneys, where urine is produced. Most of the time, oxalate is removed in the urine, but if the urine becomes saturated with oxalate, stones can develop. *Surprising ways to stop stones from forming…*

Step #1: Add just two daily servings of fruit and vegetables to your diet. When researchers at the University of Washington recently analyzed the diets of more than 80,000 postmenopausal women, they found that women who consumed the most fiber, fruits and vegetables had a 6% to 26% lower risk of developing kidney stones than women who ate the least. Good news: Just two additional servings a day were enough to make a big difference.

Simple way to get two more fruit/veggie servings daily: Have an extra apple and a handful of carrot sticks.

Step #2: Consume calcium. You might be wondering why foods that contain calcium—a main constituent of kidney stones—would help reduce your risk of developing the stones.

Here's why: Calcium gives the oxalate something to latch on to in the stomach. Otherwise, the oxalate ends up in the urine, where stones are more likely to form.

Good sources of calcium: Yogurt, kale, bok choy and calcium-fortified foods.

Exception: People who use calcium supplements may face a higher risk for kidney stones. If you use calcium supplements, take them with meals. That way, the calcium can bind with any oxalate that may be in the food.

Step #3: Go easy on oxalates. Eating oxalate-rich foods in moderation usually doesn't promote kidney stones. But if you start getting large amounts of these foods—for example, by regularly using lots of spinach or

beets in homemade juices—you might have a problem.

If you have had kidney stones—or your doctor believes that you may be at increased risk for them due to such factors as a strong family history of the condition—talk to your doctor about limiting your intake of oxalate-rich foods such as spinach…Swiss chard…rhubarb…beets…all nuts (including almond milk)…chocolate (especially dark)…and soy/tofu products.

Step #4: Eat less fish and other animal protein. Wait a minute—isn't fish good for you? Fatty, omega-3–rich fish usually is healthful, but people at increased risk for kidney stones (including anyone with a history of stones) should limit their intake of fish and any type of meat to six ounces a day.

Here's why: Protein is made up of amino acids and gets broken down into uric acid. Eating lots of animal protein acidifies the urine and can increase uric acid levels in the blood, leading to gout…or in the urine, leading to calcium-based or uric acid kidney stones.

Step #5: Drink the right beverages. Staying well hydrated is crucial—drink enough water and other fluids so that your urine is clear or light yellow. But pay attention to what you drink. One very large study showed that drinking sugar-sweetened sodas and punches increased risk for kidney stones by a whopping 33%. However, orange juice, coffee (both decaf and caffeinated) and tea decreased risk by varying amounts…beer cut risk by 41%…and wine reduced risk by 33%. Even so, these fluids should be consumed in moderate amounts.

Make lemonade: About one-third of stone formers are low in citrate (your doctor can test your levels), which is a known stone inhibitor. Since lemons have more citrate than any other citrus fruit, low-citrate patients may benefit from drinking a mixture of one-half cup of fresh or bottled lemon juice and seven-and-one-half cups of water (sweetened to taste). Consume the entire batch throughout the day to keep a steady stream of citrate flowing through the kidneys.

Step #6: Watch your salt intake. Sodium causes the kidneys to excrete more calcium into the urine, and many studies show that increased salt consumption raises the likelihood of kidney stones. Don't get more than 2,000 mg of sodium per day.

Step **#7: Get moving!** You might not think that exercise would affect your risk for kidney stones, but it does. A new study showed that even a small amount of physical activity reduced risk for kidney stones in women with no history of stones by 16%. Moderate activity (four hours of gardening or three hours of walking a week) reduced risk by 31%. There's no added benefit from very strenuous exercise.

Physical activity, especially weight-bearing exercise, may increase calcium absorption into bones, which means less calcium is excreted in the urine.

Soda and Your Kidneys

David Shoham, PhD, MSPH, assistant professor, department of preventive medicine and epidemiology, Loyola University Health System, Maywood, Illinois.

There's just nothing to be gained from drinking soda. Think about it—people don't hesitate to drink what is basically a bubbly brew of water, sugar (mainly high fructose corn syrup or HFCS), food coloring and assorted chemicals, packed with calories and lacking in nutritional value. Carbonated soft drinks are the single largest source of calories in the American diet, according to the Center for Science in the Public Interest, providing about 7% of our total calorie intake. In addition to staining, eroding and decaying our teeth, soft drinks are associated with an increased risk of obesity, a risk factor for type 2 diabetes and possibly osteoporosis. Now there is a new health problem to add to that list—kidney damage.

More Soda = More Sugar = More Risk

In a study of 9,358 adults (mean age 45), women who reported drinking two or more sugary sodas within the last 24 hours were nearly twice as likely to have albuminuria—excess levels of a protein in the urine that is a possible sign of kidney damage. More research is needed to determine if the association with kidney damage is due to sugar in general...HFCS in particular...or some shared lifestyle characteristics of soda drinkers.

Heres what we know so far...

• **The widespread use of high fructose corn syrup**—popular with manufacturers because it is cheap, sweet and extends shelf life—has been prevalent over the same time period there's been a significant rise in diabetic end-stage renal or kidney disease. The body processes HFCS differently than regular table sugar, and in so doing may cause harm to the kidneys.

• **Mercury has been detected in many products containing HFCS.** Mercury is involved in the manufacturing process for most commercial HFCS—and mercury is a risk for kidney disease.

• **Other ingredients in soda,** such as phosphorus in colas, may contribute to kidney stones, which are a risk factor for chronic kidney disease.

Men did not have this problem (more research is needed to learn why). Neither did people of either gender who drank diet soda, which is one reason why investigators believe HFCS may be responsible. Results of this research were published in *PLoS ONE*.

Drink Water

To protect your kidneys, your best bet is to simply drink water instead of soda, advises lead researcher David Shoham, PhD, MSPH, of the Loyola University Health System in Illinois. Soda just isn't worth it.

Do You Have a Gallstone and Not Know It?

Sarah Brewer, MD, MSc, general practitioner, registered nutritionist and registered nutritional therapist with a private practice in Guernsey, Channel Islands. Dr. Brewer is also the author of *Overcoming Gallstones: Nutritional, Medical and Surgical Approaches.*

You probably don't give much thought to your gallbladder—that four-inch, pear-shaped sac tucked beneath your liver. When it's working properly, it stores a liquid (bile) that plays an important role in digesting dietary fats.

But for more than 25 million Americans, this organ harbors one or sometimes even hundreds of gallstones. These hard deposits of cholesterol, calcium and/or other substances can be as small as grains of sand or as large as golf balls.

The good news is that gallstones usually cause no symptoms or only a single "attack" marked by abdominal cramps that may be accompanied by nausea or vomiting.

What to watch out for: Because the gallbladder can be removed relatively easily via minimally invasive laparoscopic surgery, some doctors recommend removal for patients who would do just as well with nonsurgical approaches.

A Safer Approach

Even though gallbladder removal (using laparoscopy or the traditional "open" approach) can be necessary or even lifesaving in some cases (see page 202), it's wise to consider whether you can avoid surgery. Not having a gallbladder can lead to such problems as poor digestion of dietary fats.

If your gallstones are "silent" (they have not caused you discomfort but were detected during an imaging test for another condition), or you've had just a single painful episode, your best bet is usually to wait it out—if the symptoms get worse, you might need surgery.

A Hysterectomy May Raise Kidney Cancer Risk

According to a recent study, researchers compared rates of a common kidney cancer in about 185,000 women who had undergone hysterectomies with about 657,000 who had not.

Result: Those who had undergone hysterectomies were up to 50% more likely to develop kidney cancer—with women age 44 or younger when they had the hysterectomy at highest risk.

Theory: Hysterectomy may alter urine flow, setting the stage for kidney cells to become cancerous.

If a doctor recommends hysterectomy for a noncancerous condition: Discuss kidney cancer risk and other nonsurgical options for treating your problem.

Daniel Altman, PhD, associate professor of medical epidemiology, Karolinska Institute, Stockholm, Sweden.

More often, you can stop gallstones from growing (or forming in the first place) with the following simple steps...

• **Lose weight—and lose it slowly.** People who are overweight or obese are far more likely to develop gallstones than those who are lean. They are also more likely to have one or more painful episodes.

In people who are overweight, bile (the digestive fluid that's stored in the gallbladder) tends to contain more cholesterol—the main constituent in about 70% of gallstones. Weight loss is among the most effective ways to prevent gallstones, but only if you lose weight at a reasonable pace—for example, no more than two pounds a week.

Here's why: Studies have shown that faster weight loss can trigger an increase in stone formation and/or symptoms because the gallbladder doesn't empty completely on diets that cut too many calories (for example, less than 1,500 calories daily for men and less than 1,200 calories daily for women). Stored bile becomes "stagnant" and is more likely to form stones.

• **Cut fat—but not too much.** Doctors used to recommend low-fat diets for weight loss. It makes sense to eat less fat because a diet that's high in cholesterol and saturated fat can increase stone formation—especially if you're not getting much fiber, which acts like a sponge to mop up fats.

But not getting enough fat has the same effect as consuming too few calories—it allows bile to "sit" in the gallbladder. That's why I recommend a Mediterranean-type diet that contains healthful fats (such as olive oil, fatty fish and nuts) along with plenty of fruit and vegetables.

Also helpful: Supplements that contain milk thistle and/or globe artichoke.* Follow label directions. These supplements stimulate bile production and reduce the concentration of cholesterol and other stone-causing substances.

• **Get more omega-3 fatty acids.** Omega-3s, found in fatty, cold-water fish, reduce the amount of cholesterol in bile—by up to 25%, according to research.

Important: Eat fish. You'll get all the omega-3s that you need from two to four weekly servings of fish. Good choices include salmon, kippers, sardines and mackerel. Compared with fish consumption, the evidence is not as strong for taking fish oil supplements to reduce gallstone risk.

• **Eat high-fiber foods.** A Harvard study analyzing long-term fiber intakes of nearly 70,000 women found that every 5 g increase in daily fiber reduced the need for gallbladder surgery by an average of about 10%. Eat at least five daily servings of high-fiber foods. Good options: Beans (such as kidney and soybeans)…whole grains (such as oats)…and fresh vegetables (such as dark greens).

*If you take a prescription drug or have a chronic medical condition, check with a doctor or pharmacist before trying supplements. People with a history of hormone-related cancer, such as prostate or breast cancer, should not take milk thistle. Those with a ragweed allergy should not take milk thistle or artichoke supplements.

• **Load up on vitamin C.** Research has shown that women who consume the most vitamin C–rich foods are less likely to have gallstones or gallstone-related symptoms than those who get the least of these foods. Women who got even more vitamin C from supplements were 34% less likely to have problems than women who didn't take a supplement. Vitamin C is also believed to reduce gallstone risk in men.

My advice: In addition to consuming vitamin C–rich foods (such as citrus fruits and berries), take 500 mg of vitamin C four times daily (to maintain steady blood levels and maximize absorption). The "ester-C" form of vitamin C is nonacidic and easier for the body to absorb—and less likely to cause diarrhea at the doses recommended here.

• **Get extra magnesium.** Many Americans don't get enough of this important mineral. Low magnesium has been linked to elevated LDL "bad" cholesterol, high blood pressure—and a higher risk for gallstones. A large study that followed more than 42,000 men for 16 years found that those with the highest magnesium intakes (more than 409 mg daily) were 33% less likely to develop gallstone disease than those with the lowest levels (less than 288 mg daily).

My advice: Regularly consume magnesium-rich foods, such as beans, nuts, brewer's yeast, salmon, leafy greens and dark chocolate. If you are not sure that you're getting enough, take 150 mg to 300 mg daily of a magnesium citrate supplement, which is the most readily absorbed.

• **Enjoy a little coffee.** One study linked two to three cups of coffee a day to a 20% lower risk of developing gallstones. Decaf coffee, caffeinated tea or soft drinks did not have this protective effect—perhaps because of their lower amounts of caffeine, a compound that increases the flow of bile.

When You Do Need Gallbladder Surgery

Gallstones rarely cause problems when they stay put. They usually cause symptoms, such as fever, abdominal pain, nausea or vomiting, when they migrate into other areas, such as the small ducts that lead to the intestine.

Most people need surgery to remove the gallbladder only if their symptoms are frequent (two or more episodes) or unusually painful…if they develop cholecystitis, an infection/inflammation that occurs when a stone blocks the cystic duct…or if a stone lodges in the duct leading to the pancreas. In these cases, surgery is advisable because the risk for complications, such as jaundice and chronic cholecystitis and pancreatitis, is high. Whether it's minimally invasive (laparoscopic) or "open," surgery to remove the gallbladder carries a risk for infection or the accidental severing of the bile duct. If surgery is advised, look for a surgeon who has significant experience performing this operation.

No More UTIs!

Tomas L. Griebling, MD, MPH, the John P. Wolf 33° Masonic Distinguished Professor of Urology at The University of Kansas (KU) School of Medicine in Kansas City. He is a professor and vice-chair in the department of urology and faculty associate in The Landon Center on Aging. He has published more than 200 articles in peer-reviewed medical journals.

Anyone who has ever had a urinary tract infection (UTI) knows that it's extremely unpleasant. The first clue may be that your urine is smelly and/or looks cloudy. You could also suffer burning or pain during urination, have blood in your urine and a fever or chills. To make matters worse, many people suffer repeated UTIs, and some doctors don't do much more than prescribe an antibiotic each time.

Good news: Studies now show that there are some surprisingly simple steps you can take to help guard against UTIs—whether you have suffered them repeatedly or never even had one.

Women and Men Get UTIs

Even though UTIs are commonly considered a "women's problem," men develop them, too.

What men need to know: About 12% of men will suffer a UTI at some point in their lives, but men over age 50 are at increased risk. Common causes include *prostatitis*, a bacterial infection of the prostate gland that can also enter the urinary tract…and the use of urinary catheters in medical procedures.

What women need to know: More than 50% of women will experience a UTI at some point in their lives, and one-third of them will suffer recurring infections. Women are more prone to infection around the time of sexual activity due to the spread of *E. coli* bacteria to the vagina. In postmenopausal women, lower levels of estrogen decrease the amount of Lactobacillus, a "good" bacteria that grows in the vagina and serves as a natural defense against UTIs.

Symptoms are sometimes puzzling: Diagnosis of a UTI can be difficult in older men and women because they often don't suffer the classic symptoms but instead have atypical symptoms such as lethargy, confusion, nausea, shortness of breath and/or loss of appetite. If you suspect a UTI, ask that your doctor perform a urine culture.

Stop a UTI Before It Starts

When a woman (or man) suffers from recurring UTIs (three or more infections in a one-year period), these steps will help break the cycle…

•**Go to the bathroom often.** Many people hold their urine longer than they should. This is a bad idea because the bladder may distend, making it more difficult to empty the bladder and preventing bacteria from being flushed out. To protect yourself, try to urinate roughly every four waking hours.

Important: People who are rushed when they are going to the bathroom may not fully empty their bladders. Take your time when urinating.

Helpful: When you think you are finished, give yourself another moment to see if there's any urine remaining before leaving the toilet.

•**Drink a lot of water.** You probably know that drinking water is a good way to help flush bacteria from the urinary tract. However, few people drink enough—you need to consume eight to 10 eight-ounce glasses of water each day. Water is best because it's pure and has no calories. Caffeine, soda and alcohol can aggravate the bladder.

Other preventives include…

•**Yogurt.** A 2012 study suggested that *lactobacilli,* found in probiotic supplements and yogurt, may be an acceptable alternative to antibiotics for the prevention of UTIs in women (with recurring infections, medication may be used for this purpose). The additional lactobacilli are believed to displace *E. coli* and stimulate the immune system to fight back against the infectious bacteria.

My advice: Consume a cup of yogurt each day—it should be low in sugar (avoid any yogurt that lists sugar as the first or second ingredient) and make sure it contains live cultures. Or take two probiotic capsules each day containing *Lactobacillus rhamnosus* GR-1 and *Lactobacillus reuteri* RC-14—the probiotic strains used in the study mentioned earlier. Probiotic supplements with these strains include Pro-Flora Women's Probiotic from Integrative Therapeutics, IntegrativePro.com… and Ultra Flora Women's from Metagenics, *Metagenics.com.*

•**Cranberry juice or cranberry supplements.** Research has been mixed, but several studies have shown that drinking at least one to two cups of cranberry juice daily may help prevent UTIs. Just be sure to drink real cranberry juice—not cranberry juice cocktail, which has lots of sugar, is diluted with other juices and provides minimal amounts of the actual berry that contains protective compounds known as proanthocyanidins.

You may want to try a cranberry supplement if you have diabetes (even real cranberry juice contains carbohydrates) or if you don't like cranberry juice. Do not exceed label instructions on dosage—research suggests that high doses may increase the risk for kidney stones.

•**Estrogen creams.** For postmenopausal women, a small amount of estrogen cream applied inside the vagina several times per week has been shown to significantly reduce the risk for recurrent UTIs. The cream thickens the walls of the urinary tract, making it more difficult for bacteria to penetrate.

Important: Most women who take estrogen in pill or patch form can safely add an estrogen cream—the amount absorbed into the bloodstream is negligible. Women with a history of uterine cancer or certain breast cancers may not be suitable candidates for any form of estrogen therapy. Ask your doctor.

When You Need an Antibiotic

If the steps above do not prevent recurring UTIs, you may need a long-term course (six months or longer) of a low-dose antibiotic. To minimize the development of bacterial resistance, it's wise to start with a milder antibiotic, such as *sulfamethoxazole* and *trimethoprim* (Bactrim), if possible. However, more powerful antibiotics, such as *ciprofloxacin* (Cipro), may be needed to help prevent or treat stubborn infections.

Important: Many women self-diagnose a UTI, call up their doctors and receive a prescription for an antibiotic when in fact they may have a condition, such as vaginitis, that mimics UTI symptoms. Urinalysis and/or a urinary culture is necessary to get an accurate diagnosis.

Standard Test for Urinary Tract Infection May Be Inaccurate

Nearly 25% of women who had signs of urinary tract infections (UTIs) had no evidence of bacteria in their urine when tested with the midstream urine culture, currently the standard test for detecting infection.

E. coli, the most common bacteria that causes UTIs, often is present in such low amounts that they are missed by labs, which test only for high quantities.

If you think you have a UTI: Ask the doctor to request that the culture be tested for small amounts of E. coli.

Thomas M. Hooton, MD, professor of medicine at University of Miami Miller School of Medicine and lead author of a study published in *The New England Journal of Medicine.*

The Baffling Bladder Condition Antibiotics Can't Cure

Kristene E. Whitmore, MD, professor and chair of urology and female pelvic medicine and reconstructive surgery at Drexel University College of Medicine, and medical director the Pelvic and Sexual Health Institute, both in Philadelphia. She is coauthor of *Overcoming Bladder Disorders. pelvicandsexualhealthinstitute.org*

Perplexing, painful and inconvenient, the chronic condition interstitial cystitis/painful bladder syndrome (IC/PBS) affects women more than nine times as often as men. Its symptoms, including bladder pain and frequent urination, often are mistaken for those of a bladder infection—yet tests reveal no bacteria, and antibiotics bring no relief.

Though IC/PBS affects up to 6% of American women, its cause is a mystery.

What is known: The bladder wall becomes inflamed and super-sensitive...pinpoints of bleeding and ulcers often appear...stiffness and scarring may develop.

Many women suffer for years without a proper diagnosis, taking antibiotics for infections that they do not actually have. This delay causes needless pain...raises the odds of becoming resistant to antibiotics...and increases the risk that an IC/PBS–triggered inflammatory reaction will spread to other organs. In severe cases, surgery may be needed to remove part or all of the bladder.

IC/PBS cannot be cured—but treatment can relieve symptoms and reduce complications.

Getting Diagnosed

If you have symptoms that suggest IC/PBS, visit your doctor. If no infection is found or symptoms persist despite treatment, consult a urologist or urogynecologist.

IC/PBS symptoms...

- **Bladder pain or pressure**
- **Frequent urination (more than eight times in 24 hours)**
- **Urgent need to urinate**
- **Discomfort, pain or pressure in the lower pelvis or vulva**
- **Pain during or after sex**
- **Flare-ups during menstruation.**

There is no definitive test for IC/PBS. Diagnosis involves excluding other conditions, such as a bladder infection, overactive bladder or bladder cancer. Testing may include blood and urine tests, bladder biopsy and cystoscopy (exam of the bladder using a viewing instrument).

Good news: For about 70% of patients, natural remedies ease symptoms with few or no side effects.

Soothing Dietary Strategies

Your diet affects how your bladder feels. Helpful...

- **Identify foods that spark symptoms.** A chief culprit is cranberry juice. Yes, this juice combats bladder infections—but with IC/PBS, you aren't fighting an infection. And cranberry juice is acidic, so it irritates a sensitive bladder.

Other top troublemakers: Alcohol...artificial sweeteners...caffeine (coffee, soda, tea)...carbonated drinks...citrus fruits, citrus juices...spicy foods...and tomato products. For a comprehensive list of problematic foods, visit the Web site of the Interstitial Cystitis Association (*www.ichelp.org/wp-content/uploads/2015/07/food-list.pdf*). To identify your personal triggers, for one month do not eat anything on the ICA list. Then, reintroduce one food from the list every three to five days. If symptoms flare up, swear off that food.

•**Drink more, not less.** You may think that limiting fluids reduces your need to urinate—but skimping on water makes urine more concentrated and thus more irritating. Drink six to eight cups of water daily—and sip, don't gulp.

•**Take supplements.** With your doctor's okay, try the following...

•Prelief (sold at drugstores) contains calcium glycerophosphate, which makes food less acidic.

•CystoProtek (sold at *www.cysto-protek. com*) has antioxidants and anti-inflammatories (glucosamine, quercetin, rutin) that help repair the bladder lining.

Note: If you take a multivitamin or other supplement that contains vitamin C, choose one with ascorbate, not ascorbic acid.

Mind Over Bladder

Try any or all of the following mind-body therapies...

•**Bladder retraining.** Urinating temporarily relieves pain, so patients use the toilet often—in some cases, up to 60 times a day—but this habit further reduces the bladder's capacity to comfortably hold urine.

Best: Try to increase your typical time between bathroom trips by 15 minutes. After two weeks, increase by another 15 minutes. Continue until you can wait at least two hours.

•**Stress reduction.** Practice relaxation techniques daily, such as deep breathing, meditation and yoga. Also consider craniosacral therapy (gentle head and spine massage).

Practitioner referrals: Upledger Institute, 800-233-5880, *www.upledger.com.*

•**Acupuncture.** This reduces IC/PBS pain for some patients.

Referrals: American Association of Acupuncture and Oriental Medicine, 866-455-7999, *aaaomonline.org.*

Medical Treatment Options

Persistent bladder pain eventually can cause pelvic muscles to spasm, worsening IC/PBS. Helpful...

•**Intravaginal Thiele massage.** To relieve spasms, a physical therapist massages muscles inside the vagina and/or rectum...and patients learn to do the procedure themselves at home. In one study, this reduced symptoms for 90% of patients.

•**Electrical nerve stimulation.** Stimulating the sacral nerves in the back with a mild current helps pelvic floor muscles function normally. If symptoms are severe, a urologist or urogynecologist can implant a nerve stimulator under the skin near the tailbone for continuous stimulation.

•**Medication.** About 5% to 10% of IC/PBS patients must resort to narcotic prescription painkillers—but these can have adverse effects, including a risk for dependence.

Better: First consider one or more of the following non-narcotic prescription drugs, discussing the pros and cons with your doctor...

•Dimethyl sulfoxide (DMSO). This pain-relieving anti-inflammatory and antispasmodic is infused into the bladder through a catheter and kept in place for about 20 minutes. The procedure typically is done once a week for six weeks. Relief lasts three to 12 months...treatment is repeated as needed. Side effects may include garlic taste in the mouth, headache and dry nasal passages. DMSO is the only drug approved for this treatment, but for some patients, other anesthetics (such as lidocaine) work as well with fewer side effects.

•*Pentosan* (Elmiron). This oral drug helps heal the bladder lining. It can thin the blood, however, so it may be inappropriate if you use a blood thinner, such as *warfarin* (Coumadin).

•*Potassium citrate* (Urocit-K). Taken orally, this makes urine more alkaline. Possible side effects include nausea, muscle weakness and irregular heartbeat.

•Urelle. This brand-name oral medication is a five-drug formulation that reduces pain and spasms. Side effects may include nausea, dizziness and blurred vision.

Lifestyle Changes

To make day-to-day life with IC/PBS more comfortable, try…

•**Modified exercise routines.** When symptoms flare up, reduce the intensity and duration of workouts—for instance, by walking instead of running. Rinse off after swimming to remove irritating chlorine.

•**Bathing.** Soak in bathwater mixed with colloidal oatmeal (sold at drugstores). Avoid bubble baths and bath oils—these can be irritating.

•**A personal lubricant for sex.** This makes intercourse more comfortable.

Try: The organic Good Clean Love line (541-344-4483, *goodcleanlove.com*).

This Supplement Can Help Interstitial Cystitis

Mark A. Moyad, MD, MPH, Jenkins/Pokempner director of preventive and complementary medicine at the University of Michigan Medical Center and the co-director of the Men's Health Program at the University of Michigan, both in Ann Arbor. He is also the author, with Janet Lee, of *The Supplement Handbook.*

There are no consistently effective medications for IC, an inflammatory bladder disorder that causes frequent and uncomfortable urination, mainly in women.

Supplement to try for IC*: Calcium glycerophosphate. It neutralizes the acidity of foods, one of the main IC triggers. Research shows that calcium glycerophosphate reduces pain and urinary urgency when taken before consuming foods that exacerbate IC symptoms.

Typical dose: Two to three tablets (the dose studied has 345 mg of calcium glycerophosphate per tablet) or one-quarter

*Check with your doctor before trying this supplement alone or in combination with a prescription medication.

teaspoon of powder (the equivalent of two 345-mg tablets) taken right before or during acidic meals. The Interstitial Cystitis Network website, IC-Network.com, lists many of the problem foods such as coffee, alcohol and artificial sweeteners.

Caution: Long-term use of this supplement could slightly interfere with absorption of some nutrients, so talk to your doctor about ways to monitor your nutrient levels.

Don't Let Your Bladder Run Your Life!

Holly Lucille, ND, RN, naturopathic doctor based in West Hollywood, California. She is the author of *Creating and Maintaining Balance: A Woman's Guide to Safe, Natural Hormone Health* and serves on the Institute for Natural Medicine Board of Directors. *Dr HollyLucille.com*

Women who scout out restrooms wherever they are may think that others don't have to worry so much about their bladders. But that's not true.

Eye-opening statistic: One in every five adults over age 40 has overactive bladder… and after the age of 65, a whopping one in every three adults is affected. If you regularly have a strong and sudden urge to urinate and/or need to hit the john eight or more times a day (or more than once at night), chances are you have the condition, too.

Postmenopausal women (due to their low estrogen levels) and men with enlarged prostate issues are at increased risk of having overactive bladder. Urinary tract infections, use of certain medications (such as antidepressants and drugs to treat high blood pressure and insomnia) and even constipation also can cause or worsen the condition.

But there is a bright side. Research is now uncovering several surprisingly simple natural approaches that are highly effective for many people with overactive bladder. *Among the best…*

207

Start With Your Diet

Most people don't connect a bladder problem to their diets. But there is a strong link. *My advice…*

• **Take a hard line with irritants.** Alcohol, caffeine and artificial sweeteners can exacerbate the feeling of urgency caused by overactive bladder. Cutting back on these items is a good first step, but they often creep back into one's diet over time.

What helps: Keep it simple—completely avoid alcohol, caffeine (all forms, including coffee, tea and caffeine-containing foods such as chocolate) and artificial sweeteners. Stick to decaffeinated coffee and herbal teas, and use agave and stevia as sweeteners.

Many individuals also are sensitive to certain foods, such as corn, wheat, dairy, eggs and peanuts. They often trigger an immune reaction that contributes to overall inflammation in the body, including in the bladder. If your symptoms of urinary urgency and/or frequency increase after eating one of these (or any other) foods, your body may be having an inflammatory response that is also affecting your bladder. Eliminate these foods from your diet.

• **Keep your gut healthy.** The scientific evidence is still in the early stages, but research now suggests that leaky gut syndrome, in which excess bacterial or fungal growth harms the mucosal membrane in the intestines, is at the root of several health problems, including overactive bladder.

The theory is that an imbalance of microbes, a condition known as dysbiosis, can irritate the walls of the bladder just as it does in the gut.

What helps: Probiotics and oregano oil* capsules. Probiotics replenish "good" bacteria, and oregano oil has antibacterial properties that help cleanse "bad" bacteria and fungi from the gut.

• **Drink up!** People with overactive bladder often cut way back on their fluid intake because they already make so many trips

---

*Talk to your doctor before trying any of these herbal remedies, especially if you take medication or have a chronic health condition. You may want to consult a naturopathic doctor. To find one near you, check *Naturopathic.org*.

to the bathroom. But when you don't drink enough fluids, urine tends to have an irritating effect because it becomes more concentrated. This increases urgency.

What helps: Drink half your body weight in ounces of water or herbal tea daily. Do not drink any fluids after 5 p.m. to help prevent bathroom runs during the night.

The Right Supplements

Cranberry supplements (or unsweetened cranberry juice) can be helpful for bladder infections, but they're usually not the best choice for overactive bladder. *My advice…*

• **Try pumpkin seed extract.** These capsules help tone and strengthen the tissue of your pelvic-floor muscles, which gives you better bladder control.

Typical dosage: 500 mg daily.

• **Consider *Angelica archangelica* extract.** This herb has gotten positive reviews from researchers who have investigated it as a therapy for overactive bladder.

Recent finding: When 43 men with overactive bladder took 300 mg of the herb daily, they made fewer trips to the bathroom. This study was about bladder capacity, not the prostate, so women can benefit too.

Typical dosage: 100 mg daily.

Other Ways to Bladder Control

• **Kegel exercises,** which help strengthen the pelvic-floor muscles, are essential for getting control of overactive bladder symptoms. Unfortunately, most people who try doing Kegels end up doing them the wrong way.

How to do Kegels: Three to five times a day, contract your pelvic-floor muscles (the ones you use to stop and start the flow of urine), hold for a count of 10, then relax completely for a count of 10. Repeat 10 times. If you're a woman and aren't sure if you're contracting the right muscles, there is a possible solution.

Recent option for women: A medical device called Apex Pelvic Floor Muscle Stimulator acts as an automatic Kegel exerciser. It is inserted into the vagina and electrically stimulates the correct muscles ($299 at *Pour-Moi.com/apex* or at *Amazon.com*—cost may be covered by some insurance plans). Check with your doctor to see if this would be an appropriate aid for you.

Kegels can easily be part of anyone's daily routine—do them while waiting at a red light, after going to the bathroom or while watching TV.

•**Try acupuncture.** An increasing body of evidence shows that this therapy helps relieve overactive bladder symptoms. For example, in a study of 74 women with the condition, bladder capacity, urgency and frequency of urination significantly improved after four weekly bladder-specific acupuncture sessions.

•**Go for biofeedback.** Small electrodes are used to monitor the muscles involved in bladder control so that an individualized exercise program can be created. Biofeedback is noninvasive and is most effective when used along with other treatments. To find a board-certified provider, consult the Biofeedback Certification International Alliance, *BCIA.org*.

The "Other" Bladder Problem

Michael B. Chancellor, MD, urologist and director of neuro-urology at the Beaumont Health System in Royal Oak, Michigan. He is coauthor of *Atlas of Urodynamics* and a founding member of the Congress of Urologic Research and Education on Aging Underactive Bladder, which is spearheading research on novel therapies for treating UAB.

Ask anyone who is health conscious to name some common bladder problems, and you can bet that "overactive bladder" will be near the top of the list.

What few people realize: An estimated 20 million Americans are living with a different condition, which actually has the opposite effect on the bladder, but the problem is not getting diagnosed or treated by most doctors.

Known as underactive bladder (UAB), this disorder can make something as simple as going to the bathroom a chore...damage the kidneys...and even land a person in a nursing home.

Red Flags of UAB

UAB occurs when the bladder loses its ability to contract and fully empty. Part of what makes this condition so vexing is that the symptoms can come and go, and they often mimic those of other diseases, such as prostate enlargement and urinary tract infections—both of which can cause frequent urination, another UAB symptom.

With UAB, sufferers have a hard time telling when their bladders are full. When they do have the urge to urinate, it may be painful, the urine may dribble or it may not come at all. In fact, it may take several minutes to start a stream of urine. They also may feel that there's urine left behind and end up heading to the bathroom again a short time later.

Of course, when the bladder does not completely empty, urine builds up. This can lead to embarrassing episodes of leakage from overflow incontinence...recurring urinary tract and kidney infections...and, in severe cases, kidney damage.

What Causes UAB?

As we age, the muscles of the bladder lose some of their elasticity and ability to contract. However, UAB is not a normal part of aging.

When messages between the brain and the bladder are short-circuited in any way, your body doesn't register the normal urge to urinate when the bladder is full.

This breakdown in communication may be triggered by a stroke, Parkinson's disease, acute urinary tract infection, radiation therapy to the pelvic area, nerve damage after pelvic surgery or even a herniated disk. In people under age 40, multiple sclerosis is a common culprit, as is diabetes, which can damage peripheral nerves in the lower spinal cord that supply the bladder.

Even overactive bladder can be a trigger: In some cases, overactive bladder thickens the bladder wall in a way that interferes with the bladder's ability to contract during urination…leading to underactive bladder.

Certain medications can also lead to UAB: These may include antidepressants, antihistamines, blood pressure drugs and cholesterol-lowering statins.

Do You Have UAB?

If you're suffering from any of the symptoms of UAB, see your primary care doctor soon. He/she may refer you to a specialist—either a urologist or a uro-gynecologist, who treats urologic problems in women.

To find out whether you have UAB, the specialist will take your medical history…do a physical exam…and order blood and urine tests to see how well your bladder and kidneys are functioning. A cystoscopy, ultrasound or CT scan might also be ordered to determine whether your bladder muscles and nerves are working normally.

Helpful: Keeping a diary that lists how often and how much you urinate (using a measuring cup) can give your doctor valuable information. For a free online diary to track your bladder activity, go to *UroDaily.com.*

How to Cope with UAB

Doctors are still clearly defining UAB and working to understand what therapies are most effective. But if you've got this condition, you want help now! The research is ongoing, but here are some ways to cope with the condition—go ahead and bring up these approaches with your doctor. *Not all physicians are familiar with them…*

• **Double-voiding.** This technique gives you extra time to empty your bladder.

What to do: After urinating, stay at the toilet for a few additional minutes. After this short break, try to urinate again. If your bladder has not fully emptied, you will often be able to pass more urine.

• **Triggered-reflex voiding.** This involves the use of various stimulation techniques to trigger the brain signals that jump-start contractions of the bladder and the flow of urine. The technique may work for anyone with UAB but can be especially useful for a person with a spinal cord injury who still has some reflexes but may not be able to feel whether the bladder is full.

What to do: Rub the area just above the pubic bone…tug on your pubic hair…or (for men) gently squeeze the head of the penis. Test different trigger zones to see which one might work for you.

• **Medications.** Men with UAB may get relief from a drug often used for prostate enlargement, such as *doxazosin* (Cardura). It helps a man empty his bladder by relaxing the muscle of the urethra (the tube through which urine flows).

• **Catheterization.** This is another way to empty the bladder. With self-catheterization, you insert a catheter, a strawlike tube, into your urethra to drain urine from your bladder. For people who are unable to do this, an "indwelling" catheter can be inserted into the urethra by a health-care professional to automatically drain urine into a pouch for a set period of time. However, if the catheter is not changed every two to four weeks, it can injure the urethra and/or cause infection.

For people who can't tolerate an indwelling catheter, a suprapubic catheter may be used. It requires a surgical procedure to insert it through a small hole in the abdomen directly into the bladder.

• **Surgery.** When the therapies described above are not effective or practical, the only option is surgery—either to enlarge the bladder by using a small section of the stomach or bowel that helps the bladder to stretch more easily…or to insert a mesh stent that allows the bladder to empty into a pouch outside the body.

Promising new approach: Stem cell therapy is being studied as a possible treatment for UAB. Researchers theorize that transplanting stem cells to help the bladder regenerate new, fully functioning tissue could be an effective solution for UAB sufferers.

Is a Full Bladder Interrupting Your Sleep? You're Not Alone

Amy Hsu, MD, fellow, division of geriatrics, San Francisco VA Medical Center.

Mary Townsend, ScD, associate epidemiologist, Brigham and Women's Hospital, Boston.

Obstetrics & Gynecology.

Many women have to get up more than once a night because of a full bladder, a new study finds.

Researchers found that of over 2,000 women aged 40 and up, one-third said they routinely got up at least twice a night to use the bathroom. Doctors refer to that as nocturia, and it can be a sign that you're drinking too much tea or coffee at night—or a signal of a serious health condition.

"Traditionally, nocturia has been considered a part of other urinary tract disorders," said lead researcher Amy Hsu, MD, a fellow at the San Francisco VA Medical Center.

But in this study, 40% of the women with nocturia reported no other urinary tract symptoms, such as daytime overactive bladder or urine leakage.

That suggests nocturia often cannot be attributed to those conditions, according to Dr. Hsu, who reported the findings in the January 2015 issue of *Obstetrics & Gynecology*.

Mary Townsend, ScD, a researcher at Brigham and Women's Hospital in Boston, said nocturia is increasingly being recognized as a condition unto itself.

"And this study supports that view," said Dr. Townsend, who was not involved in the research.

Dr. Hsu's team found that, not surprisingly, nocturia was more common among relatively older women. For every five-year increase in age, a woman's risk rose by 21%. Nocturia was also more common among women who'd had a hysterectomy, hot flashes or had used vaginal estrogen to treat menopause symptoms.

Bladder problems are common after hysterectomy, and other studies have found a link to nocturia. As for hot flashes, they are notorious for keeping women up at night—which could be one reason for the connection to nocturia, according to Dr. Hsu.

On the other hand, relatively few women in the study were actually bothered by their nighttime trips to the bathroom. Only one-quarter said they were at least "moderately" bothered.

Should You Pay Attention to Nocturia?

So is nocturia only an issue if it "bothers" you?

"That's a good question," Dr. Hsu said. "If it really doesn't bother you, and you're able to go right back to sleep, then it may not be a problem."

That's especially true, she noted, if you can attribute the nocturia to something benign—like drinking liquids close to bedtime.

However, Dr. Townsend said nocturia can be a symptom of certain health conditions that boost the body's urine production, like diabetes or heart failure. "So, there are still reasons to pay attention to nocturia, even if a woman isn't bothered by it," she said.

Nocturia can also affect people with certain conditions that disrupt sleep, Dr. Townsend said—including sleep apnea and restless legs syndrome.

Even if nocturia is a woman's only symptom, it can still be significant. "We know that nocturia can lead to lower sleep quality," Dr. Townsend said. "Poor sleep can negatively affect your mood or daytime functioning, including your productivity at work."

And for older women, she noted, getting up at night could lead to a fall and potentially serious injury.

"So women with nocturia—especially those whose symptoms are affecting their mood or ability to function during the day—

should be encouraged to talk to their health care provider," Dr. Townsend said.

Treatment for Nocturia

Treatment for nocturia might include tackling the underlying cause—such as untreated diabetes—or simple lifestyle changes or pelvic floor physical therapy. And if necessary, Dr. Hsu said, there are medications that can help regulate urine production or calm an overactive bladder.

"I think women should be aware that this condition is common, and not something to be embarrassed about," Dr. Hsu said. "You're not alone."

Two of Hsu's co-authors on the study have received research funding from companies that make drugs for urinary tract disorders.

The Bladder and Bowel Foundation has more information on nocturia at *http://www. bladderandbowelfoundation.org/bladder/ bladder-problems/nocturia.asp*.

Keep Your Bladder Healthy

Jamison Starbuck, ND, naturopathic physician in family practice and a guest lecturer at the University of Montana, both in Missoula. She is past president of the American Association of Naturopathic Physicians and a contributing editor to *The Alternative Advisor: The Complete Guide to Natural Therapies and Alternative Treatments.*

If you're age 50 or older and haven't had a bladder infection, count yourself lucky. The reality is that these infections are among the most common complaints of the AARP crowd.

Here's why: With age, women—and men—are at increased risk because tissues in the bladder weaken, making it more difficult for it to fully empty…so bacteria have more time to proliferate and cause a urinary tract infection (UTI). As we age, our immune systems also don't work as well.

Interestingly, the symptoms of bladder infection become less apparent with age. Instead of the burning, cramping pain and bloody urine that generally accompany a UTI in younger people, only a modest increase in urinary frequency and a dark urine color may indicate a bladder infection once you're middle-aged or older. After about age 70, confusion, agitation, balance problems and falling may be a physician's only clues of a bladder infection.

Fortunately, there are some highly effective natural approaches to help prevent UTIs. *My favorite UTI-fighting strategies…*

• **Stay hydrated.** You must drink a minimum of two quarts of plain water daily—no matter what other beverages you consume. If you take a prescription medication, you may need even more water. Diuretics and some other drugs will make you lose water, so you'll need to drink more than usual. Discuss this with your pharmacist.

• **Use good hygiene.** OK, you might find this is a little embarrassing, but make sure that you wipe from front to back after a bowel movement…wash your genitals before and after sex…and change your undergarments regularly, particularly if you have incontinence or are sedentary (small amounts of stool on underwear can increase infection risk).

• **Load up on cranberry.** Everyone knows that cranberry is supposed to be good for the bladder, but recent research made some people doubt its effectiveness. One study found that cranberry may not be very effective at preventing UTIs. But don't write off cranberry. The same research showed that compounds in cranberry do prevent infections by making it difficult for bacteria to stick to the walls of the bladder. Because most brands of cranberry juice (perhaps the most convenient form of the fruit) have added sugar to make them less tart, I usually advise people who develop more than one bladder infection a year to take 600 mg of a freeze-dried cranberry extract daily.

Caution: People with a history of calcium oxalate kidney stones or who take *warfarin* (Coumadin) or regularly use aspirin should avoid cranberry—it can increase stone risk and interact with these medications.

• **Get more probiotics.** The beneficial bacteria found in yogurt and other cultured foods, such as kefir and miso, reduce risk for bladder infection. Eat one cup of plain yogurt, kefir or miso soup daily or take a probiotic supplement.

• **Do Kegel exercises.** Women—and men—listen up! Strong pelvic muscles allow for more complete bladder emptying and reduce infection risk.

What to do: At least once daily, contract and release the muscles of your pelvic floor (the ones that stop urine flow) 10 times while seated or standing.

Coffee Protects Against Liver Cancer

Carlo La Vecchia, MD, department of epidemiology, Istituto di Ricerche Farmacologiche "Mario Negri," and department of clinical sciences and community health, Università degli Studi di Milan, Milan, Italy. His study was published in *Clinical Gastroenterology and Hepatology.*

The poor neglected liver. People tend to worry about their hearts, their lungs, their stomachs—but the liver gets little TLC, despite being essential for cleaning the blood, storing energy and aiding digestion. Good news: You can show your liver a little love by doing something that's also immensely enjoyable…drinking coffee.

That's right—coffee is linked to a reduced risk for liver cancer, the world's third-most-deadly type of cancer. Here's the scoop from a recent meta-analysis, including the amount of coffee that seemed to give drinkers the most protection.

Researchers from Italy combined the results from 16 high-quality studies that examined the association between coffee consumption and the most common form of liver cancer, hepatocellular carcinoma (HCC). Together, the studies from around the world included 3,153 cases of HCC. *Here's what the researchers found…*

• **Coffee drinkers in general had a 40% lower risk for HCC than people who did not drink coffee.**

• **"High coffee consumption" was linked to a 56% reduction in risk for HCC.** The studies varied in how they defined "high coffee consumption," with most considering high consumption to be three or more cups per day…but in five studies, high consumption meant just one or more cups per day.

• **Alcohol consumption, hepatitis and liver disease**—known risk factors for liver cancer—did not appreciably modify the apparent benefits of drinking coffee.

The meta-analysis did not differentiate between regular and decaffeinated coffee (though the researchers noted that most data referred to regular coffee), nor could it examine whether adding cream and/or sugar to coffee made any difference in terms of liver cancer risk.

How might coffee protect the liver? There are several hypotheses that could explain this. Coffee contains various minerals and antioxidants—including chlorogenic acid, cafestol and kahweol—that may inhibit the development of liver cancer. Coffee also reduces the activity of certain enzymes that may play a role in the development of several liver diseases. And some studies show that coffee consumption is inversely related to diabetes and cirrhosis, both of which are known risk factors for liver cancer.

The Breakthrough That Can Save Your Liver and Your Life

Jonathan Fenkel, MD, assistant professor of medicine at Thomas Jefferson University in Philadelphia, where he directs the Jefferson Hepatitis C Center and is the associate medical director of liver transplantation.

As more and more people are getting tested for hepatitis C, new advances are making it easier than ever to eliminate the virus and its potential to cause dead-

Coffee and Tea Are Good for the Liver

Caffeine has been found to stimulate the metabolization of lipids (fats) stored in liver cells and decrease the fatty liver of mice. People at risk for or diagnosed with nonalcoholic fatty liver disease could benefit from drinking up to four cups of coffee or tea a day.

Study by researchers at Duke-NUS Graduate Medical School's Cardiovascular and Metabolic Disorders Program, Singapore, and Duke University School of Medicine, Durham, North Carolina, published in *Hepatology*.

ly diseases such as cirrhosis and liver cancer. In case you missed it, in 2012, the CDC advised that everyone born between 1945 and 1965 get tested for hepatitis C—along with people of any age who have risk factors.

Why the CDC took action: Even though hepatitis C can strike at any age, more than two million US baby boomers are infected with the virus—and most don't realize it or even think they're at risk.

But the fact remains that anyone can be infected with hepatitis C. People at greatest risk include those who received blood transfusions before 1992 (when screening became more advanced) or anyone who used self-injected drugs with possibly contaminated needles. In some cases, people are believed to have become infected with the virus while getting tattoos or piercings done with contaminated ink or equipment or when being stuck with an infected needle in a health-care setting.

You can be vaccinated for hepatitis A and B, but there is no vaccine for hepatitis C.

An Exciting Advance

Antiviral medication and immune therapy that requires self-injections have long been the main treatments for chronic hepatitis C. However, these drugs often cause grueling side effects, such as debilitating fatigue, headaches, depression, muscle aches and anemia. Also, the drugs need to be taken for at least 24 weeks or up to 48 weeks.

What's new: The FDA has recently approved two new medications that block enzymes that the hepatitis C virus needs to survive. Now patients are given a two- or three-drug cocktail that includes a new drug—*sofosbuvir* (Sovaldi) or *simeprevir* (Olysio)—combined with the antiviral ribavirin and sometimes interferon, which tends to have the most side effects. For the first time, some patients may be eligible for interferon-free therapies if they have a favorable hepatitis C genotype.

With the new regimen, 80% to 90% of patients will be completely cleared of the virus and often in as little as 12 weeks. Previous combination therapies had cure rates of 40% to 80%. Plus, even with interferon, the side effects of the new drug cocktail, such as stomach upset, fatigue and headache, last about half as long as they do with older regimens.

Who Needs Treatment?

Some experts argue that the high cost of the new medication—a full course of treatment can cost roughly $100,000—means that it should be given only to those who have already developed liver disease.

My advice: Everyone with chronic hepatitis C should consult a doctor who is familiar with the risks and benefits of treatment, because even if your liver is healthy, you may still benefit from treatment, especially if the virus is causing joint pain, rashes, kidney disease or certain types of cancer such as lymphoma. Check with your insurance company to see if treatment is fully covered.

Timing Is Flexible

Because chronic hepatitis C progresses slowly, you could potentially wait months or even years before starting treatment. Interferon-free treatments are expected to be available within the next year or two, so some doctors advise patients to delay getting treatment—both to avoid the side effects of interferon and to take advantage of an all-oral treatment plan (interferon is given by injection once a week). To determine the treatment schedule that's best for you, discuss all the options with your doctor.

Follow-up Care

Even when hepatitis C is cured, many patients still have liver damage—and a higher-than-average risk of developing liver cancer.

How I advise my patients: Get screened (with ultrasound) for liver cancer one year after treatment and every few years after that. Those who have cirrhosis will need an ultrasound every six months and an upper endoscopy every two to three years. A low-sodium (less than 2,000 mg a day) diet is also recommended, and raw shellfish, which can cause sepsis, should be avoided.

If you have liver damage: Don't drink alcohol. If you take *acetaminophen* (Tylenol) for pain, don't use more than 2,000 mg daily.

Also, make sure your vitamin D levels are checked at your annual physical—liver damage can cause vitamin D deficiency.

A Lethal Virus

Because hepatitis C has an uncanny ability to elude the immune system, most people exposed to the virus develop a chronic infection that, without treatment, never goes away.

Between 5% and 20% of people with chronic hepatitis C develop liver scarring (cirrhosis)—typically decades after the initial infection. Hepatitis C also is the leading cause of liver cancer and liver transplants in the US.

Testing You Need

A simple blood test reveals if you ever have been exposed to the hepatitis C virus, but a second test is needed to determine if you're still infected.

Shocking: About half of individuals who test positive on the first test do not follow up with the second test, meaning that they probably won't get the treatments that can save their livers—and their lives.

TEST #1: An initial antibody test will reveal if you've been exposed to the virus at any time in your life. If the test is positive, you'll need a second test (see below). If test #1 is negative, you can relax and will not need testing again unless you're possibly exposed to the virus in the future (for example, you find out that you have shared a razor or toothbrush with someone who has hepatitis C). Even if results were negative to test #1, test again in six months if you have hepatitis risk factors.

TEST #2: A viral load assay, also a blood test, will reveal if the infection is chronic (still active in the body). If it is, discuss treatment options with your doctor and be tested for the strain—or genotype—of the virus, which will help determine the most effective medication.

The Truth About Herbal Supplements and Your Liver

Andrew L. Rubman, ND, naturopathic physician and founder and medical director of the Southbury Clinic for Traditional Medicine, Southbury, Connecticut. *SouthburyClinic.com*

Like synthetic prescription drugs that change body chemistry, herbal products also can hurt your liver, especially if they contain impurities...aren't really what they claim to be...or are just not used properly. Some herbs have been associated with liver injuries so often that they've been banned in the United States. But, in these cases, was the herb itself really bad or were other factors causing the problem?

Although some of the concerns we are seeing about herbal supplements and liver toxicity are valid, most herbal products pose no harm when taken properly. "Properly" means at the right dosages, for the right reason and for the right length of time. But the trend, unfortunately, is not making herbal supplements look good. Research compiled from a large database that tracks liver injuries caused by either prescription drugs or herbal supplements shows that the proportion of liver injuries associated with herbal and dietary supplements has increased over the past 10 years from 7% to 20%.

One study based on data from this research summarized the dangers of several different herbs and herbal formulations implicated in liver injuries. Here's the lowdown on seven commonly known herbs that were on the list. Some of these herbs definitely should be avoided...others used with caution...and others have just gotten a bum rap...

• **Comfrey.** Comfrey has been traditionally used, often in the form of a tea, to soothe an upset stomach. It also has been used topically to treat wounds and skin inflammation because it is rich in tannins and other substances that promote skin repair. But because comfrey contains pyrrolizidine alkaloids, compounds that are toxic to the liver, products containing it that are meant to be drunk or eaten are now banned for nonprescription use in the United States.

Comfrey is now available only in the form of creams and ointments for treatment of skin wounds and inflammation, and because its harmful alkaloids can penetrate the skin, consumers are warned to not overdo use of these products—do not use on open wounds or broken skin and do not use for longer than 10 days at a time or for more than four to six weeks total in one year.

But the concern about comfrey's liver-harming properties might be overblown. Other compounds in the herb that are beneficial to the liver may offset the dangers of the pyrrolizidine alkaloids. Although the herb could probably be safely used while in the care of a naturopathic doctor who would monitor liver health, there are certainly plenty other safer remedies for soothing an upset stomach.

• **Kava.** Kava comes from the root of a type of pepper plant. On the tropical islands of the Pacific Ocean where the plant is native, kava has been used as a mild intoxicant, similar to alcohol. In Western herbal medicine, however, it has found a place, in pill form, in the relief of anxiety and insomnia. Liver damage, including hepatitis and liver failure, has been associated with kava use. This has led several countries, including the United Kingdom, Poland and France, to restrict or ban it. But researchers have been debating whether kava is, indeed, toxic or whether nontraditional ways of preparing it are causing liver injury.

It's neither banned nor restricted in the United States. Although the FDA acknowledges that kava is useful for managing anxiety, it has issued a warning that it has been linked to serious liver damage.

Kava's predicament is a perfect example of why herbs should be used in their traditional ways. When extracts are prepared in the traditional manner from the entire plant, they are generally safe, but when an isolated chemical from the plant is commercially sold in capsule form, problems can occur. Why? Because other beneficial parts of the plant that act in a check-and-balance way are left out. For this reason, I prefer the kava extract manufactured by Eclectic Institute in Sandy, Oregon, which is produced using the original extraction method. This brand of kava is widely available in nutrition stores and online through *Amazon.com*, *Vitacost.com*, and other sellers.

• **Green tea extract.** Green tea extract is on store shelves everywhere, frequently marketed as a weight-loss product. But when green tea extract is taken while fasting, as some people using weight-loss supplements may be doing, the liver may be overwhelmed by the high volume of antioxidant compounds, resulting sometimes in serious liver injury.

Taking weight-loss or other potent supplements while fasting is unwise. When someone adopts an unusual diet or fasts, the body's metabolism is thrown off. The change can cause the liver to go into overdrive to adjust. In the case of green tea extract, the same compound that is protective for someone with a normal metabolism can harm someone whose metabolism is not working at its best. Green tea extract, thus, is normally safe when taken in between meals but should not be part of a fasting or cleansing regimen.

• **Germander.** Germander actually refers to about 250 species of plants in the mint family that have been used to treat high blood pressure, gout, diabetes and other conditions, but it is known to be potentially poisonous to the liver. It should be used only under direct supervision of a naturopathic doctor or other knowledgeable health-care provider who can monitor the supplement's impact on the liver. He cautioned that germander has been finding its way into weight-loss supplements and is also often added to supplements made from skullcap—an herb belonging to the mint family—or even substituted for skullcap in supplements claiming to contain skullcap. This unethical behavior by some supplement companies has put skullcap into a predicament. See the next section for details.

• **Skullcap.** Skullcap, also called asafetida, produces stalks of delicate flowers—usually purple although violet and red varieties also exist. American skullcap (*Scutellaria lateriflora*) is generally used to calm the nerves and relax muscles. Chinese skullcap (*Scutellaria baicalensis*) is used to treat allergies, infections, inflammation and headaches. Some studies have suggested that skullcap can cause hepatitis, but it's not known whether the blame lies with the herb itself or with one of the other products it is often mixed with (or replaced by)—namely germander.

Skullcap is really just an innocent bystander, guilty only of being associated with or replaced by germander. In this instance, reading labels is not enough. Choosing high-quality supplements and not any eye-catching bottle on a store shelf is essential for your safety. Products manufactured by Eclectic Institute and HerbPharm, are among those I use in my clinical practice.

• **Celandine.** From the poppy family, celandine has traditionally been used as a mild sedative and treatment for digestive problems. Blockage of bile ducts and other liver problems can develop in people who regularly use the herb for too long (three months or more). How celandine does its damage, which goes away once celandine use is stopped, isn't known.

I have yet to encounter problems with celandine in my practice, but I prescribe the herb only in moderation and not on a regular basis. It should be used only under the guidance of a naturopathic physician who will decide what the appropriate dosage for an individual patient is and how long it should be taken.

• **Chaparral.** High in antioxidants, chaparral refers to the leaves of the creosote bush, which is an evergreen shrub native to southwest deserts. Chaparral has been used to treat bronchitis, skin conditions and pain, but it very commonly causes bile ducts to become blocked after three weeks of use. Although the damage usually clears up quickly after chaparral is stopped, severe liver damage, including cirrhosis (a common cause for liver transplantation), has been associated with chaparral. As with green tea extract, an overload of an antioxidant compound may be behind the liver damage caused by chaparral. This is another herb that should be taken only under the guidance of a knowledgeable health-care provider.

Staying Safe

How would you know if a supplement is hurting your liver? Fatigue, loss of appetite, looking sick and pale and/or noticing a strong body odor can be signs of liver trouble. You may become gassy, and your stools may be paler than usual. If you have any of these symptoms, stop taking the supplement and make an appointment to see your doctor as soon as possible. In extreme cases, jaundice may occur. Signs of jaundice include itchiness, yellow eyes and skin, dark urine, and yellow stools. If this happens, get to a doctor—or hospital emergency room—immediately.

The liver is a very resilient organ. If a drug or supplement harms the liver, the damage is frequently—but not always—reversed once you stop taking the offending drug or supplement. One way to avoid liver problems that might be set off by herbs and herbal supplements, in addition to taking swift action if the symptoms described above occur, is to not be like the approximately 40% of supplement users who hide use from their doctors. Tell your healthcare provider about everything you're taking so that your doctor will know what to do to prevent complications—such as not prescribing a drug that might interfere or interact with a supplement.

Most importantly, buy your herbs and supplements from a licensed naturopathic doctor. Naturopathic practitioners have access to the best, professional-grade products that are free from contaminants and sneaky substitutions. And naturopathic professionals can best advise you about the safe and effective use of a botanical remedy.

Chapter 10

PROTECT YOURSELF FROM KILLER INFECTIONS

How to Wreck Your Immune System

Nobody wants to spend time sick in bed feeling miserable with a cold, the flu or any other illness. *But here's the catch:* Even if you stay well rested, exercise and eat healthfully, you still could be sabotaging your immune system. Most people are unknowingly making it harder for their bodies to fight off illnesses. *How to stop hurting your immune system...*

•**Skip the germ-killing soaps.** Studies now show that triclosan, the key ingredient in many antibacterial hand soaps (as well as some shaving gels, shampoos, cosmetics, deodorants and other personal-care items), fuels the growth of antibiotic-resistant bugs in the public at large. With frequent use, triclosan also can hurt you personally by setting up your body to develop a secondary "superinfection" that can occur as a complication of colds, the flu or viral pneumonia.

Among the best ways to prevent colds and the flu: Vigorous, frequent hand-washing with plain soap is all you need, but here's the key—you need to scrub long enough (count to 20).

If you like the reassurance offered by a hand sanitizer, products with at least 60% alcohol, such as Purell or Germ-X, are widely recommended. However, the alcohol in such hand sanitizers can lead to dry, cracked skin, which provides an entry point for bacterial or fungal skin infections. Alcohol-based products are supported by strong research, but if dry skin is a problem, rely on hand-washing and/or a hand sanitizer that contains natural antibacterial plant oils such as citrus, oregano, rosemary and/or thyme.

Good choice: CleanWell, $10.99 for three one-ounce spray bottles, *CleanWellToday. com.*

•**Take a pass on sugar.** Sugar, refined carbohydrates and high- fructose corn syrup can impair the effectiveness of our immune cells. As soon as you notice cold or flu symptoms, cut these foods out of your diet.

Beware: The caramelized sugar found on cinnamon rolls, donuts or sticky buns is particularly harmful to our immunity. Certain

Robert Rountree, MD, family physician in private practice and owner of Boulder Wellcare in Boulder, Colorado. He is coauthor of numerous books, including *Immunotics: A Revolutionary Way to Fight Infection, Beat Chronic Illness and Stay Well.* He is also medical editor of the journal Alternative and Complementary Therapies and a faculty member at the Institute for Functional Medicine, based in Federal Way, Washington.

molecular structures in this type of sugar resemble bacteria, and our immune system receptors mistakenly bind to them, interfering with their ability to respond effectively to true infections.

If you need a sweetener: Try raw honey, which has immune-building properties.*

• **Watch out for pesticides.** Most nonorganic produce gets showered with pesticides, which damage your immune system.

What to try instead: Load up on fresh, organic fruits and vegetables to arm your immune system with disease-fighting vitamins and nutrients. Organic berries, citrus fruits, grapes and spinach are especially rich in antioxidants that support immune function. When fresh berries aren't available, try frozen organic berries. You can save money by opting for nonorganic citrus fruits and other peelable items (such as bananas) that are less likely to harbor dangerous pesticides than produce without peels.

Power Up Your Immunity

Many people rely on well-known immunity boosters such as vitamin C and/or echinacea, but you're likely to get better results from using the following on a daily basis as a preventive during cold and flu season (or year-round if you work directly with the public)…**

• **Probiotics.** By far, probiotics are the best way to enhance your immunity. These "good" bacteria, including Lactobacillus and Bifidobacterium, reside in your digestive tract, where they keep intestinal microbes in check and elevate your number of infection-fighting T cells.

Fermented foods, such as kefir, yogurt, kimchi, sauerkraut and kombucha, are all naturally rich in probiotics. Aim for two (four- to six-ounce) servings a day.

In general, however, probiotic supplements are more potent and may be more reliable than probiotic-rich foods. If you opt for

*Infants under age one and people who are allergic to pollen or immunocompromised should not consume raw honey.

**Consult your doctor before trying dietary supplements—especially if you take prescription medication and/or have a chronic medical condition.

a supplement, use a combination of Bifido-bacterium and/or Lactobacillus species.

A probiotic found in studies to boost immunity: Culturelle, $39.99 for 80 capsules, Amazon.com.

• **N-acetylcysteine (NAC).** The body easily converts this amino acid into a usable form of glutathione, an immunity-protecting antioxidant that itself is poorly absorbed from the gastrointestinal tract.

Scientific evidence: Italian researchers found that taking 1,200 mg daily of NAC throughout flu season reduced the frequency, severity and intensity of flu-like symptoms.

Typical dose: 600 mg to 1,200 mg daily as a preventive…at the first sign of infection, increase the dose to 3,000 mg daily (taken in doses of 600 mg each throughout the day).

• **Elderberry syrup.** When used within the first 48 hours of feeling flu-ish, this syrup (made from naturally antiviral elderberries) has been shown to relieve symptoms four days faster than a placebo.

If you are not taking elderberry syrup as a daily preventive, start using it within the first two days of developing cold or flu symptoms. Follow label instructions.

Good choice: Sambucol Black Elderberry Immune System Support, $19.99 for 7.8 ounces, *Drugstore.com.*

Don't Go It Alone!

What do close relationships have to do with immunity? A lot, according to research.

When researchers exposed 276 adults to a rhinovirus (a cause of the common cold), subjects with only one to three relationships (such as fulfilling marriages or friendships with colleagues, neighbors and religious community members) were four times more likely to get sick than those who had more than six relationships.

Possible explanation: Social interactions help ease the negative effects of stress—a known threat to immunity.

The Jekyll-and-Hyde Bacteria

Martin J. Blaser, MD, Muriel G. and George W. Singer Professor of Translational Medicine and director of the Human Microbiome Program in the departments of medicine and microbiology at New York University School of Medicine, New York City. He is author of *Missing Microbes: How the Overuse of Antibiotics Is Fueling Our Modern Plagues*.

Doctors have long been prescribing antibiotics to anyone with gastric discomfort, including ulcers. The goal was to eliminate the bad guy—the H. pylori bacteria. But over time, scientists have discovered that the bad guy actually is a good guy as well. On the one hand, H. pylori increases your risk for ulcers and then later for stomach cancer, but on the other hand, it is good for the esophagus, protecting you against GERD and its consequences, including a different cancer, and it may even protect against asthma and weight gain.

We talked with renowned scientist Martin J. Blaser, MD, who has studied H. pylori for nearly 30 years and is the author of the recent book *Missing Microbes. Here he explains what this means for you…*

Microbes in Decline

Antibiotics are effective at killing bacteria and stopping infections. But they're not very discriminating. Each dose kills many different organisms, including ones that you may need to stay healthy.

In 2010, health-care practitioners in the US prescribed 258 million courses of antibiotics—about 833 prescriptions for every 1,000 people. The average child in the US receives about 17 courses of antibiotics before he/she is 20 years old.

Do we need all of these drugs? Absolutely not. In Sweden, where doctors are slower to write prescriptions, antibiotic use is only about 47% of US levels. Swedish children, in the first three years of life, are receiving less than one-and-a-half courses of antibiotics versus about four in US children—and the death rate in Swedish children is lower than in US children.

In the US, doctors routinely prescribe antibiotics for infections that usually are caused by viruses (which aren't affected by the drugs) or for conditions that usually get better with no treatment.

Result: Many people no longer have the bacteria that they may need to stay healthy. *Examples…*

Heartburn and Cancer

In the 1980s, researchers discovered that most ulcers were caused by H. pylori, a common stomach organism. Doctors can test for it using a blood test or a stool test. Now ulcers are routinely cured with antibiotics that kill the bacterium.

The catch: The same microbe that causes ulcers is simultaneously protective. Researchers speculate that diminished populations of H. pylori—caused by improved sanitation as well as antibiotics—could explain why heartburn, known as gastroesophageal reflux disease (GERD), now affects about 18.6 million people in the US.

What's the connection? In the past, most people lived with H. pylori all their lives. It gradually damaged stomach cells and reduced acid levels. Less acid meant that GERD

Ask Your Doctor to Clean This

Stethoscopes can transfer bacteria from one patient to another. Bacteria were found on the part of the stethoscope that touches patients' skin. Some were contaminated with the deadly methicillin-resistant *Staphylococcus aureus* (MRSA).

Self-defense: Ask the doctor to clean the stethoscope with alcohol before using it to examine you.

Study by researchers at University of Geneva Hospitals, Switzerland, published in *Mayo Clinic Proceedings*.

was less common, and less severe, than it is today.

This paradox is one of nature's trade-offs. People who take antibiotics to eliminate H. pylori won't have ulcers, but they're twice as likely to develop GERD. They also have an increased risk for Barrett's esophagus, tissue damage that can lead to esophageal cancer.

You should take antibiotics if you've been diagnosed with an ulcer. But the majority of patients with ulcerlike symptoms don't actually have ulcers. They're far more likely to have non-ulcer dyspepsia, a condition that isn't helped by antibiotics.

Obesity

There's some evidence that the nation's obesity epidemic is caused in part by antibiotics. In laboratory studies, mice given antibiotics have increases in body fat even when their diets stay the same. Livestock producers routinely give antibiotics to uninfected animals not to ward off illness but because it increases their body weight.

The same bacterium that causes ulcers (and protects against GERD) also appears to regulate the activity of two stomach hormones—ghrelin, a hormone that triggers appetite when your stomach is empty, and leptin, a hormone that signals the brain when it's time to stop eating.

Children who get the typical courses of antibiotics may grow up without any H. pylori in their stomachs. This could increase their appetites by causing ghrelin levels to remain steady even after they've already eaten.

Antibiotics are just one factor that could affect bacteria and, in turn, contribute to obesity. Another is the increasing use of Cesarean-section childbirths. When researchers reviewed data from 15 separate studies with more than 38,000 participants, they found that babies delivered by Cesarean section—who aren't exposed to the same bacteria as those delivered vaginally—are 26% more likely to be overweight as adults.

Probiotics Help Cure H. Pylori

Standard "triple therapy" (proton pump inhibitor, *amoxicillin* and *clarithromycin*) for *Helicobacter pylori* (H. pylori) infection (which can cause ulcers) worked better when a probiotic was added in a study of 804 adults with the infection. After taking a probiotic that contains Lactobacillus and Bifidobacterium, twice daily for six weeks, 88% had no H. pylori infection versus 73% who didn't take probiotics.

Goran Hauser, MD, PhD, gastroenterologist, Clinical Hospital Centre, Rijeka, Croatia.

Asthma and Allergies

Many patients with GERD also develop wheezing, constricted airways and other asthmalike symptoms. Once again, a missing bacterium might be to blame. In one study, researchers collected blood samples from more than 500 people. They found that those who tested positive for H. pylori were 30% less likely to have asthma than those who didn't have H. pylori.

It is possible that stomach inflammation triggered by some strains of H. pylori triggers the activity of immune cells that help prevent asthma and allergies. Also, it is possible that the higher acid levels (discussed above) in those without H. pylori could lead to asthma symptoms.

Antibiotic Caution

Antibiotics can be lifesaving drugs. I don't advise people to never take them. But doctors need to prescribe antibiotics more judiciously.

Important...

• **Don't insist on antibiotics just because you (or your child) has an ear, sinus or upper-respiratory infection.** The vast majority of these infections are caused by viruses. Even when bacteria are to blame, the infections usually clear up on their own. Ask your doctor if he/she is sure that an infection needs to be treated.

•**Ask for a narrow-spectrum drug.** Doctors often prescribe high-powered, broad-spectrum antibiotics (such as the Z-Pak) because they knock out many common infections. But the broad-spectrum drugs also kill more innocent organisms.

When possible, it's better to take a narrow-spectrum antibiotic (such as penicillin) that's less likely to kill beneficial organisms. It's not a perfect solution, because all antibiotics kill multiple strains of bacteria. But "targeted" drugs may be somewhat less likely to cause long-term problems than broad-spectrum antibiotics.

On the horizon: In 1998, I predicted in the *British Medical Journal* that we would one day be giving H. pylori back to our children. Since then, the support for this idea has only grown deeper, but we are not there yet.

Is It Safe to Kiss Someone with Cold Sores?

A cold sore is a group of small blisters around the mouth, usually caused by the herpes simplex 1 virus. Most initial infections occur in childhood. The virus is stored in an underlying nerve under the skin, and recurrences can emerge periodically, usually around the border of the lip, after a cold, stress or a sunburn.

When a cold sore is present, close contact (kissing or sharing objects such as lip balm) should be avoided until the sore is completely healed. Even when there's no apparent cold sore, an infected person can spread the infection. But by adulthood, most people have been exposed to the virus, which builds their immunity so they may not get cold sores.

Lynne J. Goldberg, MD, professor of dermatology and pathology & laboratory medicine, Boston University School of Medicine.

Acupuncture for Sepsis

A nimals given acupuncture were more likely to survive sepsis—a major cause of hospital deaths—than those that weren't treated.

Why: Acupuncture may reduce out-of-control inflammation, the hallmark of sepsis.

Nature Medicine.

Follow Up on Blood Infection

F ollow up to get the best infection treatment.

New study: 38% of patients with a bloodstream infection got the wrong treatment or were initially given an ineffective antibiotic while the cause of the infection was being investigated.

Most common types of infection: Staph and E. coli. If you develop a bloodstream infection, ask your doctor to review your updated blood culture results if symptoms don't improve within 24 hours.

Deverick J. Anderson, MD, MPH, associate professor of medicine, Duke University School of Medicine, Durham, North Carolina.

Watch Out for Bacteria Hot Spots!

Cindy Owen, MD, assistant professor of dermatology and the residency program director in dermatology at the University of Louisville School of Medicine in Louisville, Kentucky.

S tinky underarms aren't unusual, but when one man's stubbornly smelly armpits lasted for four years, doctors knew something was, uh, fishy.

According to a report appearing in a recent issue of *The New England Journal of*

223

Medicine, the 40-year-old's underarm hairs were infected with bacteria known as *Corynebacterium tenuis*.

The hair shafts were covered with—beware: what follows is pretty gross!—a creamy, yellow substance that emitted an irrepressible odor.

This man's case is a stark reminder that our skin is crawling, usually unbeknownst to us, with hundreds of types of bacteria. And some of these stealthy germs can lead to serious illnesses such as sepsis (a potentially deadly inflammatory response throughout the body) and pneumonia.

Where Bacteria Live

The good news is, most skin bacteria, which outnumber our body's own cells, are harmless and even protect skin cells from more dangerous microorganisms.

For example, harmless *Staphylococcus epidermidis* takes up space on our skin that the insidious *Staphylococcus aureus*—usually called "staph"—would otherwise colonize. Scientific research is increasingly indicating that the vast majority of skin bacteria inhibit disease-causing agents or even "educate" the immune system to help us fend off illness.

Harmful bacteria, however, tend to congregate at certain skin sites that are either moist or oily. Here are four of the most common "hot spots" for harmful bacteria—and the red flags that mean you should get to a doctor…

Hot Spot #1: Tip of the nose. The anterior nares (the ends of the nostrils) are the most common site for colonized methicillin-resistant *Staphylococcus aureus*, or MRSA, highly dangerous bacteria that can cause sepsis and even death. MRSA also can colonize in areas inside the nose.

About 2% of people carry MRSA (often harmlessly) on their skin—it also can congregate in adults in the armpits and groin area.

What to look for: Constant irritation at the tip of the nose, which may include tiny skin cracks called fissures, can clue you in to MRSA's presence. Another tip-off is the development of numerous or recurrent boils

anywhere on the body. If you develop one of these signs, see a doctor.

Hot Spot #2: Between the toes. The webby region between the toes and the cuticle areas on toes and fingers can harbor *Pseudomonas aeruginosa* bacteria, which can cause an infection of the toes and feet, especially in people who sweat a lot or are active and wear closed-toe shoes. The infection may cause pain and difficulty walking and can result in cellulitis (an infection just below the skin surface) or sepsis in people with weak immunity.

What to look for: A discharge that may stain socks a green color and a sweet, grape-like odor.

Hot Spot #3: Armpits. The Corynebacteria causing the 40-year-old man's long-term odor have a fondness for armpits and the groin area, coating the hair shafts with a "cheesy" yellow paste. The infection, called trichomycosis axillaris, is most common in tropical or other warm climates. Similar bacteria can cause infections of the feet.

What to look for: A noticeable smell, and if the feet are infected, small, "punched out" pitting of the soles.

Hot Spot #4: Scalp/hairy areas. While the scalp is the most reliably hair-covered spot on our bodies (or so we hope), hair follicles cover almost our entire bodies. In men, of course, the hair tends to be more visibly abundant—for example, on the chest, back and face.

Densely packed areas of hair follicles can be the target of *Propionibacterium acnes*, which plays a role in the development of inflammatory acne that's typically far worse than a blackhead or two.

What to look for: Pustules and/or large, painful bumps grouped on the face, chest or back.

How the Mystery Ended

And what about the man with the smelly armpit infection? After the hair was shaved, he received an antibiotic for the infection and topical aluminum chloride to curb his armpit sweating, which had created the ideal home for the bacteria.

Remember: Most bacteria are beneficial. Still, it's wise to inspect your skin regularly for the red flags of infection described in this article. Avoid antibacterial soaps unless directed by your doctor. These soaps disrupt the normal skin barriers that protect us from invading bacteria and other pathogens. Plain soap and water are usually the best way to wash.

To Banish a Boil

A nasty collection of pus under the skin, known as a boil, is an infection typically resulting from Staphylococcus aureus, more commonly referred to as "staph."

Recurrent boils, however, can signal infection with MRSA, a drug-resistant form of staph that can cause pneumonia or severe infections of the blood, bones, heart valves or lungs. Boils can occur anywhere on the body but are more common in the armpits, groin and the area between the genitals and anus.

Important: Seek medical attention for boils larger than one-half inch in diameter, which should be professionally drained. The same goes for boils with red streaks around them, which can be a sign of dangerous blood vessel involvement…boils that continue to enlarge…if a fever develops or lymph nodes enlarge…or if the boil is near the anus.

Also, see a doctor about any boil on the spine or face. Boils on the spine can lead to a spinal cord infection, and those in the triangular area between the eyes, cheeks and lip can trigger a dangerous brain infection.

Most other boils are small and can be treated at home.

What to do…

• **Apply a compress soaked in warm salt water three times per day for 20 minutes.** Use a fresh washcloth each time.

What not to do…

• **Never squeeze or pop a boil, which can spread the infection.**

• **Do not stick a needle or other object into a boil**—this can cause dangerous bleeding or spread the infection.

Strange Lump on Tailbone

If you have a painful lump just above your tailbone, you could have a pilonidal cyst, a deep infection beneath the skin, usually located near or above the tailbone, that can cause some pain. The cyst is often clogged with hair and can ooze pus or blood. Some pilonidal cysts may get better naturally, but most need to be lanced, drained and allowed to heal. Recurring infections are generally treated with additional surgeries, sometimes requiring reshaping of the furrow between the buttocks (called a cleft lift) to try to prevent further cysts.

Your lump should be evaluated by a colon and rectal surgeon. In the meantime, keep the area clean and use a specially designed pillow that relieves pressure on the tailbone, such as a coccyx cushion, available at Walmart, CVS and other stores.

Sandy Fischler, founder and executive director, Pilonidal Support Alliance, Long Beach, California.

Avoid Bacterial Infections from Dermal Filler Injections

Morten Alhede, PhD, postdoctoral researcher, department of international health, immunology and microbiology, Faculty of Health Sciences, University of Copenhagen, Denmark. His research was published in *Pathogens and Disease.*

Nearly two million visits to cosmetic dermatologists are made each year for dermal filler gel injections for fuller, luscious lips or smooth, wrinkle-free skin. But as dermal filler gel injections become more popular, dangerous side effects become more common, too. In fact, serious side effects from dermal filler gels have tripled since 2005, according to the FDA.

To make matters worse, some estheticians and dermatologists are in denial about the cause of some of these side effects. Rather than admitting that they are caused by bacterial infection—as research is showing—they are blaming them on allergic reactions and treating with them corticosteroids, which can interfere with the skin's ability to fight off infections, making the situation worse. But when the right precautions are taken, bacterial infections associated with dermal filler gel use can be avoided.

Dermal Filler Gel...a Bacterial Orgy?

A group of Danish researchers have taken up the task to prove that bacterial buildup is what's causing some of the bad reactions, such as swelling and the appearance of pustules or subdermal bumps, that sometimes happen at the site of the gel injection. This group recently confirmed earlier research that some dermal filler gels are the perfect breeding ground for biofilms, bacteria that clump together to live and thrive when they find the ideal environment.

First, the researchers examined what happened when three different popular dermal filler gels—one meant to have relatively temporary effects (Restylane, which lasts less than 12 months), one semipermanent (Radiesse, which lasts from one to seven years) and one permanent (Aquamid)—were mixed with three different common skin bacteria—*Pseudomonas aeruginosa, Staphylococcus epidermidis* and *Propionibacterium acnes*, and left to incubate. Within 24 hours, all three gels showed dense bacterial colonies that only grew bigger over the next 24 hours...showing that the gels were a good habitat for biofilm growth.

The researchers then tested whether the gels might not only be good media for bacterial growth but also might help the bacteria grow resistant to antibiotics—a potential double whammy for people unlucky enough to have this bacterial party injected under their skin. And what they found was that after 72 hours of growth in the cosmetic gels, two of the bacterial strains—P. aeruginosa and S. epi-

dermidis—were reduced but not completely cleared up when exposed to antibiotics.

When the researchers then injected mice with gels that had either P. aeruginosa or S. epidermidis added to them, bacteria grew only in mice that were injected with the permanent filler. When this experiment was repeated, but with some mice receiving antibiotics two hours before the injection and others seven days afterward, the pretreated mice were spared from infection but the mice treated seven days after being infected were dealing with an antibiotic-resistant infection. To quickly get a handle on how these results in mice translated to what might happen in humans, researchers studied the medical records of 657 people who had received dermal filler gel injections at one cosmetic dermatology center. The researchers compared records from 2001 to 2006, which was before the center began to pretreat patients with antibiotics, with records from 2007 to 2011, when pretreating became the standard protocol. The results...incidence of signs of infection after the procedure dropped from 7% to 2%.

Pretreatment Is the Key

The take-home message is that simply piercing the skin with the dermal filler injection needle can potentially allow normal skin bacteria to mix with the filler gel and grow into a problem. To combat this, the study researchers strongly recommend that folks going in for dermal filler gel injections receive antibiotic therapy in preparation for the procedure or have antibiotics injected with the filler as a preventive measure.

While commercials often present dermal filler injections as little more than lunchtime spa treatments, it's wise to not forget that they are medical procedures that carry risks—some known and some perhaps not known yet. If you are considering having dermal filler injections, go to a medical doctor for the procedure—preferably a board-certified cosmetic dermatologist or plastic surgeon—and discuss your concerns about possible bacterial infection with him or her. A well-trained physician will know what type of antibiotic treatments are best to prevent skin infections.

Protect Yourself From Germy Airplanes

Up to 20% of airplane passengers report coming down with a cold in the weeks after travel. Researchers recently found that some germs can live for up to one week on armrests, plastic tray tables and in seat pockets. *Examples...*

Methicillin-resistant Staphylococcus aureus (MRSA), which can cause life-threatening infections, and *Escherichia coli*, often the cause of severe diarrhea and vomiting.

Since most of the infections you are likely to pick up on these surfaces are transmitted via your hands, the best way to protect yourself is to bring a small, two-ounce bottle of alcohol-based hand sanitizer on the plane with you and use it frequently. You can also bring disinfecting wipes to use on tray tables and armrests. For example, Ebola is considered to be an airborne virus but can live on surfaces for several hours. The Centers for Disease Control and Prevention (CDC) recommends the above hand-hygiene practices for all airline passengers.

Charles Gerba, PhD, professor of microbiology and environmental sciences, The University of Arizona College of Public Health, Tucson.

Air-Travel Health Myths Debunked

Roundup of travel and health experts, reported in *USA Today.*

Myth: Cabin air is full of germs. **Reality:** Aircraft are equipped with HEPA filters to clean the air. The problems lie on chair upholstery, tray tables, armrests and toilet handles where bacteria such as MRSA and *E. coli* can live for up to one week.

Myth: Bagged pillows and blankets are safe to use.

Reality: Pillowcases on bagged pillows are rarely changed, and blankets should be used only on your lower legs—not near your eyes, nose and mouth.

Myth: The aircraft is cleaned between flights.

Reality: Airplanes typically are wiped down after every 30 days of service or at 100 flying hours, but the FAA doesn't regulate cleaning, so frequency and thoroughness vary.

Myth: There is nothing you can do to protect yourself in an aircraft cabin.

Reality: Use alcohol-based hand sanitizer...wipe the armrest and tray table with disinfectant wipes...stay hydrated...use tissues to open bathroom doorknobs and touch toilet handles...don't touch your eyes because tear ducts are a fast route to the nose and throat.

The Germiest Spots in Public Places

Philip M. Tierno, Jr., PhD, microbiologist and director of clinical microbiology and diagnostic immunology at New York University Langone Medical Center and a professor in the departments of microbiology and pathology at New York University School of Medicine, both in New York City. He is author of *The Secret Life of Germs.*

You're not paranoid—germs really are out to get you. But not from the much publicized diseases such as Ebola. The real risk comes from mundane microbes lurking where you might not expect them. *Here's where they are and what to do about them...*

Lying in Wait

About 80% of all infections are caused by touch—either from direct contact or from touching a contaminated surface. And when you're in a public place, just about every surface is contaminated.

When researchers at University of Arizona applied a noninfectious virus to an office door—a virus that was not naturally present in the office—the virus was detected on more than half of the office surfaces (and on the hands of office workers) within just four hours.

Don't count on people washing their hands. Researchers observed the hand-washing habits of nearly 4,000 people in public restrooms. They found that about 10% didn't wash at all. Among those who did, about two-thirds didn't use soap, and only 5% washed long enough to thoroughly remove harmful organisms.

Public Offenders

Bacteria and viruses can survive on hard surfaces for anywhere from a few hours to several days—and sometimes longer when they're protected by a sheen of hand lotion or residue from a greasy meal. *Watch out for…*

•**Coffee-cup lids.** A University of Arizona professor found that about 17% of disposable coffee-cup lids placed on cups by coffee shop workers were contaminated with fecal bacteria.

Solution: Skip the lid, or pour the coffee into your own thermos cup.

•**Office coffeepot handles.** The pots usually get rinsed out, but the handles are rarely cleaned.

Solution: Wash your hands after pouring your coffee, or use a disposable wipe to wipe down the handle before using.

•**ATM machines.** A British study found that ATM machines were heavily contaminated with bacteria at the same levels as nearby public toilets.

Solution: Bring a disposable wipe to wipe the keypad or touch screen, or clean your hands with a disposable wipe immediately after using the machine.

•**Supermarket checkout conveyor belts.** Juices from raw poultry and beef, which may be contaminated with dangerous bacteria, including salmonella and *E. coli*, may leak onto the belts. Other food-related bacteria end up

there, too. A study by Michigan State University tested 100 belts in 42 grocery stores. All 100 belts were found to have mold, yeast, the disease-causing bacteria *Staphylococcus aureus* (staph) and other bacteria.

Solution: When you get home, wash your hands before opening cabinets and the refrigerator. Wash them again when you're done unpacking your groceries. Put packaged raw meat and poultry in plastic bags before you refrigerate or freeze it. Wash off the tops of cans before you open them.

•**Public telephones.** Though pay phones have all but disappeared, you still find telephones for public use in office lobbies, conference rooms, hotel lobbies, etc. They're rarely cleaned.

Solution: Use a disposable wipe to clean the mouthpiece…the part that presses against your ear…and the buttons before using public phones.

Hotels

•**Bathtubs.** Don't be fooled by the gleaming white porcelain and legions of bustling hotel maids. When we took cultures from hundreds of apparently clean bathtubs, about 60% were contaminated with staph.

Rinsing a tub doesn't help because staph survives in biofilm, an invisible coating that forms in tubs and keeps the bacterium moist and viable.

Solution: You need mechanical action to remove biofilm. If you know that you'll want to take a bath in your hotel, bring a small scrub brush and a few ounces of bleach. A solution of one part household bleach to nine parts water and a few drops of soap (such as the shampoo or shower gel at the hotel) will kill most microbes within a few seconds, and the brush will remove them.

•**Pillows.** Pillows are rarely laundered. When I travel, I always bring protective covers (look for antiallergy pillow casings). I wash them each time I return home.

Also: Just about everyone knows (or suspects) that the bedspreads used in most ho-

Watch Out for Restroom Hand Dryers

Restroom hand dryers spread more germs than paper towels do. Researchers placed a harmless type of bacteria on the hands of study subjects to imitate poorly washed hands and found bacteria levels around high-powered "jet air" dryers were 27 times higher than levels near paper-towel dispensers…and 4.5 times higher than levels around warm-air dryers. Nearly half the bacteria around dryers remained for five minutes after the units were used—and some bacteria still could be detected after 15 minutes.

Study by researchers at University of Leeds, UK, published in Journal of Hospital Infection.

tels aren't laundered anywhere near as often as the sheets.

Solution: Remove the bedspread and toss it in a corner. To stay warm, request additional blankets, which are laundered more often than bedspreads.

•**Carpets.** The carpets in public places can harbor some 200,000 bacteria per square inch—thousands of times more than live on the average toilet seat. Since carpets aren't deep-cleaned very often, they provide a veritable buffet for bacteria and other organisms.

Solution: Higher-end hotels often provide a pair of disposable scuffs or slippers. Wear them! Or bring your own slippers or flip-flops.

Restaurants

•**Tables.** Does the server wipe your table before you sit down?

Bad news: The damp wiping cloths should be sanitized between uses but often aren't. They can harbor astonishing amounts of bacteria. One study found that 70% of wiped restaurant tables were contaminated with *E. coli* and other fecal bacteria.

Solution: When you go to a restaurant, wipe the table yourself with a sanitizing wipe.

•**Toilets.** The top of the toilet seat might be sparkling clean, but most germs are underneath. Your fingertips are contaminated when you raise or lower the seat.

Solution: Use a disposable wipe or a thick layer of toilet tissue to lift the seat.

Also important: Close the lid, if the toilet has one, before you flush. Flushing an old-style toilet can spray bacteria-laden droplets up to 20 feet—the newer, low-flush toilets will spray no more than one foot.

Superbug Found in Homes

Methicillin-resistant *Staphylococcus aureus* (MRSA) once was confined to hospitals and nursing homes, but it has been found in homes—specifically, strain USA300, the primary cause of community-acquired MRSA infections throughout the US. MRSA is resistant to common antibiotics and can cause pneumonia, blood infections and other serious illnesses. The infection is spread through skin-to-skin contact or by sharing personal hygiene items, such as razors or towels.

If you have a MRSA infection: Keep the wound covered, and wash your hands frequently to prevent MRSA from spreading to family members. Wash bedding and clothes with hot water.

Study led by researchers at Columbia University Medical Center, New York City, reported in Proceedings of the National Academy of Sciences.

Popular Meat Substitute May Contain Salmonella

Tempeh, made from fermented soybeans and often used in place of meat, has been linked to a salmonella outbreak among 100 people in five states last year. The tempeh had been unpasteurized and made with tainted ingredients imported from Indonesia.

Let Microwaved Meals Sit

Frozen meals need standing time to finish cooking. When researchers investigated a salmonella outbreak that was caused by frozen entrées, they found that 12% of the people infected did not follow the package directions and skipped the standing time before eating. Letting the meal rest after taking it out of a conventional oven or a microwave allows it to finish cooking properly.

Morbidity and Mortality Weekly Report by the Centers for Disease Control and Prevention.

Self-defense: Tempeh should be treated like a meat and thoroughly cooked. Knives and hands should always be thoroughly washed after touching tempeh.

Study by researchers at North Carolina Division of Public Health, Raleigh, published in *Emerging Infectious Diseases*.

Plastic Versus Wood Cutting Boards

Both plastic and wood cutting boards are OK to use.

The difference: Plastic is easier to sanitize (just throw it in the dishwasher) but develops more grooves and scratches where bacteria can grow because moisture can be trapped. Wood is tougher to sanitize, but a hardwood will not have as many scratches (and they close up). Capillary action within the wood grain actually sucks bacteria deep into the wood, and as the wood dries, the bacteria die. Bamboo (a grass) also can be a good choice, since it is typically hard and resistant to bacteria. However, some bamboo boards are soft and should be avoided. Using different cutting boards for different foods helps avoid cross-contamination.

Benjamin Chapman, PhD, associate professor of food safety, North Carolina State University, Raleigh.

Ward Off Food Poisoning Naturally

Activated charcoal—available at drugstores, natural-food stores and stores such as Target and Walmart—traps toxins and other substances and removes them from the body. To prevent food poisoning or lessen its severity, take two capsules of activated charcoal as soon as possible. Repeat every 30 minutes for several hours.

Also helpful: Probiotics. Take a standard dose—read the label for the correct dosage—every hour for several hours as soon as possible. Don't take probiotics at the same time as activated charcoal. Schedule the doses for in between the charcoal doses.

Important: Consult a health-care provider if you have pain or fever for more than 24 hours after eating contaminated food.

Jamison Starbuck, ND, naturopathic physician in family practice and guest lecturer at the University of Montana, both in Missoula. She is past president of the American Association of Naturopathic Physicians and a columnist for *Bottom Line/Health*.

Is Gym Equipment Germy?

Yes! In a study in the *Clinical Journal of Sports Medicine*, cold viruses were found on 63% of equipment in fitness centers. And 80% of infectious diseases are transmitted by contact—either direct (such as kissing, coughing or sneezing) or indirect (for example, touching a contaminated surface, such as gym equipment, and then touching your eyes, nose, mouth or a wound, which are considered portals of entry for germs).

Always make sure to wash your hands with soap and water for at least 20 seconds before eating or drinking anything or before touching those portals of entry. If you're not near a sink, use a hand sanitizer that contains at least 60% alcohol.

Philip M. Tierno, PhD, clinical professor of microbiology and pathology, New York University School of Medicine, New York City.

Is It OK to Pee in the Pool?

Jonathan Vapnek, MD, associate clinical professor of urology, Icahn School of Medicine at Mount Sinai Hospital, New York City.

As disgusting as it may sound, urinating in a swimming poll should not cause health problems for other swimmers. Healthy urine does not contain bacteria or anything else that could make someone sick. The water will dilute the urine, and chlorine removes most germs. Surprisingly, one in five adults admitted in a survey to urinating in swimming pools, so chances are your son isn't the only one secretly doing this.

A bigger problem is fecal contamination, which can lead to diarrhea, respiratory illness and skin, ear and eye infections if someone swallows or comes into contact with even a tiny amount of pool water. Anyone who has had diarrhea in the past two weeks should avoid swimming pools, according to the Centers for Disease Control and Prevention. Tiny amounts of fecal matter contain germs such as *Cryptosporidium* that could take days for chlorine to kill.

To avoid spreading germs, make sure everyone showers before using the pool.

Vaccinate the Babies

Vaccinating babies against rotavirus, which causes stomach illness, prevents older children and adults from developing the potentially fatal infectious disease. The Centers for Disease Control and Prevention (CDC) recommends that all children be vaccinated against the disease starting at two months. Adults generally do not need to be vaccinated against the rotavirus.

Study by researchers at the division of viral diseases, CDC, Atlanta, published in *The Journal of the American Medical Association.*

Don't Let Your Pet Make You Sick

William Schaffner, MD, professor of preventive medicine and infectious diseases, Vanderbilt University School of Medicine, Nashville, and past president of the National Foundation for Infectious Diseases, Bethesda, Maryland.

One of the most popular stories that Daily Health News ever brought to readers was about injuries and illnesses you could get from your pet cat. It covered how to avoid those injuries and illnesses and how to do right by kitty, too. The article went viral. And that's a good thing! But, even though it was incredibly popular, the article offended loads of people. They couldn't believe that cat bites or scratches could lead to limb-threatening infections or that cats could pass other types of infections to people or vice versa. Because the article was so popular and because some people questioned why cats were being "singled out," we decided to look into the human health issues that might be related to living with other animal friends, including dogs, birds, fish and reptiles.

To start, let's acknowledge that, generally speaking, most house pets are wonderful and extremely safe to share space with. In fact, despite the fact that more than half of all American households have at least one

Bacteria in Your Contacts Case

Bacteria can survive in contact lens solution for hours. *Pseudomonas aeruginosa* bacteria can cause corneal ulceration that can result in vision loss. In a test of nine strains, most were killed within 10 minutes of being placed in contact lens solution. But strain 39016 survived for more than four hours.

Craig Winstanley, PhD, professor, department of clinical infection, microbiology and immunology, University of Liverpool, UK, and leader of a study presented at a recent meeting of the Society for General Microbiology.

animal living with the family, infections and injuries caused by pets are relatively uncommon. But there are some things you need to watch out for, according to William Schaffner, MD, professor of preventive medicine and infectious diseases at Vanderbilt University School of Medicine in Nashville.

Slitherin' Friends

Take reptiles, for instance…lizards, snakes, turtles and the like. The biggest concern, according to Dr. Schaffner, is *Salmonella*, a bacterium that can cause a serious intestinal illness in humans. Although any animal can carry the bacteria, lizards, turtles and other reptiles are most "guilty." Not that it's the creature's fault…it is just a simple reality. Studies show that up to 90% of reptiles shed Salmonella. This makes pet reptiles potentially hazardous to your health. So much so that Dr. Schaffner discourages anyone with young children in the home from having them.

"Reptiles shed the bacteria in their feces, and it then can grow and contaminate their living spaces. The bacteria are then transmitted to anyone handling these pets," he explained. If you keep reptiles, you need to be extra diligent about keeping the pet's living space—and your hands—very clean to help avoid Salmonella infection. And this is why children are especially at risk for infection. Children frequently handle their pet reptiles and rummage around their tanks and cages. And we all know that most children don't really know when to wash their hands after touching this or that—and they're constantly putting their fingers in the noses and mouths. A perfect storm for Salmonella infection.

Tweety Birds

After enraging many readers by telling them not to sleep with their cats in our cat-dangers article, dare we tell them not to kiss and cuddle their pet birds…and to wear face masks when cleaning cages? Birds such as parrots, parakeets, cockatoos and lovebirds are common carriers of the bacterium *Chla-*

mydophila psittaci, which can cause parrot fever—a type of pneumonia in humans.

C. psittaci is excreted in a bird's feces and nasal discharge. The bacteria become airborne when the cage is cleaned or the bird flies around. If enough of the airborne bacteria is breathed in by a human or gets in a person's mouth or nose from kissing and cuddling the bird, then parrot fever can develop. And while the pneumonia that parrot fever causes is treatable, an infected person may not be prescribed the proper antibiotic (tetracycline or doxycycline) unless he or she knows to tell the doctor that a pet bird lives in the home and may be the source of the infection, said Dr. Schaffner.

Fishy Friends

Pet fish aren't exactly cuddly, and they're mostly just something to look at, but pet fish can and do transmit disease—namely infection from the bacterium *Mycobacterium marinum*. This pathogen can infect you through tiny nicks and scratches in your skin when you clean the fish tank. The result is a painful skin infection that's not easily recognized by the average busy doctor unless you know to tell your doctor that you may have got it from cleaning a fish tank, said Dr. Schaffner. It can be treated with antibiotics. But to stay on the safe side, wear long rubber gloves when cleaning a fish tank and rinse the gloves thoroughly with clean water before taking them off. (If you are allergic to latex, you can find latex-free gloves.)

Your Best Friend

Then, of course, there are dogs. Each year, about 4.5 million people in America are bitten by them, sending 885,000 people to their doctors for medical attention. Although rabies virus infection is rarely a concern thanks to vaccination efforts, unvaccinated dogs can be infected by wild animals—most commonly bats, said Dr. Schaffner. He urges readers to make sure that their dogs are up-to-date with rabies vaccinations even if the dogs are kept indoors…you never know when Spot will sneak out or have a run-in with a rabid raccoon or bat that broke into the attic.

While rabies may be the least of your worries because your dog is vaccinated, dog bites and scratches can still transmit other harmful bugs. For example, the bacterium *Pasteurella multocida*, normally found in the mouths of healthy dogs (and cats), can cause soft-tissue infection, septic arthritis and bone infections in humans. That's serious stuff. Similar to what our expert said in our article on cats, Dr. Schaffner recommends that you get to a doctor for an antibiotic if you get a deep bite or scratch from a pet dog. Treatment will help prevent a possible *P. multocida* infection.

As for fleas and ticks that latch onto dogs (and cats)…they can transmit Lyme disease, Rocky Mountain Spotted fever and a potentially lethal tick-borne disease called babesiosis to humans. So protect yourself and your dog by treating the dog's coat with a flea and tick spray, powder or shampoo once a month, said Dr. Schaffner.

Who's Most At Risk

Because children naturally want to handle pets and don't often think about hand hygiene (or any hygiene!), they are most prone to the injuries and infections we've discussed. It is important to teach them how to handle pets respectfully to avoid bites and scratches and to wash their hands frequently, said Dr. Schaffner. Another group of people who are most at risk for infections from pets are those with compromised immune systems. This group includes anyone receiving chemotherapy or other immunosuppressive drugs, recipients of a bone marrow or organ transplant, and people infected with HIV, warned Dr. Schaffner. "The emphasis should be on hand washing. But people who have profoundly suppressed immune systems should not be taking care of animals at all because the risk of infection is too great," he said.

To read how your cat can harm your health, visit *BottomLineHealth.com* (search "ways your cat can make you sick").

Can Bedbugs Give You Deadly Chagas Disease?

Jerome Goddard, PhD, extension professor, medical and veterinary entomology, department of biochemistry, molecular biology, entomology and plant pathology, Mississippi State University, Starkville, and affiliate faculty, department of medicine, The University of Mississippi Medical Center, Jackson.

If the idea of bedbugs doesn't already give you the heebie-jeebies, news blasts from the National Institutes of Health, Scientific American, Newsweek and other Internet sources are stirring a pot of frenzy with headlines such as "Bedbugs…Linked to Deadly Chagas Disease in US"! It's all in the wake of research showing that the critters invading our bedrooms and even the nicest hotels can carry a dangerous parasite that causes a tropical illness called Chagas disease, which can cause serious heart or respiratory problems decades after infection occurs, and it kills about 50,000 people every year. Sounds gruesome…but, that said, your true level of risk of Chagas disease from bedbugs doesn't match the hype that even the government is hawking.

Don't Panic

The health alerts that flooded the Internet were the spin of a lab study by researchers at the University of Pennsylvania. They found that bedbugs allowed to feed off mice infected with the tropical parasite *Trypanosoma cruzi*, which causes Chagas disease, became infected themselves. When the infected bedbugs were then allowed to feed off healthy mice, those mice became infected, too. But while the study showed that infected animals could infect bedbugs and vice versa in a laboratory, it did not prove that infected mice—or bedbugs—are actually running around and spreading Chagas disease in the US.

Jerome Goddard, PhD, a professor of entomology at Mississippi State University, agreed. He explained that although the study about bedbugs and Chagas disease was scientifically

233

sound and enlightening as scientific experiments go, no human cases of Chagas disease have yet been traced back to a bedbug infestation. News outlets are simply making a big stink about it to catch more eyeballs (and advertising dollars).

The real carriers of Chagas disease are the tropical pests called kissing bugs.

If you are now concerned about whether you should panic about kissing bugs, know that they particularly like to take up residence in poorly constructed homes made of mud, adobe clay and straw and are primarily native to South and Central America, Mexico and some southwestern parts of the United States. Most Americans live in homes made of lumber, brick, concrete and plaster, so Chagas disease infection may be more of a concern for "adventure" vacationers who like rugged travel in the tropics.

Bedbug Vigilance

Until there is evidence that Chagas disease is actually being spread by bedbugs, ignore the hyped headlines. Dr. Goddard categorizes bedbugs as mostly harmless "nuisance pests"—but that doesn't mean we have to endure them. Here is Dr. Goddard's advice on protecting yourself from bedbugs.

Lyme Disease May Be Sexually Transmitted

Researchers found Lyme bacteria in all of the vaginal secretions from female study participants and in almost half of the semen from male participants with Lyme disease. Identical strains of the bacteria were found in married couples having unprotected sex, suggesting that sexual transmission occurs. If you are concerned about Lyme disease, talk to your doctor about being tested and treated.

Study led by Marianne Middleveen, MD, veterinary microbiologist, Alberta, Canada, published in *Journal of Investigative Medicine.*

When It's Not Just Lyme Disease

Richard I. Horowitz, MD, an internist and integrative-medicine practitioner who is the medical director of the Hudson Valley Healing Arts Center in Hyde Park, New York. Dr. Horowitz is the author of *Why Can't I Get Better: Solving the Mystery of Lyme & Chronic Disease. CanGetBetter.com*

When it comes to tick-borne infections, Lyme disease is the one that gets all the attention.

What most people don't realize: A single tick bite can transmit many disease-causing organisms. These so-called "coinfections" often persist even after a person takes antibiotics (the standard treatment for Lyme).

Unfortunately, most doctors assume that people who test positive for Lyme disease have only Lyme—and they don't have an answer if these patients fail to get better.

A hidden threat: Despite treatment, about 25% of patients with early Lyme disease go on to develop a persistent infection that doesn't adequately respond to antibiotics. Even when the infection appears to be gone based on blood tests, these patients can suffer headaches, joint pain, fever, difficulty concentrating and other symptoms that can last for months or even years.

I call this condition Lyme-MSIDS (Multiple Systemic Infectious Disease Syndrome).* Many doctors believe that Lyme and other tick-borne infections are unlikely to persist after a monthlong course of antibiotics. However, based on my 27 years of experience treating Lyme patients, I'm convinced that Lyme-MSIDS does occur and that patients can remain ill due to overlapping chronic bacterial and parasitic infections.

What you need to know...

*If you've been treated for Lyme and your symptoms don't improve, you may want to see a Lyme-MSIDS specialist. To find such a doctor in your area, consult the Lyme Disease Association, *LymeDiseaseAssociation.org*, or the International Lyme and Associated Diseases Society, *ILADS.org*.

Hidden STD

Nearly 400,000 Americans have chlamydia and don't know it. A new government report estimates that 1.8 million people in the US have the symptomless sexually transmitted disease, but only 1.4 million infections have been reported.

Study by researchers at US National Center for HIV/AIDS, Viral Hepatitis, STD and TB Prevention, a division of the Centers for Disease Control and Prevention, presented at the STD Prevention Conference in Atlanta.

What to Look For

If you have Lyme-like symptoms that don't improve after a month of antibiotic treatment, ask your doctor to check for simultaneous infections. Even if you have tested negative for Lyme, you could still be infected with a similar organism that causes Lyme-like symptoms but isn't detectable with the standard tests for Lyme.

Tick-borne Coinfections...

•**Babesiosis.** This parasitic infection is spreading rapidly in the US. Babesiosis has been reported across the country from the East Coast (New York) to the upper Midwest and West Coast (Washington State and California). It typically causes malaria-like symptoms—such as chills, sweating and fever—that occur intermittently, sometimes for years. It also can cause shortness of breath and an unexplained cough.

How it's diagnosed: Blood tests that check for the infecting organism (Babesia). It's important to test for different Babesia species—and do DNA and RNA testing if Babesiosis is suspected, but the antibody titer is negative.

Typical treatment: I often rotate combinations of different antibiotics with antimalarial drugs and herbs.

Example: Clindamycin (Cleocin) combined with *atovaquone* (Mepron) and *azithromycin* (Zithromax) and/or *sulfamethoxazole/trimethoprim* (Septra) with the herbs artemisia and cryptolepis. I have found these regimens help reduce Babesia symptoms.

Also helpful: Curcumin, the yellow plant pigment in the spice turmeric. It reduces inflammation that may be caused by Babesiosis as well as Lyme disease. If you want to try a curcumin supplement, follow label directions.

•**Ehrlichiosis/Anaplasmosis.** This is a bacterial infection that typically causes a high fever accompanied by severe headaches, muscle pain and fatigue. It's among the most common coinfections found in Lyme patients.

How it's diagnosed: Antibody blood tests help to diagnose Ehrlichiosis/Anaplasmosis, but a low white blood cell count, low platelet count and elevated liver enzymes are also signs that the infection is present.

Typical treatment: Doxycycline or other tetracycline antibiotics.

•**Bartonella.** Also known as cat scratch disease, this bacterial illness was once thought to be transmitted to people only from cat scratches or bites. It is now known that Bartonella also can be spread by ticks, fleas and biting flies.

A classic Bartonella infection usually causes a rash or papule (a small, red, raised bump on the skin), along with swelling of the lymph nodes, but patients who also have Lyme-MSIDS usually have more intense symptoms. For example, they may not have a rash but could experience seizures and severe nerve pain, burning, tingling or numbness as well as severe memory and concentration problems.

How it's diagnosed: Antibody blood tests as well as DNA and RNA testing.

Typical treatment: Doxycycline, combined with rifampin or other medications such as a quinolone antibiotic like Cipro.

Act Quickly

The majority of patients with Lyme disease will recover completely—and quickly—when they take antibiotics within two to four weeks after a bite from an infected tick.

If you do not get better within a month after taking antibiotics, and the additional testing shows that you do not have a tick-borne coinfection, it's possible that blood tests missed the infection, you have one or more other tick-borne coinfections and/or you're still infected with the Lyme bacterium and need further treatment.

Helpful: Because inflammation can cause—or increase—the symptoms of Lyme and other tick-borne infections, I often advise patients to take small doses of *naltrexone* (ReVia). This prescription medication, which is also used for alcohol/opiate dependency, reduces inflammation and helps regulate an overstimulated immune system.

Naltrexone can be combined with over-the-counter anti-inflammatory supplements, including the antioxidant glutathione (liposomal is best for absorption), which helps reduce fatigue and pain, and green tea extract and resveratrol.

Sudden Rheumatoid Arthritis Symptoms? It Might Be Chikungunya Virus

Jonathan J. Miner, MD, PhD, fellow, rheumatology division, Washington University School of Medicine, St. Louis.

Y ou may not yet have heard of chikungunya virus, but chances are you will be hearing a lot about it…and soon. It was nonexistent in the Western hemisphere until December 2013, but in just over a year, more than one million cases were reported, mostly in the Caribbean and South and Central America—and now it's here in the United States. The virus, which is transmitted by mosquitoes, can cause symptoms that mimic rheumatoid arthritis—and those symptoms can last for months to years. Plus, treating the infection as if it were rheumatoid arthritis might do more harm than good! Here's what you need to know about this new viral threat—and how to tell whether your "arthritis" might actually be a case of chikungunya infection…

Rheumatoid Arthritis Or Chikungunya?

First of all, don't panic. Chikungunya virus, often referred to as "CHIKV," is not a lethal illness. The most common symptoms are joint pain and fever. Symptoms can also include headache, joint swelling and muscle pain in the first seven to 10 days of infection. In most people, the more severe symptoms, such as flu-like fever and achiness, last for about a week or so and pass. But joint symptoms in particular can persist for 12 to 15 months in up to 60% of those infected and up to three years for some, according to Jonathan Miner, MD, PhD, a fellow in the rheumatology division of Washington University School of Medicine in St. Louis and a key US researcher of CHIKV infection.

As mentioned, some CHIKV symptoms, such as joint achiness and swelling, are similar to those of—and easily confused with—rheumatoid arthritis. But unlike rheumatoid arthritis, with CHIKV, joint pain and inflammation occur very suddenly, in the same way flu symptoms occur, in many joints all at once instead of gradually over months or years, said Dr. Miner.

How It Got Here

First described in Tanzania in the 1950s, CHIKV spread from Africa to Asia and Eu-

---

Danger after Visiting the Doctor

C. difficile, which can cause deadly diarrhea, used to be a problem primarily in hospitals, but now patients are becoming infected after visiting doctor and dentist offices. Antibiotics can suppress the normal bacteria in the colon, allowing C. difficile to flourish.

Self-defense: Take antibiotics only when needed. Wash hands with soap and water—do not rely on alcohol-based gels, which are not effective against C. difficile.

L. Clifford McDonald, MD, medical epidemiologist. Study published in *The New England Journal of Medicine*.

rope before hitting the Caribbean and South America and, ultimately, the United States. Most of the nearly 2,500 reported cases in the United States in 2014 were linked to travel to other affected areas, but 11 cases were reported in nontravelers in Florida. This means that mosquitoes in parts of the southern United States are now carrying the virus.

The only factor currently limiting the virus's spread in the United States, according to Dr. Miner, is the type of mosquito that is, so far, carrying the virus our way—an insect known as the yellow fever mosquito. It is native to the Caribbean, Florida, the Gulf Coast and parts of Texas. If the virus mutates to jump from the Caribbean yellow fever mosquito to the American Asian tiger mosquito, found throughout much of the continental United States, the number of cases might rival that of West Nile virus, which caused a panic about a decade ago. And it is likely to happen eventually, said Dr. Miner...the virus is also spread by the Asian tiger mosquito in the Eastern hemisphere.

Proper diagnosis hinges on giving your doctor appropriate details about your symptoms and travels, said Dr. Miner—such as whether your joint pain and swelling developed slowly over several months...or developed after traveling to places where the virus is actively spreading, such as the Caribbean. If you only visited places such as Canada or most of the United States where CHIKV outbreaks are rare or have not yet occurred, infection is very unlikely, he said.

The problem is that CHIKV, generally speaking, has not necessarily been on an American rheumatologist's radar, which is why you ought to be well informed about it. A rheumatologist might treat the joint symptoms of CHIKV in the same way as rheumatoid arthritis—with immunosuppressive drugs. This may not be so bad when the residual symptoms of joint pain and swelling persist after the body has otherwise fought off the viral infection, but such treatment will thwart your body's natural efforts to fight off the virus during the early stages of infection. And your body's natural efforts are all you've

What to Do About the Measles

• **Get tested if you're not sure about your vaccination status...**Adults born in 1957 (about the time the measles vaccine began to be widely used) or later who have no record of vaccination or memory of having measles as a child should get a blood test to determine immunity. If none is found, they should have at least one dose of the MMR (measles-mumps-rubella) vaccine, according to the CDC. (Those born before 1957 are presumed to have had measles and are considered immune.) Measles is highly contagious, so anyone without immunity is at risk of contracting the disease. Complications from measles can include pneumonia and encephalitis.

Aaron E. Glatt, MD, executive vice president, Mercy Medical Center, Rockville Centre, New York.

• **But if you know that you were vaccinated...**Adults don't need to be revaccinated against measles. Although measles is on the upswing in the US, people who have been vaccinated—even decades ago—have lifelong immunity.

William Schaffner, MD, professor of preventive medicine, Vanderbilt University School of Medicine, Nashville.

got...there is no medical remedy for CHIKV infection. Treatment is similar to that of the flu bug, according to the US Centers for Disease Control and Prevention: Get plenty of rest, drink fluids to prevent dehydration and take aspirin, ibuprofen, naproxen or acetaminophen for pain and fever relief.

"During the first week of infection, levels of the virus are high in the blood. This is when the body's immune response is extremely important. It has to be allowed to fight off the virus," said Dr. Miner. "I think it's fair to say, therefore, that taking immunosuppressive drugs when symptoms first appear is likely to be dangerous."

In fact, people with weakened immune systems, including infants, people older than 65 and people who have serious medical conditions, such as high blood pressure, heart disease or diabetes, are known to be at greater risk for more severe and prolonged symptoms from CHIKV. And if you already have arthritis, the virus may worsen your condition. On the up side, if you've been infected with CHIKV, your body becomes immune to reinfection if you should happen to again be bitten by an infected mosquito.

Safe Travels

If you're traveling to the Caribbean or an area with locally transmitted cases of CHIKV, it goes without saying that you should use mosquito repellent and wear long-sleeved shirts and long pants if the weather permits. Also keep the windows of your lodging closed or screened at night, and use the air conditioner to keep the mosquitoes out and the room air temperature and humidity at levels that discourage presence of mosquitoes.

In addition, keep abreast of which travel areas are more affected than others, said Dr. Miner. One Caribbean island may be having more of an outbreak than another at any given time. You can find up-to-date information on the number of CHIKV cases by region on the websites of the the Centers for Disease Control and Prevention and the Pan American Health Organization.

Better C. *Diff* Cure

*C*lostridium difficile (*C. diff*) infections, which cause severe, sometimes deadly diarrhea, have been treated with fecal transplants—inserting feces from a healthy donor into the patient's gastrointestinal tract to rebalance the gut.

Problem: Fresh donor feces may not be available.

Solution: When frozen feces were given (through colonoscopy or a nasogastric tube),

70% of C. diff patients got better after just one treatment and 90% recovered after a second dose. Currently available at some major medical centers, a frozen fecal capsule is now being developed for widespread use.

Ilan Youngster, MD, clinical fellow, Division of Infectious Diseases, Boston Children's Hospital.

Treat Skin Infection in One Dose

*N*ew antibiotic treats serious skin infections in just one dose, says William Schaffner, MD. Potentially dangerous skin and soft-tissue infections, such as MRSA (methicillin-resistant *Staphylococcus aureus*), often require a week or more of twice-daily antibiotic infusions at a health-care facility. The new IV drug *oritavancin* (Orbactiv) is equally effective—but it is so fast-acting, potent and long-lasting that it needs to be given only once.

William Schaffner, MD, is professor of preventive medicine and professor of medicine in infectious diseases at Vanderbilt University School of Medicine, Nashville. He is a board member and former president of the National Foundation for Infectious Diseases. *NFID.org*

Superbug Danger from a Common Procedure

Lawrence F. Muscarella, PhD, biomedical engineer and health-care safety expert who advises hospitals about gastrointestinal endoscopy and infection control. Based near Philadelphia, he writes the blog "Discussions in Infection Control." *EndoscopeReprocessing.com*

*I*n February 2015 a "superbug" infected several patients (two of whom died) during a common medical procedure at a California hospital. The bacterium can't reliably be stopped by any antibiotic and is fatal in at least 40% of cases.

The patients were infected by duodeno-scopes that are used to diagnose and treat problems of the liver, bile ducts and pancreas. Within the past two years, 135 scope-related infections were reported to the FDA. The true number is likely higher because many infections, particularly those caused by less virulent organisms, are never reported.

The scopes have an adjustable tip that is controlled by an "elevator wire." This part of the device tends to collect biological material (including bacteria) that's difficult to remove even when the devices are cleaned.

Here's how to protect yourself if you need a procedure involving a duodenoscope...

Request that the scope be tested. Some hospitals are doing this now. The scopes are cleaned, disinfected, sampled for bacteria and then quarantined in storage until their safety can be assured.

Ask about ethylene oxide (EtO) steril-ization. With this method, a gas is used to sterilize scopes. It's a time-consuming step, however, that isn't available in most hospi-tals. Ask for it.

If your doctor doesn't address your con-cerns, or if the medical center doesn't have the enhanced testing or sterilization method mentioned above, consider going somewhere else.

Chapter 11

UNDOING PAIN AND AUTOIMMUNE DISEASE

Conquer Pain Safely

What's the first thing you do when you're hurting? If you're like most people, you reach for aspirin, *ibuprofen* (Advil, Motrin), *naproxen* (Aleve) or a similar non-steroidal anti-inflammatory drug (NSAID). Each day, more than 30 million Americans take these popular medications. Another roughly 7 million take a different class of painkiller, *acetaminophen* (Tylenol) each day (see end of article).

The risks most people don't think about: Even though NSAIDs are as common in most American homes as Band-Aids and multivitamins, few people realize that these medications often cause stomach and intestinal bleeding that leads to up to 20,000 deaths every year in the US. And while previous studies have suggested that these drugs also threaten heart health, an important new meta-analysis found that the risks are more significant than once thought. In fact, ibuprofen and other NSAIDs—taken in doses that many people consider normal—increased the risk for "major vascular events," including heart attacks, by about one-third.

Safer Pain Relief

The good news is, it's still fine to take an NSAID for arthritis, a headache or other types of short-term pain up to two or three times a week. It is also safe, with your doctor's approval, to take a daily low-dose aspirin (81 mg) to prevent heart attacks and stroke.

What not to do: It is never a good idea to depend on these drugs to relieve chronic pain. As a doctor who specializes in treating arthritis pain, I rarely recommend these medications for long-term use because there are safer analgesics that are just as effective.

My favorite alternatives to oral NSAIDs (ask your doctor which might work best for your pain)…

Analgesic Creams

You've probably seen over-the-counter pain-relieving creams, such as Zostrix and Capzasin. These products contain capsaicin, which causes a mild burning sensation and appears to reduce substance P, a neurotransmitter that sends pain signals to the brain. Capsaicin products work well for some

Vijay Vad, MD, sports medicine physician and researcher specializing in minimally invasive arthritis therapies at the Hospital for Special Surgery in New York City. He is the author of *Stop Pain: Inflammation Relief for an Active Life. VijayVad.com* people suffering from osteoarthritis or rheumatoid arthritis, back pain, shingles and diabetic nerve pain (neuropathy). *Many people, however, get better results from…*

•**Voltaren Gel.** In the heart study mentioned earlier, oral *diclofenac* (Voltaren) was one of the riskiest NSAIDs. But a topical version, Voltaren Gel, which is available by prescription, is less likely to cause side effects, even though it's just as effective as the tablets. Voltaren Gel is good for pain in one joint, but if your pain is in several joints, supplements will offer more relief.

How it's used: Apply the gel (up to four times a day) to the area that's hurting—for example, your knee or wrist.

Helpful: Apply it after a bath or shower, when your skin is soft. More of the active ingredient will pass through the skin and into the painful area. Voltaren Gel should not be combined with an oral NSAID.

Pain-Fighting Supplements

If you need even more pain relief, consider taking one or more of the following supplements. Start with the first one, and if pain has not decreased after eight weeks, add the second, then wait another eight weeks before adding the third, if necessary.

Important: Be sure to check first with your doctor if you take blood thinners or other medications because they could interact.

•**Curcumin.** There's been a lot of research on the anti-inflammatory and painkilling effects of curcumin (the compound that gives the curry spice turmeric its yellow color). One study found that it reduced pain and improved knee function about as well as ibuprofen.

Typical dose: 1,000 mg, twice daily.

•**Fish oil.** A huge amount of data shows that the omega-3 fatty acids in fish oil have analgesic and anti-inflammatory effects.

Scientific evidence: One study found that 60% of patients with neck, back and joint pain who took fish oil improved so much that they were able to stop taking NSAIDs or other medications.

Typical dose: 2,000 mg daily.

•**Boswellia.** Boswellia (or frankincense) is an herbal medicine that reduces both pain and inflammation. It's effective for all types of joint pain, including osteoarthritis and rheumatoid arthritis.

Scientific evidence: In one study, patients with knee arthritis took boswellia or a placebo for two months, then switched to the opposite treatment for another two months.

Results: The people taking boswellia had less pain and more knee mobility than those taking placebos.

Typical dose: 300 mg to 400 mg, three times daily.

How to Use Tylenol for Pain

If you prefer an oral medication over the options in the main article, ask your doctor about switching from NSAIDs to *acetaminophen* (Tylenol). It's not an anti-inflammatory, but it's an effective pain reliever that doesn't cause stomach upset or bleeding—or trigger an increase in cardiovascular risks. I've found that people who limit the dosage of acetaminophen are unlikely to have side effects.

Caution: Taking too much of this drug can lead to liver damage, particularly if it's used by someone who consumes a lot of alcohol or has underlying liver disease, such as hepatitis.

My recommendation: No more than 2,000 mg daily of acetaminophen (this dosage is lower than the limits listed on the label).

Important: In calculating your total daily dose, be sure to factor in all sources of acetaminophen. More than 600 prescription and over-the-counter drugs, including cold and flu medications and allergy drugs, contain the active ingredient acetaminophen. For a partial list of medications that contain acetaminophen, go to *KnowYourDose.org/*common-medications.

To be safe: Get a liver function test (usually covered by insurance) every six months if you regularly take acetaminophen.

The Amazing Pain-Relieving Diet

Heather Tick, MD, Gunn-Loke Endowed professor for integrative pain medicine at the University of Washington, Seattle, where she is a clinical associate professor in the department of family medicine and the department of anesthesiology and pain medicine. She is the author of *Holistic Pain Relief: Dr. Tick's Breakthrough Strategies to Manage and Eliminate Pain.*

Chronic pain (that which lasts for longer than six months) can occur anywhere in the body—in the muscles…joints…head…stomach…bladder…and so on. And though some people find it hard to believe, there are more Americans affected by pain—whether it is from arthritis, headaches, nerve damage or some other condition—than diabetes, heart disease and cancer combined.

What's the answer? Fortunately, there is a variety of highly effective, evidence-based ways to turn your diet into a pain-fighting machine.

Heal Your Digestive Tract

Pain anywhere in the body is almost always accompanied, and made worse, by inflammation. The inflammatory response, which includes the release of pain-causing chemicals, can persist in the body for decades, even when you don't have redness or other visible signs.

Common cause: A damaged mucosa in the innermost lining of the intestines. The damage can be caused by food sensitivities…a poor diet with too much sugar or processed foods…or a bacterial imbalance, among many other factors. A weakened mucosal lining can allow toxic molecules to enter the body, where they then trigger persistent inflammation.

If you suffer from chronic pain—particularly pain that's accompanied by intermittent bouts of constipation and/or diarrhea—your first step should be to heal the damaged intestinal tissue. *To do this…*

• **Eat a variety of fermented foods.** They are rich in probiotics, which will help the mucosa heal. Most people know that live-culture yogurt is a good source of probiotics…but yogurt alone doesn't supply enough. You can and should get more probiotics by eating one or more daily servings of fermented foods such as sauerkraut or kimchi (Asian pickled cabbage).

Because highly processed fermented foods—such as canned sauerkraut—will not give you the live probiotics you need, select a product that requires refrigeration even in the grocery store. You also can take a probiotic supplement, which is especially important for people who take antibiotics or who don't eat many fermented foods.

• **Cut way back on sugar.** A high- or even moderate-sugar diet, which includes the "simple sugars" in refined carbohydrates such as bread and other baked goods as well as white rice, many breakfast cereals and most juices, increases levels of cytokines, immune cells that cause inflammation.

• **Limit red meat.** Red meat, especially the organic, grass-fed kind, does have valuable nutrients and can be part of a healthy diet. But eaten in excess (more than three ounces daily), red meat increases inflammation. Other good protein sources include lentils, beans and tempeh.

Eat Other Foods That Turn Off the Fire

Avoiding inflammatory foods is only half the equation—the other half, if you want to reduce pain, is to eat foods that can reduce the inflammation in your body.

If you are expecting an exotic recommendation here, sorry—because what you really need to eat to reduce inflammation in your body is lots and lots of vegetables—raw, steamed, sautéed, baked or roasted. Vegetables contain cellulose, a type of fiber that binds to fats and some inflammatory substances and carries them out of the body in the stools. The antioxidants in vegetables, such as the lycopene in tomatoes and the indole-3-carbinol in crucifers such as broccoli, cabbage and Brussels sprouts, further reduce inflammation.

Helpful: It's good to avoid sweets, but make an exception for an ounce or two of dark chocolate daily. Chocolate that contains at least 70% cocoa is very high in antioxidants. It reduces inflammation, improves brain circulation and lowers blood pressure, according to research. And because it's a sweet treat, it will make it easier for you to say "no" to the nasty stuff like cake, cookies and ice cream.

Don't Forget Spices

Turmeric and ginger are great spices for pain relief and can replace salty and sugary flavor enhancers. Ginger tea is a delicious pain fighter. Also, garlic and onions are high in sulfur, which helps in healing.

Coffee: Yes…But

Even though some people can stop a migraine by drinking a cup of coffee when their symptoms first start, too much coffee (the amount varies from person to person) can have a negative effect on other types of pain. It increases the body's output of adrenaline, the stress hormone, as well as inflammation. It also masks fatigue, so you're more likely to push yourself too hard.

Do not drink more than one or two cups of coffee daily.

Women Report Feeling Pain More Intensely Than Men

In a recent study, in which participants with painful conditions rated their pain levels from one to 10, women felt pain, such as lower back pain and/or osteoarthritis, more intensely than men did.

Study of more than 11,000 people by researchers at Stanford University School of Medicine, Stanford, California, published in *Journal of Pain*.

This Supplement May Shrink Painful Fibroids

Andrew Rubman, ND, medical director, Southbury Clinic for Traditional Medicines, Southbury, Connecticut. SouthburyClinic.com.

Fibroids are benign tumors that usually grow on the muscular wall of the uterus. They are not cancer. Up to 80% of women get them by age 50. Most don't even know it because they don't cause symptoms. But when they do, watch out. Excessive menstrual bleeding, prolonged periods and severe pain are common symptoms. When fibroids disrupt life, you want relief—yesterday. Medical solutions include taking drugs that block hormones in the short term as well as surgical interventions up to and including hysterectomy. These not only have risks and side effects but, except for hysterectomy, they often don't solve the problem permanently—fibroids grow back.

Naturopathic physician Andrew Rubman, founder and medical director of the Southbury Clinic for Traditional Medicine in Southbury, Connecticut, believes that there is a better way to prevent and treat fibroids and, perhaps, avoid the knife. He often recommends the supplement Fibrovera to his patients. (Dr. Rubman endorses the product but receives no financial compensation from the manufacturer.)

How Fibroids Grow

Before we get to solutions, let's look at how fibroids grow. Essentially, it's the natural process of wound healing and scarring gone awry. "Uterine fibroids and even dense breasts contain dysfunctional tissue made up of a great deal of fibrin—scar tissue," explained Dr. Rubman. "Fibrin is a nonvital material, a temporary fix. If the body has inflammation that persists beyond a certain point, it'll throw in a little fibrin to stabilize it in order to come back to the problem to fix it later." Fibrin is involved in creating blood clots that stop bleeding when you are injured, for example, so it has a beneficial purpose, he explained. "But if the inflammation isn't controlled, fibrin keeps on getting heaped up."

Hormonal imbalances contribute to the development of excess fibrin. A leading hypothesis is "estrogen dominance," in which a woman's body produces too much estrogen and too little progesterone. This hormonal imbalance can trigger inflammatory responses including excess fibrin deposition, which can accumulate as abnormal tissue growth in the uterus as well as the breasts. "It creates an environment that will generate scar tissue like fibroids or dense breasts," he explained.

How Fibrovera Works

Fibrovera was designed to address many of the underlying conditions that give rise to fibroids. It is a formulation of botanicals and enzymes that supports hormonal balance, reduces inflammation and helps the body break down and rid itself of excess fibrin, a process called fibrinolysis. *Active ingredients include...*

• **Diindolemethane (DIM).** This is a compound found in cruciferous vegetables (such as broccoli) that improves estrogen metabolism and helps to prevent the conversion of testosterone into estrogen. It is available as a separate supplement.

• **Dehydroepiandrosterone (DHEA).** This steroid hormone may help the body produce more progesterone. While high doses can cause side effects such as irregular periods, the very low dose included in Fibrovera is safe for long-term use, said Dr. Rubman. It works synergistically with DIM to help with hormonal balance.

• **Enzymes.** Fibrovera contains several enzymes that help break down fibrin, including serrapeptase (originally found in silkworms), bromelain (from pineapples), papain (from papayas) and nattokinase (from fermented soybeans).

• **Calcium and magnesium.** These essential minerals play a role in reducing pain.

• **Gamma linoleic acid (GLA).** This fatty acid is a strong anti-inflammatory and helps relieve the severe PMS-related symptoms that are common in women with fibroids.

• **5-hydroxytryptophane (5-HTP), a vitamin B-6 precursor to the brain neurotransmitter serotonin.** Too little serotonin may interfere with progesterone synthesis. Fibrovera also contains pyridoxal-5-phosphate (P5P), another vitamin B-6 precursor that helps in the synthesis of serotonin.

• **Dong Quai.** This traditional Chinese herb produces a relaxing effect on the muscles in the uterus.

• **Milk thistle seed, dandelion root and hyssop flower.** These botanicals support healthy liver function, improving the liver's ability to metabolize the hormones that support fibrin breakdown.

Is Fibrovera Right for You?

As with any drug or supplement, there are caveats. While there is research behind many of the ingredients in Fibrovera, the product itself has not been studied directly for the reduction of uterine fibroids. While Dr. Rubman is aware of no side effects with Fibrovera, he cautions that the supplement may be inappropriate for anyone who is taking a blood-thinning medication or has a blood-clotting disorder. "Fibrin is important for clotting," he noted. It's always a good practice to let all your health-care professionals know of all the medications and supplements you are taking.

If you're considering Fibrovera, be sure to address lifestyle as well, Dr. Rubman emphasized, including avoidance of environmental toxins (especially endocrine disrupters such as BPA-containing plastics), an anti-inflammatory diet, exercise and stress reduction. According to the National Institutes of Health, there is evidence that some pesticides may promote growth hormones that promote fibroids...that dairy foods may be protective... and that green tea may inhibit the growth of fibroid cells.

In his own practice, Dr. Rubman has found that for some of his patients taking

Fibrovera, excessive menstrual bleeding and pain were no longer an issue, and no progesterone therapy or surgery was needed.

Injections Better Than Pills

For treating knee osteoarthritis, injections are generally more effective than pills. Injections of hyaluronic acid or cortisone usually relieve pain better than any oral medicine, including *acetaminophen* (Tylenol) and nonsteroidal anti-inflammatory drugs (NSAIDs) such as *celecoxib* (Celebrex).

But: The long-term safety and efficacy of injected corticosteroids is uncertain, and injected hyaluronic acid is expensive.

Best: Nondrug treatments such as exercise and physical therapy should be tried first.

Raveendhara Bannuru, MD, PhD, director of Center for Treatment Comparison and Integrative Analysis and researcher at Center for Arthritis and Rheumatic Diseases, both at Tufts Medical Center, Boston.

Knee Surgery Warning

Common knee surgery may lead to arthritis.

Recent study: All 31 knees operated on to repair tears of the meniscus (cartilage that stabilizes the knee joint) developed arthritis within one year, compared with 59% of the 165 knees that didn't have surgery. Talk to your doctor about whether surgery is really necessary and whether physical therapy, including targeted muscle exercises, is a better option for you.

Frank Roemer, MD, associate professor of radiology, Boston University School of Medicine and University of Erlangen–Nuremburg, Germany. His study was presented at a meeting of the Radiological Society of North America.

Rheumatoid Arthritis Surging Among Women

Eric L. Matteson, MD, chair of rheumatology, Mayo Clinic, Rochester, Minnesota.

When most people hear the word "arthritis," what comes to mind is osteoarthritis, the seemingly ubiquitous aching-joint condition suffered by more than a third of people over age 65. Much less common, but often more devastating, is rheumatoid arthritis (RA), an autoimmune disease that also attacks the joints affecting many in the prime of life. About three-fourths of patients with rheumatoid arthritis are women. Where incidence had been declining for nearly 40 years, researchers from the Mayo Clinic announced that it is again on the upswing, specifically among women. Between 1995 and 2005, the number of female patients diagnosed with rheumatoid arthritis climbed 50% from 36 new female patients per 100,000 to 54 per 100,000.

Natural Osteoarthritis Care

Eating foods that have been shown to lower inflammation may help relieve your pain, so make sure your diet includes plenty of these—broccoli, red grapes, tea (black or green), pineapple, blueberries, strawberries, spinach, plums, cabbage, Brussels sprouts and salmon. Supplements that may help ease osteoarthritis pain include sulforaphane, bromelain, ginger, turmeric and curcumin. Check with your doctor first—these supplements and some of the foods above may interact with certain medications, including blood thinners. Follow directions on the supplement label. Also helpful are regular—twice daily for five to 10 minutes—soaks in a warm bath or whirlpool.

Harris H. McIlwain, MD, pain specialist in private practice in Tampa, and coauthor of *Diet for a Pain-Free Life*. iPainFreeDiet.com

What's Behind the Increase?

Why the increase? Some of the growth can be accounted for by the fact that doctors now have more awareness of how to diagnose the disease. Other factors are at work too, we learned from Eric L. Matteson, MD, chair of rheumatology at the Mayo Clinic in Rochester, Minnesota. Hormones are known to play a role (since RA typically improves with pregnancy but comes back after delivery) but researchers are examining possible environmental explanations as well. For instance, researchers recently learned that there is an association between living near busy highways and development of RA.

Here's another theory: For unknown reasons, some people are prone to develop RA after exposure to particular viruses. After a virus has made the rounds and exposed large numbers of people, it may be dormant for a long period, since many people have built immunity. That immunity eventually fades—then, if the same virus returns, it once more affects many people, including some who are susceptible to developing RA. Dr. Matteson noted that such a swell in chronic diseases due to reemergence of a triggering cause, such as virus, is not uncommon.

A recent discovery is that people with RA are at higher risk for heart disease. However, this is not much of a surprise, says Dr. Matteson, since RA is an inflammatory disease—increased inflammation in the body causes more inflammation in the lining (endothelium) of the arteries including those into the heart, which leads to greater cardiovascular risk. Researchers are at work trying to identify more sophisticated inflammation biomarkers to learn more about this and other health risks that may coexist with RA.

Mainstream Treatment

Doctors used to wait till joint damage showed up on X-rays before they would prescribe drugs for RA to hold off further harm. Now, doctors prescribe these drugs as soon as the diagnosis is recognized, so patients can live longer with less pain and permanent damage. It's important to be aware of the symptoms that could indicate a diagnosis of RA and treat them early on.

While several drugs are effective, methotrexate is the anchor drug for most RA patients, Dr. Matteson said. All treatments have the same goal—to reduce signs of inflammation and free patients from joint swelling discomfort. RA drugs have many toxic side effects, so doctors typically try to find the lowest effective dose.

Natural Treatment

Dr. Matteson said there are a number of ways to ease RA through natural treatment. Since omega-3 fatty acids reduce inflammation and its associated pain, he recommends a large dosage—perhaps two to three grams per day. Exercise keeps the joints limber, increases range of motion and strengthens supporting muscle and keeps the bones strong. Research shows that yoga may be helpful in reducing discomfort, but Dr. Matteson cautions against more active and intense forms of power yoga, which can stress the joints. In his view, gentle Tai chi is ideal—patients report that it helps reduce pain and creates more comfortable stretching.

Dr. Matteson advises following a healthy diet, including avoiding foods that may provoke inflammation and choosing fresh fruits and vegetables. Turmeric has some anti-inflammatory properties and may help somewhat. While some people believe that nightshade vegetables—primarily eggplant, tomatoes, white potatoes and peppers—can exacerbate discomfort in certain sensitive patients, Dr. Matteson says he hasn't found that to be true for most of his patients.

His advice: Watch to see if these or other foods trigger discomfort and, of course, avoid any that do.

Finally, it is also important to stop smoking if you smoke, because smoking is associated with an increased risk of RA, and people who smoke and have RA tend to have worse symptoms of the disease than those who do not smoke.

Diagnosis Can Be Tricky

Typical RA symptoms include joint pain on motion, swelling, reddening and decreased range of motion of the joints of hands, especially the wrists and fingers, most especially where the fingers meet the palm (metacarpophalangeal joints) and the middle finger joints (the proximal interphalangeal joints). Rheumatoid arthritis also often affects the feet and ankles, as well as other joints. The disease can arise in children or the very old, but the median age is 56. Anyone who experiences an increase of small joint discomfort and especially with swelling in the joints and symptoms that continue for six weeks, should get an evaluation from his/her doctor or a rheumatologist.

Does Glucosamine Work?

Studies occasionally come to the surface claiming that glucosamine does not help joint pain. Are these supplements worth taking?

It depends on what kind of glucosamine you are using. Only glucosamine sulfate has been shown to be effective in reducing osteoarthritis pain. Sulfate helps the body produce cartilage. That is why researchers believe this form works better than glucosamine hydrochloride or N-acetyl glucosamine, neither of which has sulfate. Studies have shown that glucosamine sulfate reduces pain about as much as acetaminophen and the nonsteroidal anti-inflammatory drugs ibuprofen and piroxicam. But NSAIDs relieved arthritis pain in about two weeks, while glucosamine sulfate took up to 12 weeks.

David Borenstein, MD, clinical professor of medicine, The George Washington University Medical Center, Washington, DC. DrBHealth.org

Natural Relief for Fibrocystic Breasts

Cindee Gardner, PhD, DHom (doctor of homeopathy), registered and certified homeopathic practitioner, molecular biologist, herbalist and nutritional counselor in private practice in Pittsburgh. CindeeGardner.com and Homeohelpline.com

Mark Stengler, NMD, naturopathic medical doctor, Encinitas, California. MarkStengler.com

Among the challenges that come with being a woman, having fibrocystic breasts may seem like a minor one. Unless, that is, your breasts often feel achy and tender...you experience significant pain and swelling before your period...and/or your mammogram is too murky to read, requiring you to have further tests to screen for cancer.

Fibrocycstic breasts have ropy, dense tissue and lumpy, fluid-filled cysts. Frustratingly, Western medicine doesn't have much to offer other than over-the-counter pain medication and, in cases where a large cyst causes extreme pain, drainage with needle aspiration or surgery—but these won't help prevent further cysts from forming. So, it's a relief to hear that alternative therapies can ease symptoms and even help resolve the root causes that lead to fibrocystic breasts, according to Cindee Gardner, PhD, DHom, a homeopathic practitioner, molecular biologist and herbalist in Pittsburgh.

The following natural therapies have long traditions of use and (unlike drugs and surgical procedures) have no adverse side effects or risks when used as directed, so there's no harm in trying them to see if they relieve your symptoms and/or help prevent future flare-ups. The products mentioned below are available without a prescription at health-food stores and/or online...the treatments can be used alone or together in any combination. *Options...*

•**Homeopathy.** Homeopathic remedies are tailored to address a particular combination of symptoms, so choose whichever one of the following most closely matches your situation. *If...*

• **Your breasts often feel heavy, hard, stony and swollen**—try the homeopathic remedy called *Phytolacca decandra.*

• **Aching and lumpiness worsen before your period and tend to be accompanied by tearful moods**—opt for pulsatilla.

• **Cysts and soreness occur mainly in the left breast**—consider *Calcarea phosphorica.*

• **Symptom flare-ups are accompanied by itching**—use silica.

For moderate pain, Dr. Gardner recommended using a 30x or 30c remedy three times per day as needed, following the directions on the label…for severe pain, use the remedy every 30 minutes as needed, lessening the frequency as symptoms improve.

Important: When using any of the remedies above, avoid drinking strong coffee or inhaling strong scents of mint or camphor (for instance, from mothballs)—these can counteract a remedy's effects.

If a nonprescription remedy doesn't help or you need to use it more than a few days per month, it is best to consult a professional homeopath. As Dr. Gardner noted, there are about 45 different remedies for fibrocystic breasts listed in the *Homeopathic Materia Medica* (the homeopath's version of the *Physician's Desk Reference*)—so identifying the most effective one for you may require expert guidance. To find a practitioner, visit the Web site of the National Center for Homeopathy (*homeopathic.org/practitioners*) or The National United Professional Association of Trained Homeopaths (*nupath.org*).

• **Breast massage.** This practice relieves fibrocystic breast symptoms and helps prevent flare-ups because it stimulates the endocrine system to balance female hormones, keeps breast tissue from getting overly congested and reduces stagnation in the breast glands and ducts, Dr. Gardner said. She recommended massaging the breasts with a topical product called Vita-Cal with Poke, available from *Archeusonline.com*, which contains vitamins A, D3 and E and organic cold-pressed oils (sesame, avocado, mango, nut, etc.). This rich cream, which is easily absorbed through the skin, is designed to help break up cysts and relieve lymph stagnation.

At least once a week: Lie down, breathe deeply and relax. With a dab of the cream, massage each breast for five minutes or more, moving outward from the nipple and using circular motions, first in one direction and then the other.

• **Dietary changes.** Many women report that fibrocystic symptoms ease significantly when they avoid caffeine and limit high-fat foods, particularly meat and dairy products, Dr. Gardner noted. It also is helpful to drink plenty of water between meals and to increase intake of high-fiber, high-water-content foods such as fruits and vegetables.

• **Chasteberry.** Vitex agnus-castus (chasteberry) is an herb that Mark Stengler, NMD, often prescribes to his patients with fibrocystic symptoms. Vitex acts on the brain to stimulate the ovaries to ovulate, producing more progesterone and lessening estrogen dominance. Vitex is helpful for women of all ages, but do not use it if you are pregnant or taking birth control pills. *Dose:* 160 milligrams (mg) to 240 mg daily of a standardized extract. Try it for three months. If it helps, keep taking it. If you experience digestive upset, nausea or headaches, stop taking vitex.

Referrals: American Herbalists Guild, *AmericanHerbalistsGuild.com.*

More-Comfortable Mammograms

Ellen Mendelson, MD, professor of radiology at Northwestern University Feinberg School of Medicine and section chief of breast and women's imaging at Northwestern Memorial Hospital, both in Chicago.

Many women dread the brief breast-squishing discomfort of mammograms—sometimes to the point where they delay or skip the test. This is unfortunate, because mammography is the one screening test proven to reduce mortality from breast cancer. Why the big squeeze? Compressing the breast allows X-rays to penetrate better, reducing your radiation absorption and producing clearer images. *What minimizes discomfort…*

• **Breast cushions.** In studies, about 70% of patients reported significantly less pain when single-use, adhesive-backed foam cushions were attached to the mammography machine's compression plates. The cushions do not affect mammogram image quality. To find a facility that uses cushions, visit *Mammopad.com/locator.*

• **Good timing.** Schedule your mammogram for the week after your period—premenstrual hormonal fluctuations trigger fluid retention, making breasts tender. If you are postmenopausal, timing doesn't matter unless you are on cyclical hormone therapy, in which case schedule your mammogram for the first half of the cycle.

• **Limiting caffeine.** For some women, caffeine increases breast sensitivity. Avoid coffee, tea, cola and chocolate for three days before your mammogram.

• **Nonprescription pain reliever.** Take one or two tablets of *ibuprofen* (Motrin) one hour before your mammogram. Avoid aspirin—it can lead to bruising.

Caution: Some radiology centers provide a topical lidocaine cream to numb breasts. This anesthetic carries a slight risk for causing cardiac problems, however—so use it only if you really need it and wash it off when the test is done.

Relieve Genital Pain in Women

Joel M. Evans, MD, clinical assistant professor, Albert Einstein College of Medicine, New York City, and founder and director, The Center for Women's Health, Stamford, Connecticut. Dr. Evans is the coauthor of *The Whole Pregnancy Handbook. CenterForWomens Health.com*

Ladies, have you ever worn too-tight jeans that rubbed your crotch raw…developed an itchy all-over rash that really did go everywhere…or had a sore or an infection (or even a cut from shaving the bikini area) that made your private parts painful or tender?

When discomfort occurs "down there"—especially when there is an open sore or when pain is accompanied by other symptoms that could indicate an infection, such as a fever or vaginal discharge—of course you need to contact your doctor so he or she can diagnosis the complaint and prescribe treatment. To relieve simple chafing or other minor injuries or irritations, though, there often are steps you can take at home that bring relief. In some cases, the remedies suggested below also can alleviate discomfort while you wait for your doctor-prescribed treatment to take effect.

Complaint: A cut or sore in the genital area…

If you've nicked yourself shaving your bikini area or otherwise injured your genital area, you'll need to give yourself some TLC for a few days to let the problem heal—not easy in an area where everything rubs together. If you've got genital herpes, you'll have already discussed how to handle outbreaks with your doctor, such as by taking oral antiviral medication. But with herpes sores, as with cuts, it's important to keep the area very clean.

To that end, after using the toilet, wipe yourself thoroughly but gently with moistened toilet paper, then pat the area dry with clean toilet paper. Do not use disposable premoistened wipes because these may contain irritating chemicals.

To soothe sores or cuts as they heal apply a topical ointment containing aloe, calendula or shea butter twice daily. If your discomfort is severe or extremely distracting, ask your doctor about using a prescription topical cream that contains a painkilling agent, such as lidocaine, for a few days.

Complaint: External itchiness, irritation, inflammation or rash…

Chafing (for instance, from very tight pants or overzealous cycling) and allergic reactions or sensitivities (to laundry products, personal-care products, clothing fabrics, even toilet paper) are two main reasons why women can end up with a hot, itchy rash or other type of irritation in the genital area. Your first order of business is to do some detective work to figure out the cause. Go over everything you've done in the past few days that is different from your normal routine. If you identify a possible suspect, such as a new type of shower gel or new brand of laundry detergent or toilet paper, your course of action is clear—stop using it!

In the meantime, for relief, apply an ice pack to the affected region for 15 minutes or so two or three times daily. You can use an icy gel pack (available at drugstores)…create your own ice pack by placing ice chips in a plastic bag and wrapping it in a towel…or use a bag of frozen peas (peas are small enough to mold comfortably to the shape of your body). Whatever you use, do not apply the ice pack directly to the skin because this could damage the skin—instead, put a thin cloth between you and the ice pack.

It's also helpful to take a cool oatmeal bath once or twice daily—the oatmeal soothes, moisturizes and coats irritated skin. You can buy ready-made oatmeal bath products (such as Aveeno Soothing Bath Treatment Colloidal Oatmeal Skin Protectant or a similar generic brand)…or make your own by running a cup of whole oats through the blender and adding them to the bath water. Soak for 10 to 20 minutes, using only your hands to wash yourself (no soap, washcloth or loofah, which could cause further irritation). Then dry off gently but thoroughly.

Until the area is healed, wear all-cotton underwear (no thongs)…opt for thigh-high or knee-high hose rather than panty hose…and stick with loose-fitting cotton clothing as much as you can. Avoid panty liners and pads, which can trap moisture, slowing down healing.

Complaint: Internal vaginal itching or irritation…

Though a common culprit here is a recurrent or chronic yeast infection, you don't want to make assumptions. It's best not to use an over-the-counter anti-yeast product on your own because you cannot be sure that you have a yeast infection without going to the doctor. Yeast infections are often confused with bacterial infections, and the treatments are vastly different.

Until you can get to the doctor's office, for temporary relief, try taking frequent baths or sitz baths (using a plastic bowl that sits on top of your toilet seat so you can soak your pelvic area without getting your whole body wet). Use cool water, and soak for about 10 to 20 minutes two or three times daily. Bathing helps soothe the internal irritation and the itching because it dilutes the offending agent.

If it turns out that you are prone to chronic or recurrent yeast infections, for long-lasting relief, you and your doctor will need to work together to determine the underlying cause and find a solution. Your doctor also may suggest one week of nightly use of a natural douche or vaginal suppositories made with boric acid to help correct the vaginal pH.

Recommended products: Arden's Powder Vaginal Cleansing Douche and Yeast Arrest boric acid suppositories.

Important: If you notice any painless genital symptom—lesion, bump, cyst, discharge—that does not go away within a few days, contact your doctor. Certain sexually transmitted diseases and genital cancers cause no pain at the outset but absolutely must be treated.

Shingles: You Could Have It and Not Even Know It

Anne Louise Oaklander, MD, PhD, director of a diagnostic and research laboratory at Massachusetts General Hospital that studies neurological causes of chronic pain and itch and associate professor of neurology at Harvard Medical School, both in Boston.

Many people think that shingles is just a rash, so they wait for it to go away like poison ivy and sunburn do. That's a big mistake. If you suspect that you may have shingles, take action right away—it's a neurological emergency.

The rash that we see on the skin, which develops on half the body only, usually in a band around the torso or above and around the eye, is just the tip of the iceberg.* The center of the infection is deep inside the body, within sensory nerve cells close to the spinal cord or brain. In some cases, the infection can spread into the spinal cord or brain to cause myelitis or encephalitis, stroke or spinal-cord injury.

New research finding: A study published in the journal *Neurology* found that the risk of having a stroke years later was up to 74% higher in people who had been diagnosed with shingles before age 40. The virus also can cause vision loss or hearing or balance problems.

But the most common complication of shingles is post-herpetic neuralgia (PHN), where pain persists after the rash heals. The pain can be intense—some people compare it to childbirth or passing a kidney stone. It gradually improves, but that can take months or years, and sometimes it never goes away. The nerve damage that causes pain also can lead to intense itching, known as post-herpetic itch. Although both are treatable, the medications often have side effects that make them unpleasant to use.

The best way to avoid getting shingles (and its complications): Get vaccinated. For people age 60 and older, the onetime vaccination reduces the risk of getting shingles by half and reduces the chance of the persistent pain of PHN by two-thirds. It is even more effective in adults ages 50 to 60, reducing shingles risk by 70%.

Even so, a sobering new study shows that less than 7% of adults who are eligible for the shingles vaccine have received it—even though it has no major side effects.

Why are so few people getting vaccinated? One reason is that there are widespread misconceptions about who should get this vaccine. Everyone in the US has been exposed to chicken pox by his/her adult years and is at risk for shingles. However, many peo-ple think only adults in their 70s and 80s, who tend to be at greatest risk for the illness, should receive the vaccine.

The truth is, the shingles vaccine is important for people who are younger than that, but there's not a consensus even among government agencies. The CDC recommends it for adults who are age 60 and older, while the FDA has approved it for people age 50 and older. Ask your physician for his recommendation.**

To give yourself—and loved ones—the best chances of avoiding shingles, here are additional misconceptions you should know about the condition…

Misconception #1: You can't develop shingles more than once. Having shingles boosts your immunity and offers some protection against a rapid recurrence. But that "booster effect" can wane, and you can have a second attack. Furthermore, people with impaired immunity may not experience this effect and can have recurrent or prolonged episodes.

When researchers from the Mayo Clinic recently examined medical records from nearly 1,700 patients, they found that more than 6% of shingles patients had subsequent attacks. So even if you've had shingles, talk to your doctor about vaccination.

Misconception #2: The pain will end in a few weeks. Everyone with shingles breathes a sigh of relief when the painful rash is gone—usually within two to four weeks. But in some cases, the problem continues. The older you are, the longer the pain can continue. Sometimes, it never completely subsides.

Misconception #3: There's no harm in taking a wait-and-see approach. Shingles symptoms can start days or a week before the rash appears. You may notice pain or itching in a band on one side of your body before the rash appears. If pain occurs on the chest, some patients worry that they could be having a heart attack. Even without the rash, a

*To view photos of the shingles rash, to to *shinglesinfo. com.*

**Because the shingles vaccine contains a live virus, it is not recommended for people undergoing radiation or chemotherapy…those with some cancers…or patients with HIV or other conditions that affect the immune system.

one-sided area or band of pain or itching is highly suspicious for shingles, particularly in older or immunosuppressed patients.

Savvy doctors will consider starting treatment with antiviral medications even during this early "prodrome" stage, when these drugs may abort an attack.

Even when started after the rash appears, antivirals significantly reduce the severity of the rash, its pain and also the risk for PHN and other complications. So if your regular doctor can't see you immediately when you first notice symptoms, go to an urgent-care center or an emergency room.

If the doctor orders a blood test to identify shingles, ask to start antiviral medications immediately. These medications, specifically *acyclovir* (Zovirax), *famciclovir* (Famvir) or *valacyclovir* (Valtrex), can reduce the risk for PHN.

Important: Quick treatment is particularly important if the rash occurs anywhere near the eye. See an ophthalmologist immediately. Most people do not realize that shingles can cause corneal ulcers, glaucoma and even blindness.

In addition to antiviral drugs, you'll probably be given steroid eyedrops to reduce inflammation and possibly a short-term course of oral steroids. Steroids can impair immunity, so don't take them unless you've already started an antiviral drug.

Misconception #4: There's not much you can do for the painful rash. Even though antiviral medication is the main treatment, low doses of *nortriptyline* (Pamelor, Aventyl) can reduce pain. The drug also improves sleep and reduces the risk for PHN by about 50%.

Although originally marketed to treat depression, nortriptyline and other tricyclic antidepressants are unsurpassed in their ability to treat neuropathic or nerve-injury pain such as that caused by shingles. Inexpensive generics are available, and one dose lasts more than 24 hours. But they must be taken for a few weeks to fully kick in, and they can have side effects, such as dizziness and weight gain, so discuss these drugs with your doctor.

An Experimental Shingles Treatment

Transcranial magnetic stimulation, a non-invasive procedure that uses magnets to trigger firing of certain neurons in the brain, appears to relieve post-herpetic neuralgia (PHN) in some patients who suffer pain three months or longer after their shingles rash has healed.

This new approach is still in the experimental stages, but several recent studies have shown encouraging results.

Hypnotic Relaxation for Tension Headaches

Yacov Ezra, MD, assistant head of neurology at Soroka University Medical Center and a lecturer at Ben-Gurion University, both in Be'er Sheva, Israel.

In the quest to quell the pain of tension-type headaches, one crucial point often gets overlooked—up to 88% of these headaches are believed to be caused by stress. On top of that, nearly half of people suffering from chronic tension-type headaches also have depression or anxiety disorders, which painkillers don't treat.

People with tension headaches who try the technique known as hypnotic relaxation are usually surprised by the simplicity of it. In fact, it takes just a few minutes to learn the progressive muscle relaxation and focused breathing exercises underlying the technique. *How to begin…*

•**Find a quiet, private space that's distraction free.** Turn off your cell phone.

•**Get comfortable on a chair or couch (sitting or lying down).**

•**Close your eyes and empty your mind of thoughts (as much as possible).** When intrusive thoughts return, simply acknowledge them and allow them to "drift away."

•**Breathe slowly and deeply, visualizing tension leaving your body with each**

exhale. Imagine vitality entering your body with each inhale.

•**Progressively relax your body's major muscle groups,** beginning with your toes and then moving through the calves, thighs, hips, stomach, hands, arms, shoulders, neck, face and head. Stay in this relaxed state for a number of minutes, noticing the rising and falling of your chest. Now, imagine that you are at the top of a flight of 10 steps. Tell yourself that you are going to walk down the steps and count backward from 10 as you picture yourself descending each step. Feel yourself becoming more relaxed with each step.

How to create a hypnotic trance: Your next task is to self-induce a hypnotic trance using what is known as a "safe-place technique."

What to do: With your eyes closed and while breathing deeply, mentally take yourself to a place that feels calm and safe. This could be a quiet forest, a sunny beach or a serene mountaintop. What do you see, smell, hear and taste? How do you feel in this place? Engage all your senses. After a few minutes, begin repeating suggestions to yourself that reinforce a sense of well-being and lack of pain in your head.

These suggestions may include statements such as: The muscles in my head and neck are completely relaxed…my head is completely pain-free. The entire relaxation session takes only about 10 minutes. Ideally, headache sufferers should use hypnotic relaxation three times daily to guard against stressors that trigger tension-type headaches…it can also be used as soon as a headache starts to develop so the sufferer can quickly gain control over the pain. If pain medication is still needed, hypnotic relaxation will likely allow for a reduced dose.

Too Much Tension…

Up to 80% of Americans suffer from occasional tension-type headaches. About 3% struggle with these headaches almost daily.

What's causing so many tension headaches?

While the reasons vary depending on the individual, tension headaches are usually (but not always) due to tight muscles in the back of the neck and scalp. Fatigue, anxiety and emotional stress (including depression) commonly are linked to the muscle tension that can lead to these headaches. Specific stressful situations that may trigger tension headaches include conflict at home… having too many responsibilities…dealing with a chronic illness…not getting sufficient sleep…and facing tight deadlines.

Best Natural Remedies for Migraines

Jay S. Cohen, MD, author of *15 Natural Remedies for Migraine Headaches* and a member of both the psychiatry and psychopharmacology departments at University of California, San Diego.

Migraine headaches can be awful—and many people find that the side effects of the prescription medications given to prevent or treat them can be just as bad. For instance, listed among the numerous possible adverse effects for propranolol, a commonly prescribed migraine medication, are vertigo, facial swelling, receding gums, cardiac arrhythmia—and, believe it or not, headache.

However, compelling research has shown that certain natural remedies help prevent, soothe and reduce the frequency of migraine headaches—without the side effects of drugs.

Important: Check with your doctor to make sure that none of these natural treatments will interact with any other medications that you take or conditions that you have. Then I suggest working through the list to see what helps you. You also can combine remedies, such as riboflavin, magnesium and CoQ10, but always check with your doctor.

Riboflavin

Also called vitamin B-2, riboflavin occurs naturally in certain foods. It helps convert

253

food into energy...it's an antioxidant that fights free-radical damage...and it helps activate other forms of vitamin B.

How riboflavin helps migraines: It's thought that some migraines occur because oxygen is not being properly metabolized in the mitochondria (the so-called "power plants" of cells), so riboflavin's energy-boosting function may help prevent this type of migraine.

The research: The first published study evaluating riboflavin for migraine therapy reported that taking 5 milligrams (mg) three times daily over several months diminished migraine frequency—some subjects said that taking hourly doses halted acute migraines. Studies done in 1994 and 1998 found that taking 400 mg/day of riboflavin helped reduce frequency and severity of migraines, with the best results seen in the third month of therapy. A 2004 study of migraine patients who had not responded to other therapies yielded a 50% reduction in migraine frequency for patients who took riboflavin daily.

How to take riboflavin: I suggest 400 mg daily. It's safe to take riboflavin indefinitely. Some people notice improvement quickly, but others see benefits only after three or four months of taking riboflavin daily. A small percentage of people find that riboflavin makes their faces flush and/or report digestive upset—if that happens to you, you might try dividing your dose in half (200 mg, morning and night) or just take 200 mg/day.

Coenzyme Q10

Also called ubiquinone, CoQ10 is a substance that occurs naturally in the body that helps with mitochondrial function and energy production. It's also an antioxidant that may help stem inflammation.

How CoQ10 helps migraines: CoQ10 works similarly to riboflavin, supporting cellular energy production. Its antioxidant power is so strong that it's often recommended for people with certain types of heart disease and muscular and nervous system problems.

The research: Several small studies found that taking CoQ10 reduced migraine fre-

quency. In a 2002 study of 32 adults taking 150 mg/day, 61% said that the days they experienced migraines were down by 50% or more. A 2005 study found that 48% of participants experienced a 50% or greater decrease in frequency, and a 2007 study of children and adolescents had similar results.

How to take CoQ10: I typically advise patients to start with a dose of 150 mg/day and, if needed, work their way up to taking three daily doses of 100 mg (morning, noon and night). One percent of people report some stomach upset with CoQ10—if you're in that group, stop taking CoQ10.

Magnesium

The vast majority of Americans are deficient in magnesium, which is a problem because it is essential to the healthy function of muscles and the nervous system. I believe magnesium is very helpful for people with a deficiency—not so much for those whose magnesium levels already are healthy.

How magnesium helps migraines: Magnesium plays a role in many cellular processes and also is responsible for smooth-muscle activity in the nerves and arteries—both factors in migraines. Also, magnesium deficiency has been shown to cause spasms of the cerebral arteries, associated with migraine.

The research: A 1995 study reported that intravenous delivery of 1,000 mg of magnesium was effective at halting migraines. Stud-

Botox for Head Pain

Botox injections help more than just chronic migraines. They can help frequent episodic migraines, TMJ-related headaches and cluster, cervicogenic and post-traumatic headaches. In his experience, approximately 70% of patients treated with Botox for headache pain see significant improvement.

Alexander Mauskop, MD, director of the New York Headache Center and CEO of Migralex, Inc., both in New York City.

ies examining the use of oral magnesium (600 mg/day) to prevent migraines were done in 1996 and 2008 and found that it reduced both the frequency and severity of the headaches.

How to take magnesium: A good dose to begin with is 100 mg twice daily. Gradually work your way up to 400 mg/day.

5-HTP

5-Hydroxytryptophan (5-HTP) is a building block used by the body to produce serotonin, a neurotransmitter that aids cellular communication and also is associated with mood. Available in many foods, 5-HTP is produced from the amino acid tryptophan.

How 5-HTP helps migraines: 5-HTP gets converted by the body to serotonin (found in the nervous system and the gut), which is involved in the conduction of pain signals and the dilation/constriction of blood vessels—both relevant to migraine pain.

The research: A 1973 study compared the efficacy of 5-HTP therapy (200 mg/day) and a prescription medication in 20 patients and found identical results—both treatments achieved a 55% reduction in frequency, and the 5-HTP patients who continued taking the supplement reported continual improvement. Subsequent studies found 5-HTP effective at soothing the pain of migraines already in progress.

How to take 5-HTP: Begin with a small dose (50 mg to 100 mg), and if need be, work your way up to the maximum daily dosage (300 mg to 400 mg), taken at bedtime. Side effects are mild and may include gastrointestinal problems and weird dreams.

Melatonin

This sleep-promoting hormone has numerous positive effects, including suppression of the substances that promote pain. It also fosters anti-inflammatory activity, regulation of serotonin and nerve and blood vessel interaction.

How melatonin helps migraines: A theory about one possible cause of migraine relates to an imbalance in the relationship between the hypothalamus and the pineal gland that affects adequate melatonin production.

The research: A 2004 study followed 34 adult patients who were given a nightly melatonin dose of 3 mg for three months—25% stopped getting migraines altogether and 80% reported a 50% or greater reduction in frequency. A 2008 study examining children and adolescents taking 3 mg of melatonin at bedtime found a 50% or greater reduction in frequency for 71% of participants.

How to take melatonin: Start with a dose of 0.5 mg or 1 mg and go up to 2, 3 or 5 mg, depending on your reaction. Take melatonin in the evening, preventively, or as treatment for an acute migraine. Melatonin yields superior results and has far fewer side effects when compared with common migraine drugs.

Vitamin D and Migraines

Many of us take vitamin D, but one-third of American adults still don't get enough. That's bad news because it affects blood pressure and immune function. Also, low levels are linked to a range of chronic diseases including diabetes, osteoporosis, fibromyalgia and numerous types of cancer.

How vitamin D helps migraines: Though research shows the benefits of vitamin D for migraines, the actual mechanisms by which vitamin D helps prevent or treat migraines aren't well-understood. Since we do know that deficiencies affect all organ systems, it makes sense that raising levels of vitamin D would be beneficial.

The research: Studies done in 2009 and 2010 found correlations between vitamin D deficiency and chronic tension and migraine headaches—and noted improvement with vitamin D therapy.

How to take vitamin D: It's a good idea to get your vitamin D levels tested and discuss the proper dosage with your doctor based on the results. Mainstream doctors typically recommend between 200 international units

(IU) and 800 IU a day. Some alternative practitioners go far higher, to 5,000 IU/day, or even more.

5 DIY Remedies for Back Pain

Jamison Starbuck, ND, is a naturopathic physician in family practice and a guest lecturer at the University of Montana, both in Missoula.

Argh! If you've ever hurt your low back, you're familiar with that microsecond of awareness that signals something is wrong, followed by a sudden jolt of pain. You know that you're in for days, weeks or even months of painful back spasms and nagging backaches. After the initial injury, pain can be brought on even by simple tasks such as turning over in bed or getting in or out of the car.

Fortunately, there are natural back pain remedies that really work…

Back pain remedy #1: **Walking—on hills.** Here's a little secret that will make walking even more effective for low-back pain: If possible, do hill walking. Why is this better? Walking uphill requires you to lift your leg more than flat walking does. In doing this, the muscles along the spine are elongated, stretched and strengthened more effectively than with flat walking. Downhill walking is less helpful than walking uphill, though it does generally help and strengthens thigh muscles.

Important: Hill walking does not mean climbing up mountains or steep hills. If you want to try hill walking for back pain, look for rolling hills and choose a route with more up than down if possible. Walk a minimum of 20 minutes per day, four times a week. If this is painful, start with five-minute walks, spread throughout the day, and work up to 20 or more minutes per walk when you are able.

Back pain remedy #2: **Ice.** Many people think that ice helps only right after you've injured your back. This isn't so. Ice reduces

Two Drug-Free Devices Provide Migraine Relief

•**The FDA recently approved the Spring Transcranial Magnetic Stimulator (SpringTMS),** a device that a migraine patient can hold on the back of his/her head to release electromagnetic energy to the brain. In a recent study of 113 adults who have migraines with the sensory disturbance known as an aura, nearly 38% were free of pain within two hours after using the device—more than twice as many as those migraine sufferers who didn't use it.

How it works: Electromagnetic energy stimulates a part of the brain that can ease migraine pain. Side effects can include temporary dizziness.

Richard Lipton, MD, director, Montefiore Headache Center, New York City.

•**Cefaly is a headbandlike device that delivers electrical pulses to stimulate the nerves just above the eyes that are involved in migraine pain.**

Recent finding: Migraine patients who wore the device for 20 minutes a day had significantly fewer migraines and reduced their use of antimigraine medication. The device is less effective than the most widely used migraine medications, but it does not cause the unpleasant side effects, such as nausea, skin tingling and fatigue. Cefaly was approved by the FDA in early 2014. It can be purchased at Cefaly.us and from some pharmacies.

Study by researchers at Headache Research Unit, University of Liège, Belgium, published online in *Neurology.*

pain and inflammation as long as your back is still hurting.

What to do: Keep a gel pack or bag of frozen peas in your freezer. Wrap either in a thin cloth, and apply to your low back for 10 minutes only, several times a day.

Back pain remedy #3: **Stretching.** Gentle stretching is great for reducing back pain.

Instant Migraine Relief

Eliminate migraine pain with pepper. Capsaicin, an ingredient in cayenne pepper, cuts off neurotransmitters in the brain that cause headache pain.

Best: Dissolve one-quarter teaspoon of cayenne powder in four ounces of warm water. Dip a cotton swab into the solution, and apply the liquid inside your nostrils. It will burn—and by the time the burning stops, the headache pain will be reduced and sometimes gone altogether.

Eric Yarnell, ND, assistant professor, department of botanical medicine, Bastyr University, Kenmore, Washington.

Breathe deeply and stretch (reach overhead, bend forward and lean from side to side) but only as far as you can without causing pain.

***Back pain remedy #4:* Traumeel.** This ointment, which contains arnica, chamomile and other herbs in homeopathic form, is anti-inflammatory, promotes circulation and reduces pain. Apply a small amount to the painful area twice daily as needed for up to a month. Traumeel is available from naturopathic physicians' offices and over-the-counter at natural-food stores and pharmacies as well as online.

***Back pain remedy #5:* White willow bark.** This herb, which reduces pain and inflammation, contains salicin, a chemical that is similar to aspirin. I often recommend 400 mg three times daily for low-back pain relief. Like aspirin, white willow can bother the stomach, so take it with a small amount of food. Check with your doctor first if you have a chronic medical condition or take medication (especially a blood thinner, beta-blocker or diuretic).

If you follow these steps for run-of-the-mill back pain, you should feel much better within about a week.

The Right Way to Carry a Purse

Karen Erickson, DC, chiropractor in private practice in New York City. She is a faculty member at the Center for Health and Healing of Beth Israel Medical Center, also in New York City, and a spokesperson for the American Chiropractic Association. *Acatoday.org*

Backaches, headaches, neck and shoulder pain often have a common cause—that too-heavy handbag you habitually carry. It throws your posture out of alignment…causes spasms of the trapezius muscle that runs from the base of your skull to your midback…and speeds arthritic degeneration of the spine.

Solution: Lighten your load, and relieve the pain.

• **Weigh your purse.** It should weigh no more than 10% of your body weight. That's 14 pounds for a 140-pound woman.

Ideal: No more than two pounds.

• **Choose a bag made of lightweight material.** Avoid heavy leather and canvas, buckles and embellishments.

• **Switch shoulders every few minutes…** place the strap diagonally across the chest… or use a backpack that distributes weight evenly.

• **Edit your bag daily.** Weed out water bottles, magazines, seldom used keys and loose change. Carry only what's essential.

• **Get multiples of heavy items**—gym gear, makeup, hairbrush, etc. Keep the spares in your desk or car instead of carrying them around.

• **Stretch muscles.** With hands on your shoulders, trace slow, wide circles with your elbows, five in each direction. Next, shrug your shoulders up toward your ears, then drop them down. Repeat five times. Do several times daily.

• **Get a deep-tissue massage to increase circulation to muscles and remove lactic acid,** a chemical that causes soreness.

Referrals: American Massage Therapy Association (877-905-2700, *amtamassage.org*).

●**Realign your spine.** A chiropractor can help to restore the normal alignment of your spine and shoulders. Relieving purse-related pain typically takes no more than a few visits.

Referrals: American Chiropractic Association (800-986-4636, *Acatoday.org*).

Fibromyalgia: New Research Helps Unravel the Mystery

Anne Louise Oaklander, MD, PhD, associate professor of neurology at Harvard Medical School and director of a diagnostic and research laboratory at Massachusetts General Hospital that studies neurological causes of chronic pain and itch, both in Boston.

For the roughly five million American adults with fibromyalgia, the muscle soreness, body aches and telltale painful "tender points" on the shoulders, neck, back, hips, arms and legs are all too familiar.

But until very recently, the condition was a much maligned mystery illness. In fact, some doctors told patient after patient that the condition was "all in your head" because no cause could be identified.

Now: The medical naysayers are rethinking fibromyalgia because of new research showing that the condition does have an identifiable cause in some patients. Substantial numbers of people with fibromyalgia have been found to have a little-known—but testable—condition that triggers faulty signals from tiny nerves all over the body, possibly causing the symptoms of fibromyalgia.

According to several studies published in 2013, one conducted by researchers at Massachusetts General Hospital, nearly half of people with fibromyalgia have evidence of a disease called small-fiber polyneuropathy (SFPN).

A form of peripheral neuropathy, SFPN involves damage to specific nerve cells that can trigger pain and the digestive problems that often accompany fibromyalgia.

How was this discovery made? Skin biopsies were the key tests that uncovered abnormalities in the nerve cells of 40% of SFPN sufferers who were tested.

Meanwhile, researchers at Albany Medical College found another interesting piece of the puzzle—excessive nerve fibers lining the blood vessels within the skin of people with fibromyalgia. Since these fibers control the flow of blood, oxygen and nutrients to muscles during exercise, this abnormality might explain the deep muscle pain of fibromyalgia.

Even though the discoveries described above don't apply to all fibromyalgia patients, they give researchers some clues to follow toward cracking the disease's formidable mystery.

New Hope for Better Treatments

Scientists may be intrigued by this new evidence, but what does it mean for people who suffer from fibromyalgia? The most immediate—and significant—implication has to do with testing. Fibromyalgia symptoms can vary widely, so the diagnosis can be challenging even for experienced rheumatologists.

Now that fibromyalgia has been linked to SFPN, people with fibromyalgia symptoms may want to ask their doctors about testing for SFPN. A skin biopsy from the lower leg is currently the best way to diagnose SFPN. The sample can be mailed to an accredited lab—for example, at Massachusetts General Hospital—for analysis. It is usually covered by insurance.

In the meantime, the following medications (in addition to the following nondrug approaches) can help relieve symptoms of fibromyalgia…

●**FDA-approved medications.** *Pregabalin* (Lyrica), an anticonvulsant…and *duloxetine* (Cymbalta) and *milnacipran HCI* (Savella), both serotonin and norepinephrine reuptake inhibitors (SNRIs), have been shown to reduce pain and improve function for some people with fibromyalgia. Researchers do not know exactly why these drugs work, but some data suggest that they affect pain signaling in the brain and spinal cord.

•**Nortriptyline (Pamelor).** An older tricyclic antidepressant that has also been proven effective for chronic pain relief, nortriptyline is not specifically FDA-approved for fibromyalgia. But it and several other off-label medications, including the anticonvulsant *gabapentin* (Neurontin)—available cheaply as generic drugs—have strong data supporting their use for fibromyalgia.

Nondrug approaches...

Medication isn't the only treatment for fibromyalgia symptoms. *Other good options...*

•**Exercise.** Don't think this is just another plug for exercise. The research showing exercise's effect on fibromyalgia pain is very strong. Whether it's walking, strength training or stretching, exercise improves emotional well-being and lessens muscle wasting, an unfortunate consequence of avoiding exercise due to pain.

•**Vitamin D.** This inexpensive vitamin supplement has just begun to prove its mettle for some people with fibromyalgia. A study published in January 2014 in the journal *PAIN* indicates that vitamin D supplements may reduce chronic pain linked to fibromyalgia for those whose blood tests show a low level of the nutrient. The optimal vitamin D dose depends on the level of deficiency.

Promising Fibromyalgia Treatment

According to a recent study, fibromyalgia patients received a treatment called occipital nerve stimulation (ONS), in which electrodes are implanted near the occipital nerves in the neck and connected to an implanted device that delivers mild electrical current. After six months of ONS treatment, patients reported that their overall pain intensity had decreased by 44%. They also needed less pain medication and experienced less fatigue.

Mark Plazier, MD, neurosurgeon at University Hospital Antwerp, Belgium, and leader of a study of fibromyalgia patients, published in *Neuromodulation*.

Get That Eye Exam

You may know that a good eye exam can reveal more than just your eye health. But did you know that it can detect signs of multiple sclerosis, diabetes, high blood pressure, rheumatoid arthritis, high cholesterol and Crohn's disease? In a study of insurance claims, 6% of these conditions were first detected by eye doctors.

Why: The eyes contain blood vessels, nerves and other structures that can be affected by chronic illness. If you're over age 40, get an eye exam at least every two years.

Linda Chous, OD, chief eye-care officer, UnitedHealthcare, Minneapolis.

Fight Thyroid Disease Naturally

Jamison Starbuck, ND, naturopathic physician in family practice and a guest lecturer at the University of Montana, both in Missoula. She is past president of the American Association of Naturopathic Physicians and a contributing editor to *The Alternative Advisor: The Complete Guide to Natural Therapies and Alternative Treatments.*

Hypothyroidism is one of those conditions that often hovers just beneath the radar. You feel lousy, then get used to dragging yourself around and may not even think it's important enough to tell your doctor about it. Of course there's a simple blood test for hypothyroidism (underactive thyroid), and treatment—a daily synthetic thyroid replacement hormone pill, or levothyroxine—is fairly straightforward. But in my opinion, thyroid replacement hormone alone usually doesn't take care of the prob-

Your Thyroid Can Impair Your Driving

According to a recent study, adults with untreated hypothyroidism took longer to apply the brakes while behind the wheel—a delayed reaction time that was equivalent to that of drivers who were legally drunk.

Why: Thyroid hormone is needed for proper brain function.

If you have symptoms of hypothyroidism, such as weakness or cold intolerance: Ask your doctor about being tested for the condition, and be sure to take your medication if you have hypothyroidism.

Kenneth Ain, MD, professor of endocrinology, University of Kentucky College of Medicine, Lexington.

lem, because it helps patients feel better—but not great. That's not good enough!

Here's what most people don't realize: A major cause of hypothyroidism is an autoimmune condition known as Hashimoto's thyroiditis (in some cases, hypothyroidism is due to other causes such as thyroid surgery or thyroid cancer). As an autoimmune disease, Hashimoto's throws the immune system out of whack so that it goes on the attack, for unknown reasons, against the thyroid gland. This means that you've got a bigger problem than an empty gas tank—your whole body needs some tuning up. If your doctor has told you that you have Hashimoto's, talk to him/her about adding the following natural approaches to your standard thyroid replacement regimen...

1. Avoid food allergens. Food allergies are linked to autoimmune disease. Gluten and wheat allergies are particularly common in people with thyroid disease. To find out if you have food allergies (believe it or not, many people who have food allergies aren't aware of it), ask your doctor for an IgG blood test. If it's positive, avoiding the foods you're allergic to will increase your vitality and nicely augment your hormone replacement therapy.

2. Try supplements and tweak your diet. Low iodine, zinc and selenium can reduce thyroid hormone production—a bad situation when you already have low thyroid levels. That's why I prescribe low-dose supplements—300 micrograms (mcg) of iodine...30 mg of zinc...and 100 mcg of selenium daily—for my patients with Hashimoto's. (Before trying these supplements, be sure to check with your doctor—especially if you have any other chronic health condition or take medication.) Also, avoid "goitrogens"—foods that suppress thyroid function by interfering with the absorption of iodine, which plays such a key role in keeping this gland healthy. Goitrogens include raw kale and broccoli and soy (in any form). Cooked green veggies are OK—heat deactivates the goitrogenic substances.

3. Get some natural sunlight. When our eyes are exposed to sunlight, it fuels the pineal gland in the brain to produce thyroid hormone. To get this thyroid benefit, take your sunglasses off for at least 30 minutes a day when you're outdoors. (If you have an eye disease, such as glaucoma, this is not advisable.)

4. Do aerobic exercise for 20 minutes, four times a week. Moderate exercise increases thyroid hormone production and boosts the immune system by improving circulation, enhancing cardiac function and relieving stress.

5. Improve circulation to your thyroid gland. Hashimoto's often impairs blood circulation to the thyroid gland. To promote better blood flow, you can try yoga or simply do a "shoulder stand" for a few minutes every day—raise your hips and legs above your head while you lie on your back. (Don't do this if you have glaucoma, high blood pressure or neck problems.)

Diabetes Med Affects Your Thyroid

Metformin, a drug often prescribed to regulate blood sugar levels, may lower thyroid-stimulating hormone (TSH) in patients who have an underactive thyroid. Low TSH increases risk for cardiovascular problems and broken bones. Talk to your doctor before beginning metformin therapy.

Laurent Azoulay, PhD, assistant professor at McGill University, Montreal, and leader of a study of 74,300 patients over 25 years, published in Canadian Medical Association Journal.

Mysterious Thyroid Problem

Hyperparathyroidism results from a benign tumor on one or two of the four parathyroid glands.

The tumors usually have no identifiable cause. However, in about 2% of cases, parathyroid tumors develop from exposure to radiation to the neck or face 20 to 40 years earlier (for cancer treatments, for example) or even from treatments for acne and recurrent tonsillitis back in the 1950s and 1960s. Some people who had radioactive iodine destruction of their thyroid gland (for Graves' disease) develop a parathyroid tumor 10 to 30 years later. Fortunately, these tumors are nearly always benign and can be removed with a 20-minute outpatient operation.

James Norman, MD, director, Norman Parathyroid Center, Tampa. Parathyroid.com

New Thinking on MS

Rob Motl, PhD, associate professor in the department of kinesiology and community health, College of Applied Health Sciences at the University of Illinois at Urbana-Champaign.

Until recently, if you were diagnosed with multiple sclerosis (MS), treatment options were extremely limited. Doctors prescribed powerful drugs to reduce the number of new harmful brain lesions that characterize MS...to help control relapses...and to perhaps even slow progression of the disease.

Unfortunately, these medications, available only by injection, were often inconvenient to use and not always effective. Newer medications (such as Gilenya, Aubagio and Tecfidera) are now available in pill form. But is that enough?

New thinking: Even though medication is still believed to be important for most people with MS and should begin soon after diagnosis (when it is likely to be most effective), researchers are now identifying nondrug therapies that can also help.

Beyond the Rx

With MS, the immune system mistakenly attacks the myelin sheaths that insulate the nerves, resulting in weakness, tingling, spasticity (marked by stiff or rigid muscles), balance problems and dizziness.

The nondrug therapies below have been shown to help people with MS have the best possible outcomes. Try as many as possible.

•**Walking.** Inactivity is dangerous for a person with MS—it can lead to muscle weakness, shallow breathing and other problems that can be exacerbated by the illness.

In studies of people with MS, walking (a great exercise because it can be adapted to various fitness levels) has been shown to reduce symptoms of fatigue, depression and pain...and improve sleep quality. Walking also may improve cognitive functioning, which can decline with MS, and improve balance, reducing one's risk of falling.

My advice: Walk for at least 15 to 30 minutes three to five times per week. Use a cane or walker if MS symptoms include leg weakness or numbness, spasticity and/or balance problems.

•**Strength training.** Research shows that muscle-strengthening exercises increase bone health and improve bladder and bowel control—all of which can be compromised with MS.

My advice: Twice a week, use weights that target the major muscle groups (such

261

as quads, hamstrings, calves, biceps, triceps, shoulders and core). Do 15 of these exercises for each muscle group per session, and slowly add more repetitions and/or heavier weights.

Important: Speak with your physician before starting an exercise regimen. If you have problems with balance, consider working out with a physical therapist, friend or personal trainer for extra support.

• **Cooling strategies.** Increased activity and warmer temperatures can raise the core body temperature in people with MS. Even a slight increase may temporarily worsen their symptoms. With regular exercise, however, the body becomes more efficient in regulating its temperature, and heat sensitivity decreases.

My advice: While your body is becoming conditioned to respond efficiently to heat during your exercise program, take steps to prevent overheating. For example, exercise in an air-conditioned environment…use fans… wear loose-fitting clothing…and stay well hydrated. Cooling products such as vests, headbands, shirts and hats can help keep your core temperature stable.

Good cooling products include: Vests from GlacierTek (*GlacierTek.com*) or Coolture (*Coolture.net*), which range in price from $100 to $400. The cost may be covered by insurance. Cooling vests and neck, ankle and wrist wraps are also available from the Multiple Sclerosis Association of America (*MyMSAA.org*)—free to those who meet income limits.

• **Salsa dancing.** In a pilot study, people with MS who did salsa dancing for 40 minutes twice a week for four weeks improved their balance and gait and increased their activity levels. The front-to-back and side-to-side movements used in salsa dancing are believed to be especially helpful for those with MS.

My advice: If salsa dancing sounds appealing, ask your doctor whether he/she thinks lessons and regular practice sessions would be appropriate for you. Ballroom dancing

and the video game Dance Dance Revolution have also been shown to help MS patients.

• **Acupuncture.** Acupuncture has been found to help with MS symptoms such as bladder problems, sleep disorders and tingling.

My advice: If you want to try acupuncture, look for a licensed acupuncturist. To find one near you, consult the National Certification Commission for Acupuncture and Oriental Medicine, *NCCAOM.org*.

• **Massage.** In a recent study, MS patients who received a 45-minute massage twice a week for five weeks improved their physical and social functioning and suffered less depression. By relaxing the muscles and increasing blood flow, massage may also alleviate spasticity, cramping and pain.

My advice: Consider trying Swedish massage, which uses long strokes and a light touch. Avoid using a table warmer or hot packs during the session, since people with MS tend to get overheated.

Caution: Some people with MS take corticosteroids, which may increase their risk for osteoporosis. If you have osteoporosis, massage may not be advisable unless your physician recommends it.

Hope for Lupus Sufferers

Jennifer H. Anolik, MD, PhD, rheumatologist and associate professor of medicine in the immunology and rheumatology unit at the University of Rochester Medical Center, where she practices in the Lupus Clinic.

For the first time in more than 50 years, the FDA has approved a new drug for treating lupus. It's an important breakthrough because the drug, *belimumab* (Benlysta), may help reduce lupus flare-ups and could lead to more effective treatments. New treatments are needed because lupus is a systemic autoimmune disease that can affect virtually every part of the body, making it tough to treat.

Immune-suppressing medications, such as *methotrexate* (Rheumatrex, Trexall) and *azathioprine* (Imuran), may be used for more severe cases of SLE. Steroids are potent anti-inflammatories and are frequently used to treat SLE—in low doses for milder manifestations such as arthritis and in high doses for severe features such as kidney inflammation (lupus nephritis). Other immunosuppressors, including *mycophenolate* (CellCept) or *cyclophosphamide* (Cytoxan), also are mainstays of treatment for lupus nephritis.

Benlysta is the first biologic medication that was designed specifically to treat SLE. It blocks the activity of B-lymphocyte stimulator, a protein that increases the production of antibodies and SLE.

Important: This medication is an important advance, but it's effective in less than 50% of patients—and it has not yet been studied in such conditions as lupus nephritis.

Benlysta is given in a doctor's office/medical center by IV infusion. The first three doses are given two weeks apart...then, the infusions are given monthly, although the schedule may be different for some patients. Common side effects include nausea, diarrhea and fever.

The Missing Link in Lupus Care

Donald E. Thomas, Jr., MD, assistant professor of medicine at the Uniformed Services University of the Health Sciences in Bethesda, Maryland. He is the author of *The Lupus Encyclopedia.*

Lupus is a stubborn disease that most doctors treat with a variety of medications. If you're lucky, the disease can be controlled with only an antimalarial drug. Other people with lupus need a "cocktail" of powerful medications.

What most people don't realize: To control lupus, medication isn't enough. Everyone with this disease needs to also manage the triggers that cause flare-ups and can lead to

life-threatening complications. Avoiding triggers may allow lupus patients to take smaller doses of stronger immunosuppressant drugs (or even eliminate the need for them) and decrease the frequency and severity of lupus flares.

What Is Lupus?

About one and a half million Americans—mostly women—are affected with the autoimmune disease known as lupus. With this condition, the body produces antibodies, for unknown reasons, that attack the joints, skin, lungs, kidneys and/or other parts of the body.

About half of lupus patients have a mild form that affects only the joints and the skin. Others have a high risk for organ damage. Systemic lupus erythematosus (SLE), the most serious form of the disease, can affect virtually every part of the body, including not only the skin and kidneys but also the heart, brain and blood vessels.

The signs of SLE differ from patient to patient. One person might have a skin rash but no joint pain.

Someone else might have fatigue and pain but no rash. Others show early signs of heart or kidney disease. This variability makes SLE difficult to recognize—and to treat.

The Danger of UV Light

Even though most people with lupus do take the medication that's prescribed for the disease, they could benefit even more by carefully managing one of the most powerful lupus triggers—ultraviolet (UV) light.

Exposure to UV radiation—both from sunlight and indoor lighting—hurts everyone with SLE. UV light causes chemical changes in skin cells that trigger an increase in immune activity and inflammation. In about 30% of lupus patients, UV exposure causes a red rash on exposed skin (photosensitive rash). A so-called "butterfly" rash (covering the bridge of the nose and cheeks) also commonly occurs during or after sun exposure.

Those who don't get a rash may still experience some organ damage.

Even brief exposures to UV light can be dangerous. For example, with the help of her doctor, a woman who continued having symptoms even though she always applied sunscreen before going outdoors discovered that her symptoms were triggered by the light from a photocopy machine.

Best UV protection measures…

•**Apply sunscreen lotion all day, every day.** Use a water-resistant product with an SPF of 30 or higher—and make sure that it blocks both UVA and UVB radiation. Apply it every few hours.

Good products: Anthelios SX by La Roche-Posay and sunscreen brands that contain Helioplex.

Also helpful: Use Rit Sun Guard laundry treatment for your outer garments. It adds an invisible coating to clothing that blocks more than 96% of the sun's harmful rays. The treatment lasts for up to 20 washings.

•**Use sunscreen even when you're indoors or driving.** The sunlight that comes through windows can trigger symptoms. Driving with the car windows up decreases UV penetration in the car.

•**Change the lightbulbs.** Indoor lighting also emits UV radiation. Halogen lights emit the most UV light, followed by fluorescent, including both tubes and bulbs.

Best choice: UV-free LED lights, widely available at hardware stores and online.

•**Don't use the UV drying units after manicures or pedicures.** Let the nail polish dry on its own. Or use a dryer that contains a fan but no light.

What Also Helps

Avoiding ultraviolet (UV) light isn't the only self-care step to follow if you have systemic lupus erythematosus (SLE). *Three other important recommendations…*

•**Boost your vitamin D.** Most people with SLE don't produce enough of this important nutrient, in part because they avoid the sun. (Vitamin D is produced in the skin following sun exposure.) The optimal blood level for a person with lupus is around 40 ng/mL. If you've been diagnosed with SLE, your doctor probably orders blood tests four times a year. Be sure that he/she checks your vitamin D level each time, then prescribes an appropriate dose of vitamin D supplement, as needed.

•**Get more omega-3s.** Everyone with SLE should eat fish and other foods high in omega-3 fatty acids, such as flaxseed and walnuts. These healthful fats are thought to ease excessive immune activity and reduce inflammation in the body.

Also: Studies suggest that food sources of omega-3s are more effective than supplements for this disease. If you're not a fish lover, you can get more omega-3s by drinking protein shakes spiked with ground walnuts and flaxseed. One tablespoon daily of olive oil also has been found to have anti-inflammatory properties.

•**Ask about DHEA.** The naturally occurring hormone dehydroepiandrosterone (DHEA) is converted in the body into testosterone and estrogen. Many patients with SLE have levels that are lower than normal. Some patients who take DHEA may be able to reduce their doses of steroid medications—and thus reduce side effects, such as weight gain, diabetes, brittle bones, glaucoma and cataracts.

Important: Take DHEA only under a doctor's supervision, since it can raise risk for certain cancers in some people. Over-the-counter products can contain much lower amounts of the active ingredient than what's listed on the label. Ask your doctor to write a prescription, and get it filled at a compounding pharmacy.

New Crohn's/Colitis Drug

The FDA recently approved the intravenous drug *vedolizumab* (Entyvio) for ulcerative colitis and Crohn's disease patients who have not responded to standard medications. In clinical trials of 2,700 patients with either of these inflammatory bowel conditions, about 50% of symptoms eased for at least a year. When given at least every eight weeks, Entyvio blocks certain inflammatory cells from entering areas in the gastrointestinal tract. Side effects may include headache, joint pain and liver damage.

Stephen Hanauer, MD, medical director, Digestive Health Center, Northwestern University Feinberg School of Medicine, Chicago.

Supplements to Help Crohn's

Since many people with Crohn's disease, a chronic gastrointestinal condition, cannot properly absorb crucial nutrients from food, you may need a daily multivitamin that contains zinc, vitamins B-12 and D, as well as a calcium supplement.

Probiotics, especially Saccharomyces boulardii and Lactobacillus, and the supplements curcumin and N-acetyl glucosamine have been shown to reduce Crohn's symptoms in small studies. Herbs can also help reduce inflammation in the digestive tract. Try slippery elm, which helps protect the digestive lining. Follow label directions.

Talk to your doctor before taking any of these supplements because they can interact with medication, including drugs commonly prescribed to treat Crohn's disease.

Lucy Rojo, ND, an integrative physician in private practice in Palm Desert and Anaheim, California. DrLucyRojo.us

Herbal Relief for Painful Mouth Sores

Eric Yarnell, ND, associate professor in the department of botanical medicine at Bastyr University in Kenmore, Washington, and a private practitioner at Northwest Naturopathic Urology in Seattle. He is the author or coauthor of 10 books on natural medicine, including *Nature's Cures: What You Should Know*. DrYarnell.com

The inside of your mouth hurts like crazy, so you stand in front of a mirror and open wide. Do you see white, lacy, raised patches...red, swollen, tender spots...and/or open sores? If so, you may have oral lichen planus (LIE-kun PLAY-nus), an inflammatory disease that affects more women than men and often arises in middle age. Lesions usually appear on the inside of the cheeks but also may develop on the tongue, gums, inner lips and throat. The disorder causes burning pain...a metallic taste in the mouth...sensitivity to spicy foods...dry mouth...and/or bleeding gums.

Oral lichen planus is not contagious. It occurs when the immune system attacks the cells of the mucous membranes in the mouth. The exact reason for this attack is unknown, but outbreaks can be triggered by allergies (for instance, to a food or dental product)...a viral infection (such as hepatitis C)...certain vaccines and medications (including nonsteroidal anti-inflammatory drugs)...or stress.

When outbreaks are linked to an allergy or drug, identifying and avoiding the offending substance can resolve the problem. However, in many cases, oral lichen planus is a chronic condition in which flare-ups continue to come and go indefinitely, with lesions lasting for days, weeks or even months. Since there is no known cure, treatment focuses on alleviating discomfort and promoting the healing of lesions.

Problem: Steroid medication helps but has potentially serious side effects. And once steroid treatment is halted, lesions may return.

Intriguing alternative: Herbs. Eric Yarnell, ND, an associate professor in the department of botanical medicine at Bastyr University, says that while the herbs below have not been proven to cure oral lichen planus, they can ease discomfort...and some patients who use herbal treatments experience quick resolution of symptoms and remain free of recurrences for long periods of time, Dr. Yarnell said.

Important: Certain herbs can have side effects, so work with a health-care provider knowledgeable about herbal medicines, such as a naturopathic doctor. Dr. Yarnell generally prescribes a swish-and-swallow approach (taking a mouthful of a diluted herbal extract and swishing it in the mouth before swallowing it) so the herb acts topically as well as systemically—your own practitioner can advise you on this. *Ask your health-care provider about using the following...*

• **For pain—aloe vera (Aloe barbadensis).** The gel found inside the leaves of the aloe plant contains complex carbohydrates, including glucomannan, that soothe painful tissues and modulate the immune response.

• **For inflammation—turmeric (Curcuma longa).** This spice contains substances called curcuminoids that reduce inflammation via multiple pathways. It doesn't dissolve well in water, so Dr. Yarnell has patients dissolve turmeric in soymilk, nut milk or animal milk.

Caution: People who are prone to kidney stones should not use turmeric (which is high in oxalic acid)—for them, curcumin extract is better.

• **For easily irritated tissues—tormentil (Potentilla tormentilla).** Used in the form of a tincture (a medicinal extract in a solution of alcohol), this herbal preparation coats lesions, protecting them from irritation by food or compounds in saliva, Dr. Yarnell said. This remedy should not be used within 30 minutes of taking any other medications, as the herb may block absorption of other drugs.

Caution: Women who want to avoid alcohol should not use tormentil tincture.

• **For stress—licorice root (Glycyrrhiza glabra) or deglycyrrhizinated licorice (DGL).** This is an adaptogen that helps patients handle the anxiety and stress that can contribute to oral lichen planus...it also modulates the immune system. It often is used in tincture form, though patients who want to avoid alcohol should use chewable DGL tablets instead.

Caution: Licorice root remedies should not be used by patients who have uncontrolled hypertension or who are taking corticosteroids or other drugs that can deplete potassium, Dr. Yarnell said.

Note: Oral lichen planus may increase the risk for oral cancers, so it is important for patients to get regular oral cancer screenings from a doctor or dentist.

Better IBS Remedy

In a 12-week study, 275 women and men with irritable bowel syndrome (chronic abdominal pain with diarrhea and/or constipation) took 10 g daily of psyllium (a vegetable fiber), bran or a placebo. Using a standard scale, the severity of symptoms dropped by 90 points, on average, in the psyllium group, compared with 58 points, on average, for the bran and placebo groups.

Theory: Psyllium is a soluble fiber, which slows the rate at which the stomach empties—an effect that reduces IBS symptoms.

If you have IBS: Ask your doctor about taking 10 g (about two tablespoons) daily of psyllium, which can be mixed with water, taken in capsule form or added to foods, such as yogurt.

C. J. Bijkerk, MD, PhD, researcher, University Medical Center, Utrecht, The Netherlands.

Pycnogenol for Menstrual Cramps and Menopause

Mark Blumenthal, founder and executive director of the American Botanical Council and editor of *HerbalGram*, Austin, Texas. *HerbalGram.org.*

O ne supplement that can be very effective in preventing menstrual cramps is Pycnogenol, or French maritime pine bark extract. Several studies have demonstrated that Pycnogenol supplementation reduces dysmenorrhea, or pain, during menstruation

Example: A Japanese study found that women with dysmenorrhea who took Pycnogenol required painkilling medication for fewer days than those taking a placebo. Take 100 mg daily every day of the month.

Another good supplement to try: Cramp bark, an herb derived from the high bush cranberry a shrub native to Europe and Africa, which, as its name implies, reduces menstrual cramps. One good brand is Cramp Bark Extra by Vitanica (800-572-4712, *Vitanica.com, Amazon.com*). Take as directed on the label.

Fewer Menopausal Symptoms

Taiwanese researchers found that perimenopausal women who took Pycnogenol for several months experienced improvements in symptoms such as headaches, fatigue and vaginal dryness.

Pycnogenol is a well-researched botanical medicine with demonstrated safety and efficacy in study after study at the prescribed dose. Consult a physician trained in botanical medicine to determine what dosage best meets your specific menopausal symptoms. To prevent any minor stomach discomfort, it's best to take Pycnogenol with or after meals…and, as we always recommend, with doctor oversight.

What to Do About Long-Lasting Endometriosis

Andrew Cook, MD, gynecologist with a subspecialty in reproductive endocrinology, internationally respected endometriosis specialist and director of the Vital Health Institute in Los Gatos, California. He also is the author of *Stop Endometriosis and Pelvic Pain: What Every Woman and Her Doctor Need to Know. StopEndo.com*

W ith endometriosis, tissue from the uterine lining migrates outside the uterus, implanting on other pelvic structures and forming blisterlike lesions. Patients experience stabbing or aching pain in the pelvis…sex may be excruciating. Estrogen fuels the growth of endometriosis, and often symptoms are worst during a woman's period—but contrary to what many doctors believe, the disease does not always abate at midlife. "To say that endometriosis cannot be present and cause pain after menopause or hysterectomy is scientifically incorrect. In fact, 2% to 5% of postmenopausal women have endometriosis and symptoms can recur even after decades," said Andrew Cook, MD, a gynecologist with a subspecialty in reproductive endocrinology. *Reasons…*

• **Although estrogen production by the ovaries eases at midlife,** small amounts of estrogen are produced in other areas of the body. Also, endometriosis tissue itself produces estrogen, thus promoting its own growth, Dr. Cook said.

• **Endometriosis can create adhesions (areas of scar tissue) that shrink over time,** tugging painfully on organs, nerves and other internal structures. Pain from adhesions is not affected by decreasing estrogen levels.

• **Endometriosis implants (growths) are found not just on the reproductive organs,** but also on the bladder, bowel, rectum and elsewhere in the pelvic cavity. Even if you remove the uterus and ovaries, a lot of disease can be left behind—which is why a simple hysterectomy often is not an effective treatment.

For mild symptoms: One or more of the following therapies may provide sufficient relief…

•**A nutritionist can help you identify food allergies or sensitivities that exacerbate endometriosis symptoms.** For instance, Dr. Cook said, you may feel better if you avoid foods that worsen inflammation, such as alcohol, dairy, red meat, saturated fats, sugar and wheat…and increase your consumption of estrogen-balancing foods, such as apples, berries, broccoli, cauliflower, flax, green beans, nuts, peaches, salmon and turnips.

•**Bioidentical progesterone use can help counteract the effects of estrogen on endometriosis tissue for some patients.**

•**Patients with longstanding pelvic pain often develop spasms of the pelvic floor muscles (like a charley horse),** contributing to endometriosis pain. For relief, a specially trained physical therapist can perform manual massage techniques to relax the spasms.

If symptoms are severe: Unfortunately, endometriosis will not just melt away, so when a patient is truly suffering, the best option usually is surgery. But beware of any doctor who recommends burning away the endometriosis with coagulation or cauterization. This removes only the top of layer of diseased tissue—an effect Dr. Cook likened to "pulling the tops off weeds and leaving the roots behind"—so symptoms persist or return quickly.

Instead, look for a surgeon specializing in the treatment of endometriosis who can perform wide-excision laparoscopic surgery. The goal is to remove each and every bit of diseased tissue, plus a rim of normal surrounding tissue—just as is done with cancer—to ensure that no microscopic areas of endometriosis are left behind to grow again. This involves meticulously exploring all the "nooks and crannies" inside the pelvis, Dr. Cook said, and using a surgical laser to vaporize the diseased tissue as well as any scar tissue.

Best: Ask your doctor for a referral to an endometriosis specialist…or check the Web site of the support organization Endo Resolved (*Endo-Resolved.com*).

Autoimmune Disease and Endometriosis

Tine Jess, MD, researcher in the department of epidemiology research at the Statens Serum Institut in Copenhagen, Denmark, and lead author of a study on endometriosis and IBD risk published in *Gut*.

What you don't know really can hurt you. So even though the following information isn't exactly welcome, it could ultimately ease the suffering for women with endometriosis. How? By alerting them (and their doctors) to an accompanying increased risk for bowel problems, thus helping them get the treatment they need. *Here's the story…*

With endometriosis, tissue from the uterine lining migrates outside the uterus and implants on other pelvic structures. During menstruation, this displaced tissue bleeds… and the trapped blood inflames surrounding tissues, causing intense pain and internal scarring. Previous studies suggested an association between this inflammatory disorder and various autoimmune diseases. So Danish researchers decided to investigate a possible link between endometriosis and inflammatory bowel disease (IBD), an umbrella term for a group of immune disorders that affect the gut and cause abdominal pain, diarrhea and bloody stools.

The study analyzed data on 37,661 women who were hospitalized for endometriosis between 1977 and 2007. During that 30-year period, 228 of the endometriosis patients also developed ulcerative colitis, a form of IBD that affects the inner lining of the colon…and 92 endometriosis patients also developed Crohn's disease, a type of IBD that affects all layers of both the small and large intestine.

Crunching those numbers: Compared with women in the general population, endometriosis patients were 50% more likely to develop some form of IBD...while those whose endometriosis was verified through surgery had an 80% higher risk for IBD. What's more, the increased IBD risk persisted even 20 years or more after the endometriosis diagnosis.

Why this matters so much: Certain symptoms, notably chronic abdominal pain and diarrhea, are common to both endometriosis and IBD. If a doctor assumes that a patient's ongoing symptoms are solely the result of her endometriosis, he or she may fail to diagnose and treat the woman's IBD—and thus the patient will continue to suffer.

Though it is unclear why endometriosis raises the risk for IBD, researchers suggested that the two conditions might share some underlying immunological features. Or, in some cases, the IBD might be a consequence of treating endometriosis with oral contraceptives (as is commonly done), given that oral contraceptive users are at significantly increased risk for IBD.

Endometriosis patients: If you have persistent abdominal pain or other symptoms, talk with your doctor about this possible link with IBD. Bring this article to your appointment if you think it will help!

How to Cure Chronic Pelvic Pain

Geo Espinosa, ND, LAc, naturopathic doctor and acupuncturist who specializes in prostate disorders, male sexual health and chronic pelvic pain. He founded the Integrative Urology Center at New York University (NYU) Langone Medical Center in New York City. *DrGeo.com*

It is one of the most common but least talked about medical conditions. Chronic pelvic pain (CPP)—dull aching, cramping and/or sharp pains in the area between the navel and the hips—is mostly thought of as a woman's disorder. But men account for approximately 20% of the 11 million Americans who suffer from CPP.

It's a tricky condition to diagnose because the symptoms—which in women and men may include painful intercourse, difficulty sleeping, low energy and/or alternating constipation and diarrhea—can be caused by many different conditions, such as endometriosis in women. In both women and men, infection of the urethra or bladder and food sensitivities can trigger CPP.

And even though the condition is chronic—that is, lasting for six months or longer—it might wax and wane daily...or you might have a weeklong flare-up after a pain-free month.

Where to Start?

Every woman with CPP symptoms should see a gynecologist, who will perform a thorough pelvic exam to look for such problems as abnormal growths and tension in the pelvic muscles.

Examples: Ultrasound to examine the organs for abnormalities such as ovarian cysts in women and prostate enlargement in men... and laboratory tests to look for infections. In some cases, a woman may also undergo laparoscopy, the insertion of a thin tube into the abdomen to look for endometriosis.

Some patients get relief once the underlying problem is identified and treated, but many patients don't.

Reason: Within just months, CPP can trigger sometimes permanent changes in the spinal cord that allow the persistent passage of pain signals to the brain—even when the underlying cause of the pain has been corrected.

The Next Step

Patients with CPP can improve with conventional treatments (such as the use of painkillers or surgery to remove growths), but these approaches won't necessarily give them the greatest odds of adequately relieving their pain.

Better: Taking a complementary approach that combines conventional and alternative treatments.

Best therapies to try—in addition to mainstream treatments…

• **Relax trigger points.** Most women and men with CPP have one or more trigger points (areas of knotted muscle) somewhere in the pelvic area—for example, on the lower abdomen or on the upper thighs. Trigger points themselves can be excruciatingly painful and can transmit pain throughout the pelvic region.

Example: Vaginal pain could be caused by a trigger point elsewhere on the pelvis.

Massage therapists are typically trained to identify and treat trigger points. Simply pressing on one of these points for 20 to 30 seconds—and repeating the pressure several times during an hour-long massage—can relax the tension and help ease the pain. Having a weekly massage for several months sometimes can eliminate symptoms of CPP.

To find a massage therapist who specializes in trigger point treatment, go to *MassageTherapy.com*, click on "Find a Massage Therapist" and select "Trigger Point Therapy."

Drawback: Pressure on a trigger point can be painful. You can get the same relief, with less discomfort, with electroacupuncture. Two or more hair-width acupuncture needles are inserted into the skin above the trigger point. Then, a mild electrical current is administered, which causes the muscle to relax.

Treatment for CPP will typically require about six to 20 sessions of electroacupuncture. Many acupuncturists are trained in electroacupuncture. However, because the technique is less well-studied than standard acupuncture, it may not be covered by your health insurer. Electroacupuncture typically costs about $70 to $100 per session.

Electroacupuncture should not be used on patients who have a history of seizures, epilepsy, heart disease, stroke or a pacemaker.

• **Try standard acupuncture.** Even if you don't have trigger points, acupuncture is among the most effective treatments for CPP.

A study of 67 women who had bacterial cystitis (infection of the bladder wall that commonly causes CPP) found that 85% of them were virtually pain-free after receiving 20-minute acupuncture sessions, twice weekly for four weeks. Reinfection rates were also reduced.

Acupuncture is believed to help block the transmission of pain signals. It's also an effective way to reduce muscular as well as emotional stress, both of which increase all types of chronic pain. Most CPP patients will need 10 to 20 treatments. Acupuncture is often covered by insurance.

Identify food sensitivities. Many women and men with CPP are sensitive to one or more foods, particularly wheat and dairy.

What happens: When these patients eat "problem" foods, they have increased intestinal permeability, also known as "leaky gut" syndrome. Large, undigested food molecules that are normally contained within the intestine pass into the bloodstream, where they trigger the release of inflammatory chemicals that can cause pain throughout the body and in the pelvic region, in particular.

A blood test known as ALCAT (antigen leukocyte cellular antibody test) can identify specific food sensitivities. Although it is reasonably reliable, the test usually isn't covered by insurance because it is considered an "alternative" diagnostic tool. It costs about $400.

Another option: An elimination-challenge diagnostic diet.

What to do: Quit eating wheat, dairy and other likely food triggers, such as soy, wine and sugar, for 21 days. If your symptoms improve, at least one of the foods was a problem. Then, reintroduce the foods, one at a time over a period of weeks, to see which food (or foods) causes symptoms to return.

Patients may get frustrated, initially, because they feel like there are few foods left to eat, but many of the foods that they give up during the test will turn out to be harmless. Foods found to cause problems should be given up indefinitely.

• **Take probiotics.** Because infections, such as those described earlier, are a common cause of pelvic pain, patients often receive multiple courses of antibiotics. Antibiotics eliminate infection, but they also kill beneficial bacteria in the intestine. This can lead to digestive problems such as irritable bowel syndrome and leaky gut syndrome—both of which are linked to CPP.

Helpful: A daily probiotic supplement with a mix of at least 10 billion live, beneficial organisms, such as Acidophilus and Lactobacillus. A probiotic supplement should be taken indefinitely.

Also helpful: Glutamine—100 mg to 200 mg, taken twice daily until symptoms improve. It nourishes the cells that line the intestine and can help prevent leaky gut syndrome. People with liver or kidney disease should not take glutamine.

Caution: Do not take a B-complex nutrient if you're suffering from CPP. In my practice, patients who take B vitamins have more CPP symptoms for reasons that aren't clear.

Very helpful: Yoga. It is probably the best workout if you have CPP. That's because it relaxes muscle tension as well as trigger points...increases levels of painkilling endorphins...and promotes overall relaxation.

Prolapse Surgeries Work

The most common surgeries to correct pelvic organ prolapse are equally effective and safe. Pelvic organ prolapse is a weakening of the pelvic organs, most often seen in older women and those who have given birth several times. The procedures—sacrospinous ligament fixation and uterosacral ligament suspension—involve stitching the top of the vagina to ligaments inside the pelvic cavity to stop the pain and incontinence associated with the condition.

Recent finding: Both surgeries had about a 60% surgical success rate.

Study of 374 women with pelvic organ prolapse led by researchers at Women's Health Institute, Cleveland Clinic, published in *The Journal of the American Medical Association*.

Chapter 12

ALLEVIATE DEPRESSION AND EMOTIONAL UPSET

Are You "Almost Depressed"?

Most people know if they're suffering from deep depression. But what's that vaguely uncomfortable, empty feeling you may have had lately? You're not miserable, but it's as if the vitality has been sucked out of your life.

Though it often goes undiagnosed, so-called "almost depression" may have snuck up on you. It can prevent you from enjoying your leisure activities and leave you feeling unsatisfied with your family life, friendships and work.

Don't pooh-pooh it: You may be tempted to ignore these often subtle, though persistent, feelings of discontent. But don't. Almost depression can throw you into a downward spiral that deepens into serious depression—a condition that may increase your risk for chronic physical ailments such as heart disease and dementia.

The good news is that almost depression responds well to some surprising, life-affirming strategies that don't necessarily involve the conventional treatments (such as medication and/or therapy) that are usually prescribed for depression.

What you need to know about almost depression…

Looking for Clues

If you have almost depression, life may generally seem bland and gray. You haven't stopped eating, but nothing tastes very good. You still laugh at jokes…but just to be polite. These are red flags that the brain circuits responsible for processing your feelings of pleasure (the brain's "reward system") may have shifted into low gear—this is widely considered to be an underlying cause of almost depression.

Often, close friends and family members can see changes first. If you think you may be almost depressed, ask someone you trust for his/her candid opinion. For more signs of almost depression, see the list on page 273.

Getting Back on Track

If you're like most people, you can pull yourself out of almost depression—the trick

Jefferson Prince, MD, instructor in psychiatry at Harvard Medical School, Boston, and director of child psychiatry at MassGeneral Hospital for Children in Salem, Massachusetts. He is coauthor of *Almost Depressed: Is My (or My Loved One's) Unhappiness a Problem?*

is to take steps to rev up your brain's sluggish reward system. *The best ways to do that...**

• **Get up and at 'em.** Idleness due to illness or an emotional setback is a common trigger of almost depression. Fortunately, scientists are now finding more and more evidence that exercise improves mood, possibly by altering brain chemistry. In several studies, regular workouts were as effective as antidepressants. But of course, the longer you are inactive, the harder it is to get going—and a trip to the gym may sound impossible.

Best approach: Start by adding just a bit more activity to your day...the 10-minute walk you take is far better than the strenuous workout you avoid. Tomorrow, you may want to take a longer walk or do some gardening. Put yourself in motion...add a bit more activity week by week...and see what happens. It will be good!

• **Put more meaning in your life.** Do you often wonder, "What's all this for?" Almost depression can be a sign that you lack a sense of purpose in your life. Take a good look at your values. For some people, family comes first, and for others, it's career, spiritual growth or health. The key is, any of these can give you a sense of purpose.

Best approach: Identify your two or three top values. And be honest with yourself. You may think "helping others" should be your ultimate concern, but if, say, financial security actually takes priority, there's nothing wrong with making that your goal.

Then start including activities to promote these two or three values every day. Also look for small actions that promote your values. To "improve the lives of others," you don't have to volunteer at a soup kitchen—a smile or doing a favor for a stranger counts, too. Give yourself credit for these moments.

*If you suspect that you're almost depressed, and there's no improvement after trying the strategies in this article, see your doctor for advice. Many physical conditions (such as diabetes, lung disease and cancer) can cause depressive symptoms, as can some blood pressure and cholesterol drugs, antibiotics and other medications. If none of these apply to your situation, your doctor may refer you to a mental-health professional, such as a psychiatrist or psychologist.

• **Let your creativity run wild.** When you scratch beneath the surface, most people with almost depression have bottled-up emotions. Expressing these dark feelings through a creative outlet is liberating—and healing. Don't worry about being talented...just allow yourself to tap into your creative side.

To express yourself: Set aside 20 minutes to write on a computer or by hand about something that's bothering you. Don't edit your feelings—no one will see this but you. In fact, you don't ever need to look at your writing again...the benefit is in the process, not the product.

The next day, write down a story about your life. It's human nature to see life as a narrative with heroes, villains and victims. Being almost depressed puts you in a story that isn't going so well. So go ahead and rewrite your personal narrative. Create a story where the main character has problems like yours but works things out—perhaps through personal change or new insights. The character you invent may teach you some useful strategies—and you will emerge happier.

If you're more of a visual person, you can draw or paint images that will help unleash trapped emotions. Whatever approach you choose, allow your creativity to flourish.

Almost Depressed? Take the Self-Test

Do any of the following statements apply to you?

• **I get more frustrated than usual over little things.**
• **Instead of having fun with friends, I avoid them.**
• **I haven't been sleeping well lately.**
• **Nothing tastes very good.**
• **I would like to "stop the world" and take a break from everything.**
• **Nothing seems very funny (or interesting or exciting) these days.**
• **I get irritated more easily than I used to.**
• **I'm less interested in sex.**

- **I just want to be left alone.**
- **I have trouble concentrating on books or TV.**
- **I feel tired for no reason.**

If you recognize yourself in two or more of these statements, you're likely almost depressed.

6 Foods Proven to Make You Happy

Tonia Reinhard, MS, RD, a registered dietitian and professor at Wayne State University in Detroit. She is author of *Superfoods: The Healthiest Foods on the Planet* and *Superjuicing: More Than 100 Nutritious Vegetable and Fruit Recipes.*

You can eat your way to a better mood! Certain foods and beverages have been proven to provide the raw materials that you need to feel sharper, more relaxed and just plain happier. *Best choices...*

Happy Food #1: Chocolate

Chocolate can make you feel good—to such an extent that 52% of women would choose chocolate over sex, according to one survey.

Chocolate contains chemical compounds known as polyphenols, which interact with neurotransmitters in the brain and reduce anxiety. An Australian study found that men and women who consumed the most chocolate polyphenols (in the form of a beverage) felt calmer and more content than those who consumed a placebo drink.

Chocolate also boosts serotonin, the same neurotransmitter affected by antidepressant medications. It triggers the release of dopamine and stimulates the "pleasure" parts of the brain.

Then there's the sensual side of chocolate—the intensity of the flavor and the melting sensation as it dissolves in your mouth. The satisfaction that people get from chocolate could be as helpful for happiness as its chemical composition.

Recommended amount: Aim for one ounce of dark chocolate a day. Most studies used dark chocolate with 70% cacao or more.

Happy Food #2: Fish

Fish has been called "brain food" because our brains have a high concentration of omega-3 fatty acids—and so does fish. These fatty acids have been linked to memory and other cognitive functions. In countries where people eat a lot of fish, depression occurs less often than in countries (such as the US) where people eat less.

The omega-3s in fish accumulate in the brain and increase "membrane fluidity," the ability of brain-cell membranes to absorb nutrients and transmit chemical signals.

A study in *Archives of General Psychiatry* looked at patients diagnosed with depression who hadn't responded well to antidepressants. Those who were given 1,000 mg of EPA (a type of omega-3 fatty acid) daily for three months had significant improvements, including less anxiety and better sleep.

Recommended amount: Try to have at least two or three fish meals a week. Cold-water fish—such as sardines, mackerel and salmon—have the highest levels of omega-3s. Or choose a supplement with 1,000 mg of EPA and DHA (another omega-3 fatty acid) in total.

Happy Food #3: Dark Green Veggies

Dark green vegetables such as spinach, asparagus, broccoli and Brussels sprouts are loaded with folate, a B-complex vitamin that plays a key role in regulating mood. A Harvard study found that up to 38% of adults with depression had low or borderline levels of folate. Boosting the folate levels of depressed patients improved their mood.

Dark green vegetables are particularly good, but all vegetables and fruits boost mood. Researchers asked 281 people to note their moods on different days. On the days when the participants consumed the most vegetables and fruits, they reported feeling happier and more energetic. Folate certainly plays a role, but self-satisfaction may have something to do with it as well. People feel good when they eat right and take care of themselves.

Recommended amount: The minimum you should have is five servings of vegetables and fruits a day.

Bonus: Middle-aged men who had 10 servings a day showed reduced blood pressure.

Happy Food #4: Beans (including soybeans)

Beans are rich in tryptophan, an essential amino acid that is used by the body to produce serotonin, the neurotransmitter that affects feelings of calmness and relaxation.

Beans also are loaded with folate. Folate, as mentioned in the veggies section, plays a key role in regulating mood.

In addition, beans contain manganese, a trace element that helps prevent mood swings due to low blood sugar.

Recommended amount: For people not used to eating beans, start with one-quarter cup five days a week. Build up to one-half cup daily. This progression will help prevent gastrointestinal symptoms such as flatulence.

Happy Food #5: Nuts

Nuts are high in magnesium, a trace mineral involved in more than 300 processes in the body. People who don't get enough magnesium feel irritable, fatigued and susceptible to stress.

The elderly are more likely than young adults to be low in magnesium—because they don't eat enough magnesium-rich foods and/or because they tend to excrete more magnesium in their urine.

Also, many health problems can accelerate the depletion of magnesium from the body.

Examples: Gastrointestinal disorders (or bariatric surgery), kidney disease and sometimes diabetes.

Recommended amount: Aim for one ounce of nuts a day. Good choices include almonds, walnuts, cashews, hazelnuts and peanuts (the latter is technically a legume). If you don't like nuts, other high-magnesium foods include spinach, pumpkin seeds, fish, beans, whole grains and dairy.

Happy Food #6: Coffee

The caffeine in coffee, tea and other caffeinated beverages is a very beneficial compound. One study found that people with mild cognitive impairment were less likely to develop full-fledged Alzheimer's disease when they had the caffeine equivalent of about three cups of coffee a day.

Caffeine can temporarily improve your memory and performance on tests. It enhances coordination and other parameters of physical performance. When you feel energized, you feel happier. Also, people who feel good from caffeine may be more likely to engage in other happiness-promoting behaviors, such as seeing friends and exercising.

Recommended amount: The challenge is finding the "sweet spot"—just enough caffeine to boost mood but not so much that you get the shakes or start feeling anxious. For those who aren't overly sensitive to caffeine, one to three daily cups of coffee or tea are about right.

What Not to Eat

Some people turn to food or drink for comfort when they're feeling down. *Here's what not to eat or drink when you've got the blues...*

Alcohol: Alcohol is a depressant of the central nervous system. When you initially consume alcohol, it produces a euphoric effect and you become more animated and less inhibited. But as you continue drinking and more alcohol crosses the blood-brain barrier, the depressant effect predominates.

Baked goods: When you eat high-sugar, high-fat carbs such as cookies, pastries and donuts, you tend to want more of them. The food gives you a temporary "good feeling," but the excess food intake that typically results causes drowsiness and often self-loathing.

Nasal Spray for Depression

A nasal spray rapidly relieves depression. A 50-milligram dose of the intranasal spray ketamine, an FDA-approved anesthetic, was found to alleviate depressive symptoms within hours with few side effects in people with treatment-resistant major depressive disorder.

Study by researchers at Icahn School of Medicine at Mount Sinai, New York City, published in Biological Psychiatry.

Say This, Not That

Laurie Puhn, JD, couples' mediator in private practice in New York City. She is author of *Fight Less, Love More: 5-Minute Conversations to Change Your Relationship Without Blowing Up or Giving In. LauriePuhn.com*

J ust a few simple changes in what you say to your spouse can turn an unhappy marriage into a happy one. That's because most marital discontent actually isn't caused by serious differences between spouses, but by small breakdowns in communications—and these communication problems can be corrected, often quite quickly. *Five ways to do it…*

•**Compliment your spouse's character, not just his/her actions.** Commend his kindness, honesty, dependability or thoughtfulness, for example. Our studies have found that 84% of married people value compliments about their character more than other types of spousal praise (though virtually any compliment is likely to be well-received to some degree). Character compliments make spouses feel validated and appreciated on a deep level. They aren't just about something that the spouse has done or how he looks, but who he truly is at his core.

Strategy: When you compliment a deed by your spouse, link it to a positive character trait. Offer these character compliments even when you are not the direct beneficiary of his/her actions. This encourages your spouse to consider you the one person in the world who sees and appreciates who he is.

Example: "It was nice of you to make coffee for me this morning. You're a very thoughtful person."

•**Ask yourself, "Does this affect me?"** before making a critical comment. Sometimes the secret to healthy marital communication is understanding that you don't need to say anything.

Strategy: If your partner's action does not directly involve you, do not get involved. Ask yourself, "Does this affect me?" before offering your input.

Example: Your spouse shares a story with you about a disagreement he had with a coworker—and you think the coworker was right. Saying this will make your spouse feel like you're not his teammate. Instead, just express sympathy for the unpleasant interaction your spouse endured and let the moment pass. If you are desperate to share your opinion, ask permission first. Show respect with, "Would you like my thoughts on this?" If you get a no, then move on. However, showing respect by seeking permission first will make you more likely to get a yes and actually be heard.

•**Provide truly meaningful apologies when you are wrong**—don't just say, "I'm sorry." You made a mistake, but you said, "I'm sorry"—so why is your spouse still upset? As most married people already know, spouses often are not quick to forgive even when they receive a quick apology.

Strategy: A detailed apology can greatly reduce the odds of lingering anger. Say, "I'm sorry for…" then describe what you've done and why your spouse has a right to be mad about it. This establishes that you understand that you have caused pain and are not just saying "sorry" to end the conversation. Also say, "In the future, I will..." and describe how you will handle things better the next time the situation arises. If you are unsure of how to prevent the problem from recurring, seek your mate's input—"I want to make sure that this doesn't happen again. Can you help me think of a way to prevent it?" This helps rebuild your spouse's shaken trust in you. If there's something you can do to set the current situation right, say that you will do this as well.

Example: "I'm sorry for mentioning your health condition to my sister. That was something personal that you had a right to keep private. I'm going to call my sister and ask her not to share it with anyone else. And in the future, I will never discuss your medical condition with anyone without getting your permission first."

• **Figure out why the mildly annoying things your spouse does trigger more than mild annoyance in you.** We all do things that are potentially annoying to our partners. It might be leaving clothes on the bedroom floor or turning up the TV volume too loud or any of a million other missteps. But think back to early in the relationship when you felt enamored with your partner. Chances are he did annoying things then, too—only back then you probably didn't get excessively annoyed by them.

Excessive anger at a spouse's minor foibles and faux pas usually stem from feeling alone in the relationship. Your mind is making a big deal out of a small matter because it now views this small annoyance as a sign that your spouse is not truly your teammate.

Strategy: Stop pestering your partner about minor mistakes—that's only deepening the sense of distance between you. Instead, if you and/or your spouse are making a big deal about small stuff, consider it a sign that the two of you need to become teammates again. First, refocus your radar on noticing and praising the positive things your mate does, such as emptying the dishwasher. Then look for the times when your mate doesn't do the thing that annoys you and praise that, as in, "It was great to come home today and see the clean floor in our bedroom. Thank you for putting away your laundry. It made me smile." What you praise is reinforced and will be repeated more often.

Also, find time to do things that you both enjoy. Communicate with each other in positive ways, as described in this article. Feeling like teammates won't get your spouse's socks into the hamper, but it should make those socks seem like the minor matter that they really are.

• **Stop saying, "Whatever you want."** Some people imagine that letting a spouse have his way will avoid marital conflict, whether it's what to have for dinner or buying a new car. In reality, your spouse could grow resentful about always having to take full responsibility for the decision making...while you are likely to grow resentful about rarely getting what you want. And if your spouse senses your resentment, he is likely to be angry that he's getting blamed for not doing what you want when you never told him what it is you wanted.

Strategy: Both partners should offer their opinions when a decision must be made. When you don't have a strong opinion or truly wish to let your spouse choose, say that you're happy to do whatever he wants to do, then add, "But let me know if you would like my input." Do this only if you truly can accept your spouse's choice without second-guessing it later.

If you disagree on a decision, then be a detective and ask your mate neutral questions such as, "Why do you think that?" "What are your reasons for that choice?" Listen first, then share your thoughts. By seeking to learn new information from your mate, rather than assuming that you know his thoughts, you show respect. Once you've both aired your perspectives, follow up with additional questions and then brainstorm solutions together.

Walk Happily to Feel Happier

Happy people walk more quickly and in a more upright position than sad or depressed people—and they swing their arms more while swaying less from side to side.

Recent finding: Deliberately walking this way made people feel better—while walking as a depressed person made them feel sad.

Study of 39 people by researchers at Witten Herdecke University, Witten, Germany, published in *Journal of Behavior Therapy and Experimental Psychology.*

A Surprising Way to Handle Difficult People

Judith Orloff, MD, assistant clinical professor of psychiatry at UCLA. She is author of the new national best-seller *The Ecstasy of Surrender: 12 Surprising Ways Letting Go Can Empower Your Life* upon which this article is based. *DrJudithOrloff.com*

When faced with difficult behavior at work or with family and friends, most people tend to revert to automatic reactions. They cave in…get defensive or aggressive…or dig in their heels and refuse to budge.

None of these reactions produces satisfying results, but they are the only alternatives most of us are aware of.

A more effective way to deal with difficult people is to surrender—to let go of the need to control a situation and let go of the illusion that you can compel someone to change. Surrendering means accepting a person or situation as is—if you have done everything possible to create change and nothing is budging. This is very different from caving in, which means giving up your needs simply to make peace without any effort to try to create positive change.

This may sound surprising. Many people equate surrender with defeat or weakness.

However, surrender is not the same as failure or defeat. It takes great strength of character.

Surrender is an active choice to accept what life brings you, to be flexible rather than rigid and to see past a momentary block to a greater breakthrough beyond. Surrendering allows you to let go of overthinking and second-guessing.

Practicing Surrender

Surrender doesn't come naturally to most people. It needs to be learned and practiced.

Surrendering is easier to do when you are only mildly stressed. With practice, you can learn to let go even in more challenging encounters. *Simple ways to practice…*

• **Drink a glass of water or juice—slowly.** Savor the sensation of quenching your thirst. Enjoy the fact that there is nothing you have to do but sip and be refreshed.

• **Take a deep breath.** Inhale deeply, and then release your breath fully. This counteracts the stress-induced impulse to clench muscles and breathe shallowly, both of which increase resistance and tension.

• **Change what you say to yourself.** Any time you notice yourself dwelling on regrets about the past or fears about the future, bring yourself back to the present. Say, I can handle the here and now. I don't have to worry about three weeks ago or 10 years from now.

• **Observe water.** Watch the water in a fountain or creek. Notice how water doesn't keep bumping into the same boulder over and over again—it flows around the obstacle. Water can teach you how to flow.

• **Appreciate your body's natural joyful responses.** Let out a hearty laugh. Put on your favorite music, and dance around the living room. Don't choke off those urges—enjoy them.

• **Let yourself feel awe.** Look up at the night sky, and notice the vastness of the galaxy and universe around you. Like a child, allow yourself to surrender to this mystery and awe.

Difficult Situations

In most cases, difficult people aren't trying to make your life miserable—they are just preoccupied with their own frustrations and needs. *Guidelines for dealing with difficult behavior...*

• **Pause.** If you feel yourself getting angry or tense, don't say anything. Let go of the urge to express your immediate reaction. Instead, take a few slow breaths to calm your stress. Count to 10 or 20 if it helps you postpone action.

• **Listen without interrupting.** When we are upset about what someone is saying, we typically want to cut the person off in order to stop our discomfort and express our disagreement or anger. However, interruption just escalates hostility. Let go of the need to direct the discussion. Hear the other person out.

Exception: If the person is being verbally abusive, cut off the abuse at once. Verbal abuse includes personal attacks that target your worth—such as You're a terrible mother or You can't do anything right. In cases like these, break in and set boundaries in a calm voice.

Example: "That kind of statement is unacceptable. If you continue like this, I will leave the room."

• **Don't argue.** You may have the strong desire to state all the evidence that shows you are right, but defensiveness in charged situations doesn't change anyone's mind—it just fuels the conflict.

• **Empathize.** Make a genuine effort to see the situation from the other person's point of view. People who behave badly are suffering in some way. This doesn't excuse their behavior, but once you recognize that they are trying to avoid pain or anxiety, letting go becomes easier.

• **Be willing to concede a point.** Even if you agree with only 1% of what the person is saying, acknowledge that point of agreement. You can say, "That's a good point, and I'm going to think about it."

Also be willing to apologize for your own difficult behavior.

Example: "I'm sorry I snapped at you. I didn't act with love." Too many relationships disintegrate because no one will give ground. Let go of the need to protect your turf. Look at the larger picture—which is more important, this battle or the relationship?

• **Use a pleasant, neutral tone.** No matter how carefully you choose your words, they will get you nowhere if your voice has an edge of irritation, condescension or sarcasm. Practice a neutral tone by role-playing with a friend until you are able to keep the edge out of your voice.

Three Difficult Types

Here's how to deal with three common types of difficult people...

The Guilt Tripper: Blamers and martyrs activate your insecurity to get what they want. Their sentences often start with, "If it weren't for you..." or "I'm the only one..." *What to do...*

• **Be compassionate with yourself.** When you feel bad about any area of your life, work on being compassionate with yourself. By understanding your own guilt triggers, you will be better able to keep your balance when someone tries to activate them.

• **Make a matter-of-fact statement.** Tell guilt trippers that those comments hurt your feelings and that you would be grateful if they would stop making them. If you don't get emotional, most guilt trippers will lose interest in baiting you.

The Control Freak: Control freaks micromanage, give unsolicited advice, voice strong opinions relentlessly and are rarely satisfied. *What to do...*

• **Let go of needing the controller to see things your way.** Don't try to control a controller or win over the person to your way of thinking—it's a waste of time. Say, "Thank you for your input. I'll take it into consideration" or "I value your advice, but I want to work through this myself."

When NOT to Communicate

Don't have a heart-to-heart with your spouse on an empty stomach, we hear from Brad Bushman, PhD. It's better to do so after you've eaten, a recent study advises.

Details: For three weeks, 107 couples were asked to check their blood sugar before bed and then note their level of anger toward their spouses for that same day.

Outcome: Spouses of both genders were found to be more hostile on evenings when their blood sugar was lowest.

Brad Bushman, PhD, professor of communication and psychology, The Ohio State University, Columbus.

• **Be patient.** Control freaks don't give up easily, so repetition is key. Continue to be calm and pleasant even when you have to repeat the aforementioned statements many times.

The Anger Addict: Rage-aholics intimidate by accusing, yelling or cursing. *What to do…*

• **Let go of the impulse to cower or to lash out in return.** The more impulsively you react to someone else's rage, the more you reinforce the anger addict's aggressive behavior. Even if you are upset, stay as neutral as you can. Get centered before you respond.

• **Use imagery.** Picture a martial artist who finds a balanced, grounded stance and then transforms the opponent's energy by flowing with the person's movements instead of resisting them. Imagine that the person's anger can flow right through you and that you are breathing the anger out with every breath.

If the anger addict is your boss, acknowledge the person's point of view. Say, "I can see why you would feel that way." Then bring the discussion back to a solution focus. Say in a calm tone, "I have a different take that I'd like to share" or "That's fine—tell me what you need, and I'll do it."

Look for another job if you can, because being the recipient of chronic anger takes a physical and mental toll. In the meantime— or if changing jobs is not possible—remind

yourself that the rage is about the other person, not you.

If the anger addict is a spouse or family member, set limits. Say, "Your anger is hurting me. We have to find a better way to communicate" or "I care about you, but I shut down when you raise your voice. Let's talk about this when we can hear each other better." Later, when you are both calm, request a small, doable change.

Example of a small, doable change: "When we are in the midst of a disagreement, I propose that we each wait five seconds before saying anything. Would you be willing to try that?"

If the person doesn't try to change, observe how your health is affected. You may need to let go of the relationship to protect your well-being.

Play Those Uplifting Tunes

Listening to gospel and other religious music boosts mental health among older Christians in the US, a recent study shows. Benefits include improved self-esteem and life satisfaction and reduced anxiety about death.

The Gerontologist.

Anger Addiction: How to Break Free

Robert Thurman, PhD, Jey Tsong Khapa Professor of Indo-Tibetan Buddhist Studies, department of religion, Columbia University. He is the author or co-author of numerous books, including (with Sharon Salzberg) *Love Your Enemies: How to Break the Anger Habit & Be a Whole Lot Happier. BobThurman.com*

A rude salesperson treats you like dung…or a conniving coworker steals your idea…or your self-absorbed sister ruins yet another gathering…and your blood begins to boil. Your indignation mounts

(How dare they?), and soon a rush of anger is sweeping over you. Maybe you hold your tongue, and maybe you don't. But either way, your adrenaline is pumping and your heart is pounding…your emotions are running hot… and you experience a powerful sense of self-righteousness that's almost intoxicating.

That's right—your anger, in its own way, feels good.

If this sounds familiar, you may have an addiction problem—an addiction to anger. And like any addiction, this one can wreak havoc with your relationships, health and happiness.

How do you break free…so that anger no longer consumes you?

The Art of Letting Go of Anger

While no one can do the work for you, here are some suggestions that will help you address your anger addiction—and the benefits are well worth the effort involved.

Admit that your anger hurts you more than it hurts the person you're mad at. You are the one who's exploding so unattractively, damaging your own reputation…or getting stuck stewing inwardly, all your brainpower wasted on rehashing old or minor infractions. You can't concentrate, can't relax, can't sleep. Meanwhile, the source of your ire may be

feeling equally angry with you…or he may be carrying on just fine, largely untroubled by your emotional turmoil. Either way, you gain nothing. Admit it!

Acknowledge anger's power to destroy you. You may think of anger as a helpful emotion that alerts you to a situation that needs changing. Anger is seductive. It presents itself to your mind as your own helpful energy. Anger seduces you with the thought, *This is outrageous! I should explode with fury, and my fiery energy will burn away the obstacle.* But that's not what actually happens—as with other addictions, the anger rush is followed by an inevitable crash as you realize that your words or actions did not help you (or anyone).

When you're inflamed with rage, your good sense goes out the window and you are no longer the master of your thoughts, words and actions. This kind of anger destroys all in its path, not least your own emotional balance.

For instance, if you've merely indulged in an internal rant, you may be left feeling depleted and depressed, realizing that nothing has changed. If you've exploded in front of others, you may be filled with regret for the things you said or did. And the consequences can be severe. Anger not only can interfere with professional success and ruin relationships, it also has been linked to heart disease, diabetes, cancer and premature death.

Pay attention to your body's anger cues. You may think that anger surges up without warning, and that this is why you have so little control over it. But that's simply not true. Anger doesn't suddenly appear out of nowhere and explode—it arises more gradually than you may realize. The seeds of anger can be found in frustration, but many people were never taught how to catch frustration early and handle it productively before it has a chance to grow into rage.

Analyze your level of control over the situation. Exactly how you deal with the mounting frustration depends on whether you can influence the actual outcome…or whether the only aspect you can control is your own reaction to your circumstances.

Let's go back to that rude salesperson, conniving coworker or self-absorbed sister we talked about earlier. Instead of getting mad, consider what other options you might have that could improve your situation. Maybe you want to simply take your business to a different store or write a calm, carefully considered memo to your boss. Maybe you want to practice treating your sister with what I call loving-kindness, a spirit of boundless friendship. She may be so gratified when you express interest and empathy instead of irritation that she acts in a less obnoxious fashion! Think about your real goals and how to achieve them, rather than just spewing your anger all over.

Now suppose the situation is completely beyond your control—for instance, if you're stuck in traffic, so there isn't actually any particular person who is the object of your anger. In this sort of situation, what is best for you is to accept that getting angry won't help and could even lead you to do something stupid (and lead to a traffic ticket or car crash). Indulging in a road-rage tantrum only feeds your anger addiction without altering the fact that you are still stuck in traffic. In this kind of situation, defuse your anger by thinking up ways to use the time productively (here's a chance to listen to music you normally don't have much time to enjoy)…or by counting your blessings (the traffic jam could be the result of an accident, and you are not the person who's now in an ambulance). When you hone your ability to control yourself, you will no longer be a pawn to your anger addiction.

What It Means If You Talk to Yourself…

Linda Sapadin, PhD, psychologist in private practice in Valley Stream, New York, and the author of *How to Beat Procrastination in the Digital Age. Psych Wisdom.com*

N o need to worry! For the overwhelming majority of people, there is nothing wrong with talking to yourself. It

not only may relieve loneliness, it also may help you clarify your thoughts and firm up your decisions. There's only one proviso: You must speak respectfully to yourself. Cut out any negative self-talk, such as "You idiot! You should have known better!"

For productive self-dialogue: Give yourself compliments ("I'm so proud of you!") when you accomplish even a small thing like turning down a rich dessert. Motivate yourself in a kind way with language like, "Hey, guy, you've got time to organize your desk. How about it?"

For enhanced decision-making: Running through the pros and cons of a big decision out loud can help you clarify your choices and figure out what decision is best.

For goal-setting: Articulating your goal by saying it out loud focuses your attention, reinforces the message, controls any runaway emotions and screens out distractions.

Whether you're living alone or with others, you're always living with yourself. So converse, chatter and communicate respectfully with yourself. It can be a sign of good health!

In only rare cases, when you're unaware of what you're doing or talking incoherently, is talking to yourself an indication of a mental disorder.

Gentle Ways to Get Better Sleep

Jamison Starbuck, ND, naturopathic physician in family practice and a guest lecturer at the University of Montana, both in Missoula. She is past president of the American Association of Naturopathic Physicians and a contributing editor to *The Alternative Advisor: The Complete Guide to Natural Therapies and Alternative Treatments.*

W hen you're really wrestling with insomnia, it's tempting to go to your doctor and ask for one of the sleep medications we see advertised on TV—Ambien or Lunesta—or an older tranquilizing drug such as Valium. While short-term use of one of these drugs might make sense for a person who feels his/her overall health is being threatened by insomnia, I generally advise against this approach. Sure, these drugs may temporarily allow you to sleep, but they don't cure insomnia. *My advice…*

•**Do some detective work.** Thinking about your own sleep issues and making some written notes can be a big help. When do you typically go to bed? How often do you have insomnia? Do you have trouble falling asleep or wake in the middle of the night? Also, look at when your problem started to determine whether it coincided with any health issues, use of new medications or habits, such as working late hours, that could lead to insomnia.

•**Get your doctor involved.** Discuss your notes with your doctor. Chronic pain, hormonal changes (including those related to hyperthyroidism and menopause) and serious illness, such as cancer and heart or lung disease, can cause insomnia. If any of these conditions is to blame, getting proper treatment may well take care of the insomnia, too.

After you've consulted your doctor, try these gentle methods…*

•**Avoid high-protein dinners.** Protein is often hard to digest. Eating a lot at dinner can lead to gastrointestinal distress that may result in insomnia. Instead, eat foods that are easy to digest (such as soup and salad) for dinner, and have larger, protein-rich meals midday.

Also helpful: Take a 2,000-mg omega-3 supplement with your evening meal. When taken before bedtime, these healthful fats can have a calming effect on the brain, promoting sleep.

•**Try Calms Forté.** This homeopathic preparation is effective and extremely safe.

Typical dose: One tablet under the tongue at bedtime and whenever you wake up in the middle of the night (up to six tablets per 24-

hour period). Calms Forté, made by Hylands, is available at natural groceries and pharmacies.

•**Add skullcap.** If the steps above don't give you relief, you may want to also try this potent herb to relax the "busy brain" experience that often keeps people awake. I recommend using skullcap in tincture form—30 to 60 drops (one-sixteenth to one-eighth teaspoon) in a cup of chamomile or spearmint tea at bedtime.

Note: Skullcap can make some people too sleepy. If you are sensitive to medication, try just 10 drops of skullcap at bedtime—or simply drink chamomile or mint tea as a sedative.

•**Use melatonin with care.** If you'd rather try this popular sleep aid, do so thoughtfully. Melatonin is a hormone. Taking too much can trigger irritability. Melatonin supplements may also raise women's estrogen levels, increasing overall inflammation in the body. I recommend taking no more than 3 mg of melatonin in a 24-hour period and often start my patients on a daily dose of only 1 mg. Take melatonin 30 minutes before bedtime.

See the next page for an acupressure trick that will bring on a good night's sleep. Sweet dreams!

Better Sleep Remedy

Not sleeping well? Try lavender. When a bottle of lavender oil was left open within three feet of the bedsides of adults who were hospitalized, they slept significantly better and had lower overnight blood pressure.

Why: The soothing scent of lavender calms the nervous system.

To improve anyone's sleep: Use lavender oil in an aromatherapy diffuser at bedtime, or put a few drops on a cotton ball, and tuck it into your pillowcase.

Karen Davis, PhD, director of medical nursing, The Johns Hopkins Hospital, Baltimore.

*Check with your doctor before trying supplements, especially if you take medication and/or have a chronic medical condition.

Sleep Yourself Skinny

People with the most consistent bedtimes and wake-up times had less body fat than those with the most erratic sleep habits. Sleep habits were considered consistent if bedtime and wake-up time varied by one hour or less.

Best amount of time to sleep: Six-and-a-half to eight-and-a-half hours a night.

Study of 330 students by researchers at Brigham Young University, Provo, Utah, published in *American Journal of Health Promotion*.

PTSD: A Hidden Danger After a Serious Illness

Robert London, MD, practicing physician/psychiatrist for more than three decades, is on the professorial staff of NYU School of Medicine in New York City. Dr. London also developed the short-term psychotherapy unit at the NYU Langone Medical Center and ran this program for 20 years. *DrRobertLondon.com*

If you've been successfully treated for a serious illness, you're likely to feel so much relief at having dodged a bullet that you may downplay or dismiss the emotional trauma following your medical care.

An overlooked problem: Survivors of a traumatic medical situation—for example, a stay in the intensive care unit (ICU) or treatment for a heart attack or cancer—are at increased risk for post-traumatic stress disorder (PTSD).

Surprising fact: PTSD can strike weeks—or even years—after an illness. Symptoms may include nightmares, flashbacks, irritability and feeling detached (depersonalization) and emotionally numb. Ignoring PTSD after a serious medical situation carries its own risks. Without treatment, symptoms worsen, impacting the sufferer's social, family and work relationships.

Pill-Free Cure for Insomnia

Just before bed, try this acupressure trick. With your thumbs, press the soles of your feet where the heel and the arch meet. Lie on your back (on a carpeted floor is best), and bend your knees, using your right hand on your right foot and left hand on your left. Press as hard as you can for at least two minutes. You should feel the tension leaving your body.

Joan Wilen and Lydia Wilen are authors of *Bottom Line's Treasury of Home Remedies & Natural Cures*. Subscribe to their free e-letter, Household Magic Daily Tips, *MyBottomLine.com*.

How to Fight PTSD

Anyone who suffers PTSD after a serious illness—or wants to help prevent it—can benefit from one or more of the following...*

• **Cognitive behavioral therapy** typically involves weekly visits with a therapist for several months during which sufferers learn to reprocess the traumatic events by gaining a new perspective on the past trauma and improving skills to cope with the distressing thoughts that arise from it.

• **Prolonged exposure therapy** involves the patient revisiting the specific trauma in a safe environment through guided imagery until it's no longer distressing.

To find a psychologist or psychiatrist trained in these therapies, consult the Association for Behavioral and Cognitive Therapies, *ABCT.org*.

• **Hypnosis** helps people reprocess traumatic memories first by using relaxation strategies and then a series of visual images to slowly reintroduce the trauma. This is usually coupled with pleasant visualizations that reduce the anxiety of the traumatic memory. Patients generally require four to 16 sessions. To find a qualified hypnotherapist

*These therapies are generally covered by health insurance. Check with your insurer.

near you, consult the American Society of Clinical Hypnosis, *ASCH.net.*

Other therapies to consider...

• **EMDR.** With eye movement desensitization and reprocessing (EMDR), the therapist asks the patient to perform certain eye movements, such as following the therapist's finger from side to side, while the patient talks about the trauma. The exercise is then repeated, this time focusing on positive memories to help the brain reprocess the trauma so that the emotional distress is decreased. EMDR usually requires four to 12 sessions and has been approved as a PTSD treatment by the US Department of Defense. To find an EMDR-trained practitioner, consult the EMDR International Association, *EMDRIA.org.*

• **Medications.** Antidepressants known as selective serotonin reuptake inhibitors (SSRIs), which work by raising the level of the mood-boosting chemical serotonin in the brain, have been shown to help with PTSD, especially if depression is present. *Sertraline* (Zoloft) and *paroxetine* (Paxil) are two SSRIs that have been approved by the FDA specifically for PTSD.

• **Support groups.** Most PTSD sufferers find it helpful to join a support group of other people who have had similar experiences. Family members may also find comfort from support groups aimed at those caring for someone with PTSD. To find a support group near you, check the psychology/psychiatry department at your local hospital.

Specific Steps That Help

In addition to the steps above, the following strategies help prevent or treat PTSD in patients after...

• **An ICU stay.** Even though most ICU patients receive lifesaving care, ICUs are high-intensity settings with constant noise and bright lights, which can further traumatize an already vulnerable, perhaps disoriented patient. One-quarter of those admitted to a hospital ICU have symptoms of PTSD after their stays.

To prevent PTSD in ICU patients: Unlike most PTSD survivors, who have flashbacks about actual events, ICU patients often suffer flashbacks about delusions or hallucinations that occurred during their stays—a relatively common problem among these patients.

What helps...

ICU diaries, in which nurses and family members record what's happening daily while the patient is hospitalized, are one way to reduce the risk for PTSD. After discharge, the patients are given the diary to review with a nurse or family member whenever the patient feels anxious. This process helps establish what actually occurred during the patient's stay rather than focusing on the frightening details of their misperceptions.

Music therapy, which relaxes and distracts seriously ill patients during the hospital stay, helps reduce the likelihood of lasting psychological trauma. If permitted, a patient could listen to favorite music through headphones.

• **Heart attack.** Around 12% of heart attack sufferers develop PTSD, and those who do are more likely to experience a second heart attack. Some heart attack survivors may go into a state of anxiety or panic whenever they feel shortness of breath, fearing that another heart attack is on the way. This often creates a vicious circle of symptoms and worry.

To prevent heart-related PTSD: Heart patients should seek counseling to learn calming strategies such as relaxation techniques. Heart patients who have a lot of support from their families and friends—especially so that the patient can ask for help when needed—are also less likely to develop PTSD. Having this type of readily available assistance appears to reduce the feelings of vulnerability and helplessness, which so often occur in heart attack survivors.

• **Cancer.** PTSD can follow treatment for any type of cancer. As with other conditions, the more intense or frightening the situation, the higher the chance for PTSD.

To prevent cancer-related PTSD: For some patients, learning all the specifics of their disease from their doctors can help reduce anxiety, while others prefer to know as little as possible. In either case, talk to your doctor about your risk for recurrence and steps you can take to monitor for any early signs that the cancer may be returning.

As with other serious illnesses, family support is crucial in helping cancer patients readjust psychologically after treatment.

PTSD and Food Addiction

Post-traumatic stress is linked to food addiction. Women with the largest number of symptoms of post-traumatic stress disorder (PTSD) are almost three times as likely to develop addictions to food as women without the symptoms. PTSD symptoms include flashbacks, nightmares, difficulty relaxing and extreme anxiety. Mental health–care professionals who are aware that PTSD and food addiction may occur together can better tailor treatment to patients.

Study of 49,408 women by researchers at University of Minnesota, Minneapolis, published in *JAMA Psychiatry.*

Loneliness Harms Your Health

Gregory T. Eells, PhD, associate director of Gannett Health Services and director of Counseling and Psychological Services at Cornell University in Ithaca, New York. Dr. Eells is also a past president of the Association for University and College Counseling Center Directors.

Oh, those long, lonesome days...and nights! Most of us occasionally feel that way. But what if you are lonely more often than not? Plenty of people are.

Why loneliness deserves our attention: While loneliness has long been known to exact a psychological toll, studies are increasingly showing that persistent loneliness also has a profound effect on one's physical health.

Important new finding: Persistent loneliness is being linked to a growing list of health problems, including insomnia, cardiovascular disease and Alzheimer's disease. Even more startling is the fact that loneliness raises the risk for premature death among adults age 50 and older by 14%.

So for the sake of your health—and happiness—here's what you need to know about loneliness...

Are You Lonely?

While it's easy to assume that anyone who is struggling with loneliness would know that he/she is lonely, that's often not the case. For many people, that extreme sense of social disconnection—the feeling that no one really knows you and what your life is like—is so familiar and constant that they don't even realize that they're lonely. And friends and family might not necessarily recognize that a friend or loved one is lonely.

Of course, most of us do need some time by ourselves, and solitude—the opportunity to think and feel quietly without the distraction and demands of other people-—is rightly valued. But loneliness is very different.

Here are some red flags that you may be lonely: You spend hours of alone time on the computer (perhaps surfing the Internet or following the activities of "friends" on social media sites)...you have pangs of anger or envy when others around you are happy...

Internet Can Prevent Depression

The Internet prevents depression in older people. After controlling for various factors, researchers found that people over age 50 who used the Internet were one-third less likely to be depressed than nonusers. The reduced rate of depression was greatest among those who lived alone, leading researchers to believe that Internet use counters feelings of loneliness and isolation.

University of California, Berkeley Wellness Letter. *BerkeleyWellness.com* and/or you feel a vague sense of dissatisfaction even when you are spending time with other people.

Note that a romantic relationship is not a surefire defense against loneliness. Feeling uncomfortably alone and alienated is a frequent complaint of troubled couples.

Why It's Bad for You

The connection between loneliness and depression has been established for quite some time. People who have depression often withdraw from social situations and have feelings of loneliness. But only recently have researchers discovered that loneliness itself is linked to elevated blood pressure, increased stress hormones and impaired immune function.

A recent study has also found that the more lonely that people reported themselves to be, the more fragmented—and less restful—was their average night's sleep.

Loneliness also exacts a huge toll when people turn to unhealthy behaviors to avoid the pain it brings—if we don't try to drink it away, for example, then we might spend far too many hours at work to busy ourselves rather than face painful time alone.

How to Overcome Loneliness

Alleviating loneliness is like falling asleep or growing a garden—you can't force it to happen, but you can create conditions that encourage it to unfold. *Here's how…*

Secret #1: Share more about yourself. Sharing the details of your life with others and showing vulnerability will foster deep connections and minimize loneliness. This may feel risky. After all, you might run up against rejection or disapproval, but such fears are usually groundless. Nothing ventured, nothing gained!

Example: You might ask a friend to have coffee and share with him/her discipline problems you are having with your teenage daughter.

Secret #2: Make room for "small" connections. While quantity doesn't replace quality in relationships, momentary contacts do

To Stop Worrying…

Tone down extremes by writing your worries down and rewording them—instead of "Nobody likes me," you might write, "My boss does not like my report." Think of worries as trains posted on the departure board at a station—they all are there, but you need not board any of them, and as they depart, you can let them go. Set aside 20 "worry minutes" a day, and refuse to think about troubling matters at any other time—when your thoughts do drift toward something that causes anxiety, write the concern down and come back to it at the scheduled time. Make monotony your friend by slowly repeating worrying notions to yourself—expressing a negative to yourself over and over should soon make your mind wander to more enjoyable thoughts.
Psychology Today.

add to your sense of being part of the social world around you.

Exchange a few extra words with the clerk at your local convenience store, and smile at those you pass on the street. These pleasant interactions will prime you for deeper, more meaningful ones with close friends and family.

Secret #3: Be part of something big. Meaningful activity will bring you in contact with like-minded others. OK, so maybe volunteering at a soup kitchen isn't your thing. Perhaps you would rather get involved with your local political party or get involved at your house of worship.

Your local newspaper and websites such as *Meetup.com* and *Groups.Yahoo.com* are great resources for finding local groups involved in a wide variety of activities that might interest you.

Show up for whatever new activity you choose for several weeks, and if you're not feeling more connected by the end of that time, then look for something else that might be more to your liking.

Secret #4: Don't hole up by yourself when your life changes. For most people, significant changes such as job loss, the death of a loved one, divorce or retirement provide a good excuse to shut out others—and the perfect setup for loneliness. But don't let the natural tendency to withdraw at such times go on for more than a few months.

Challenge yourself to set up two outings a week with a friend, neighbor or family member to get yourself out of the house.

Secret #5: Consider getting a pet. Pets are more than mere company…dogs, cats, birds and even guinea pigs are, after all, fellow creatures that have their own feelings and are often responsive to ours. These are real connections, too.

If you don't have the time to care for a pet full time, consider sharing a pet. There are several sites (*CityDogShare.org* or *Pets ToShare.com*) that enable you to meet people near you who are interested in doing this. Or volunteer at your local animal shelter.

Both of these activities are great ways to connect with animals and animal lovers.

New Treatment for Bipolar Depression

There's a new treatment for bipolar depression—the antipsychotic drug *lurasidone* (Latuda). Bipolar depression is difficult to treat, so this new treatment offers another valuable option. Latuda can be used on its own for patients who respond well to it. Other patients may have only a partial response, in which case Latuda can be combined with medications such as lithium or valproate. Latuda is well-tolerated by most people who take it. However, some patients develop side effects such as restlessness, nausea, drowsiness, muscle twitching and slowed movements.

Robert Rowney, DO, psychiatrist in the department of psychology and psychiatry at the Cleveland Clinic.

Try Therapy First

Social anxiety is better treated with therapy than with medication.

Recent finding: Cognitive behavioral therapy can be used to help people work through their fear and avoidance of social situations, and its effects last longer after treatment than medications. Social anxiety affects up to 13% of Americans and Europeans.

Study of 13,164 people by researchers in the department of epidemiology at Johns Hopkins Bloomberg School of Public Health, Baltimore, published in *The Lancet Psychiatry.*

Being the Boss Tied to Depression Risk for Women, but Not Men

Tetyana Pudrovska, PhD, assistant professor, department of sociology, University of Texas at Austin. American Sociological Association, news release.

Being the boss at work seems to raise the odds for symptoms of depression among women, but not men, a new study finds.

Study Findings

The research included more than 1,500 middle-aged women and 1,300 middle-aged men who graduated from high schools in Wisconsin.

"Women with job authority—the ability to hire, fire, and influence pay—have significantly more symptoms of depression than women without this power," said lead author Tetyana Pudrovska, PhD, an assistant professor in the department of sociology at the University of Texas at Austin. "In contrast, men with job authority have fewer symptoms of depression than men without such power," she added.

"What's striking is that women with job authority in our study are advantaged in terms of most characteristics that are strong predictors of positive mental health," Dr. Pudrovska said.

"These women have more education, higher incomes, more prestigious occupations and higher levels of job satisfaction and autonomy than women without job authority. Yet, they have worse mental health than lower-status women," she continued.

Findings from the study appear in the *Journal of Health and Social Behavior.*

Possible Explanation For Gender Differences

"Years of social science research suggests that women in authority positions deal with interpersonal tension, negative social interactions, negative stereotypes, prejudice, social isolation, as well as resistance from subordinates, colleagues and superiors," Dr. Pudrovska explained.

"Women in authority positions are viewed as lacking the assertiveness and confidence of strong leaders. But when these women display such characteristics, they are judged negatively for being unfeminine. This contributes to chronic stress," Dr. Pudrovska said.

On the other hand, male bosses generally have less stress because they don't face the same resistance or negative stereotypes, she suggested.

"Men in positions of authority are consistent with the expected status beliefs, and male leadership is accepted as normative and legitimate. This increases men's power and effectiveness as leaders and diminishes interpersonal conflict," Dr. Pudrovska said.

Implication

The study findings show the "need to address gender discrimination, hostility and prejudice against women leaders to reduce the psychological costs and increase the psychological rewards of higher-status jobs for women," she concluded.

To learn more about women and depression, go to The U.S. National Institute of Mental Health Web site, *www.nimh.nih.gov,* and search "depression in women."

APPENDICES

Appendix I
FOOD AND FITNESS FOR ULTIMATE HEALTH

The Eat-What-You-Want Diet

Some people fast to "rest" the digestive tract, while others do so as part of a religious tradition. The last time you fasted may have been before a medical test, such as a colonoscopy.

But as a weight-loss technique, fasting has always been controversial. Its detractors claim that it shifts the body into a starvation mode that makes unwanted pounds even harder to drop.

What's gaining favor: More and more scientists are now studying fasting as a method for losing extra pounds and fighting disease. But does it work?

As one of the few scientists worldwide who has studied fasting in humans, I consider it to be the most effective—and healthful—method for most people to lose weight.* *How it works...*

*Check with your doctor before trying this diet—especially if you have diabetes. Fasting is not recommended for pregnant women.

The Simple Formula

With intermittent fasting, you eat a reduced number of calories every other day. Scientifically, this is called alternate-day modified fasting.

The principle is simple: Most people find it easier to stay on a diet in which they can eat whatever they want half of the time. In the eight clinical studies I have conducted involving about 600 people (including an ongoing three-year study funded by the National Institutes of Health), intermittent fasters typically have lost 1.5 to 3 pounds per week, depending on how much weight they had to lose.

People lose weight by eating just 500 calories one day ("fast day") and all they want and anything they want the next day ("feast day")—alternating fast days with feast days until their weight-loss goal is reached. Goal weight is maintained by increasing calories on fast days to 1,000 three days a week and enjoying feast days the rest of the time.

Why It Works

Key points about using this method to lose weight...

•**Why 500 calories?** Animal studies showed that consuming 25% of the normal calorie intake on fast days produced the best results in preventing and reversing disease.

Krista Varady, PhD, associate professor of kinesiology and nutrition at the University of Illinois at Chicago. She is also coauthor of *The Every-Other-Day Diet.*

Translating this finding to people, I calculated 25% of daily recommended calories, which resulted in a general recommendation of 500 calories on fast day using foods with optimal nutrients.

Those 500 calories are consumed with one 400-calorie meal and a 100-calorie snack, since people tend to overeat if calories are broken up throughout the day. Lunch or dinner works best for the meal—if you eat your 400-calorie meal for breakfast, you'll be too hungry later in the day.

Example of a lunchtime meal: A turkey and avocado sandwich (two slices of turkey, one slice of Swiss cheese and one-quarter of an avocado on one slice of multigrain bread) and fruit (such as one-half cup of strawberries) for dessert.

Before or after your meal, you can have a snack such as a smoothie.

Tasty option: In a blender, mix one cup of unsweetened chocolate almond milk with one-half cup of unsweetened frozen cherries and one cup of ice.

•**Hunger disappears.** After two weeks of alternate-day modified fasting, hunger on fast day disappears for most people. During those two weeks, ease your fast-day hunger by drinking eight to 10 eight-ounce glasses of water and other no-cal beverages such as coffee and tea and chewing sugar-free gum. Some people reported mild constipation, weakness and irritability, which subsided after two weeks.

•**You won't overeat on feast day.** My studies show that people almost never overeat on feast day—on average, they consume 110% of their normal caloric intake. Over the two-day fast/feast cycle, that's an average of 67.5% of normal caloric intake—a perfect formula for safe, steady weight loss but without the nonstop deprivation of every-day dieting.

•**Add exercise—and lose twice as much weight.** Every-other-day fasters can exercise on fast day without feeling weak or light-headed. Exercising before the fast-day meal is best because you'll feel hungry afterward—and can eat.

Good news: People who go on an intermittent fast and exercise (45 minutes of brisk aerobic exercise, three times a week) lose twice as much weight, on average, as people who only fast. You can exercise on both fast and feast days.

•**You won't lose muscle.** Five out of six conventional dieters who lose weight gain it all back. That's probably because the typical dieter loses 75% fat and 25% muscle—and never regains that calorie-burning muscle mass after the diet is over.

But people who lose weight using alternate-day modified fasting lose only about 1% muscle—a unique and remarkable result. And my one-year maintenance studies show that these alternate-day fasters maintain their weight. Longer-term studies are also needed.

As a Disease Fighter

People who have followed alternate-day modified fasting not only lose weight but also improve their overall health. *In weight-loss studies of 600 people that lasted up to one year, average reductions in risk occurred for…*

•**Heart disease.** Total cholesterol dropped 21%…and LDL "bad" cholesterol dropped 20 points. Triglycerides fell from 125 mg/dL (considered "normal") to 88 mg/dL (defined as "optimal").

•**Type 2 diabetes.** Glucose (blood sugar) levels dropped by up to 10% after eight weeks on the diet.

Animal studies have shown that intermittent fasting may help prevent…

•**Cancer.** The diet may also slow the growth of existing malignancies.

•**Cognitive decline.** Intermittent fasting helped protect the brains of mice genetically programmed to develop Alzheimer's… stopped the early development of nervous system problems in mice programmed to develop Parkinson's…and helped animals recover from stroke.

Weight Loss: Men Versus Women

When it comes to weight loss, men and women are not created equal. Men have an easier time losing weight because they generally have less fat and more muscle, which burns more calories.

If you're a woman struggling to lose weight, be patient. A recent study published in the *British Journal of Nutrition* followed overweight men and women on a particular diet, such as Atkins or Weight Watchers. After two months, men had lost twice as much weight as women, but by six months, both had lost similar amounts.

You can step up weight loss by making sure that strength training to build muscles is part of your exercise program.

Barbara J. Rolls, PhD, chair of nutritional sciences, The Pennsylvania State University, University Park, and coauthor of *The Ultimate Volumetrics Diet*.

3 Diet Pills That Really Work (Safe, Too)

Harry Preuss, MD, CNS, professor in the department of biochemistry, physiology, medicine and pathology at Georgetown University Medical Center, Washington, DC. He is coauthor, with Bill Gottlieb, CHC, of *The Natural Fat-Loss Pharmacy: Drug-Free Remedies to Help You Safely Lose Weight, Shed Fat, Firm Up, and Feel Great*.

Despite what you may have heard, some diet pills can help you drop pounds safely. I've spent much of my career investigating nutritional supplements to aid weight loss. Here are three that I have found to be quite effective. Try one or all three, but always check with your doctor before taking any supplement.

Garcinia Cambogia to Lose 10 More Pounds

I started conducting scientific research on *garcinia cambogia* and its active ingredient

Big Breakfast Best

Eating a big breakfast spurs weight loss. Over a 12-week period, obese women who consumed most of their 1,400 allotted daily calories during breakfast lost an average of 17.8 pounds and three inches from their waists. Women who consumed most of their calories during dinner lost an average of 7.3 pounds and 1.4 inches from their waists. Breakfast eaters also showed better glucose control and decreased triglyceride levels.

Study of 93 obese women by researchers at Tel Aviv University, Wolfson Medical Center, Holong, Israel, and Hebrew University of Jerusalem, published in *Obesity*.

hydroxycitric acid (HCA) in 2003 and wrote about it in my book *The Natural Fat-Loss Pharmacy* in 2007. But this weight-loss supplement didn't really become popular until 2012, when Dr. Oz touted it.

Garcinia cambogia is the botanical name for the Malabar tamarind, a variety of the tamarind fruit. (Tamarind, a delightfully sour spice popular in the cuisine of India, is derived from the dried rind of the fruit.) Scientific analysis of the Malabar tamarind in the 1960s and '70s showed that it is a rich source of HCA—a unique compound that lowers levels of ATP-citrate lyase, an enzyme that helps the body turn carbohydrates into fat. In other words, an extract of garcinia cambogia can help to reduce your body's production of fat.

Since that time, my research and the research of other scientists have confirmed that HCA can help people shed pounds. In one study designed to produce 100% compliance with the protocol, people taking HCA lost 12 pounds over two months, while those taking a placebo lost only three pounds. In a subsequent and similar study, HCA-takers lost 10 pounds, while placebo-takers lost 3.5. *What to look for...*

•**The right form.** HCA comes in two forms—"free" HCA, which is active in the body but tends to be unstable and to exhibit poor absorbability, and a more stable but inactive form, HCA "lactone." Formulating active HCA with certain minerals, such as potassium, magnesium and/or calcium, to create a "salt" makes the compound stable and improves absorption. The better HCA products are mixtures, such as potassium-magnesium or potassium-calcium HCA salts. For effectiveness, you also need a garcinia cambogia extract that is at least 50% HCA, with the maximum level being approximately 70%. This is why, when I have studied HCA, I mostly have used an active, stable form called HCA-SX (Super CitriMax, which includes both potassium and calcium and is 60% HCA). More recently, I studied a potassium-magnesium form of HCA with good outcomes.

Editor's note: The potassium-magnesium HCA salt that Dr. Preuss studied can be found in HCActive from Jarrow Formulas. The HCA-SX potassium-calcium HCA salt that he studied is an ingredient in several garcinia cambogia products, including those from Genesis Today, NutriGold, NutraCentials and Pure Health.

•**The right dose.** Studies show that the best single dose of the products currently on the market is 1,500 milligrams (less might not work).

•**The right time.** Take it three times a day, 30 to 60 minutes before breakfast, lunch and dinner, on an empty stomach. If you take HCA with food, it is poorly absorbed.

•**Realistic expectations.** The scale may not register any weight loss for two weeks or so because accumulation of water and glycogen (the form in which glucose is stored in the tissues) counteracts the fat weight loss.

Caution: People who are diabetic...taking a statin to lower cholesterol...or suffering from dementia should consult with their physician prior to taking this supplement.

Carbohydrate Blockers Cut Carbs with a Pill

If you're a typical American, a significant percentage of your calories are from refined carbohydrates such as sugar and white flour—calories that your body can easily store as fat. Cutting back on refined carbs is the best course of action, but that can be hard for some people because they are addicted to them. (Like other addictive substances, refined carbs stimulate the brain's pleasure centers.) To deal with carb overdosing, I recommend taking a carbohydrate absorption blocker, or carb blocker.

Made from an extract of white kidney beans (*Phaseolus vulgaris*), the supplement works by blocking the action of alpha amylase, a digestive enzyme secreted by the pancreas that breaks down carbs in the small intestine. Research shows that taking a carb blocker can cut carbohydrate absorption by 60% to 70%—in other words, taking a carb blocker and then eating two cups of pasta would be like eating only two-thirds of a cup.

There have been dozens of studies on carb blockers. In a study that I coauthored, dieters taking a carb blocker lost 6.5 pounds over one month, while those taking a placebo lost one pound. Carb blockers mainly work on starchy foods, such as bread, cake, cookies, chips, pasta, rice and potatoes. I personally reserve carb blockers for meals heavy in carbohydrates such as those at Italian restaurants.

Suggested dosage: The typical dose is 1,000 milligrams per meal.

•**Time of intake.** Take it 15 minutes before a high-carbohydrate meal. If you don't like swallowing a large pill, you can open

---

Trick to Lose Weight

To lose weight, get into daylight before noon.

Recent finding: People who spent 20 minutes outdoors in bright light in the morning had a lower body mass index (BMI) than people who got most of their light exposure later in the day.

Study of 54 people by researchers at Northwestern University Feinberg School of Medicine, Chicago, published in *PLoS ONE*. The influence of light on body weight was independent of physical activity level, caloric intake, sleep timing and age.

the capsule and sprinkle the (tasteless) carb blocker on your meal.

●**Best products.** Most of the studies on carb blockers and weight loss have been conducted using Phase 2 carbohydrate inhibitor from Pharmachem. (The FDA has approved this claim for Phase 2: "May assist in weight control when used in conjunction with a sensible diet and exercise program.") Supplements with Phase 2 include: Carb-Intercept with Phase 2 from Natrol…Phase 2 Carb Controller from Swanson…and Phase 2 Starch Neutralizer from Now.

Carb blockers can cause gastrointestinal cramps and gas, but this is rare.

Chromium for Weight Maintenance

When levels of this mineral are low, the hormone insulin does a poor job of moving blood sugar out of the bloodstream. Doctors reasoned that supplying the body with more chromium might burn up more blood sugar so that less is stored as fat. But many study results have been disappointing. In a recent review of 11 studies on chromium and weight loss published in *Obesity Reviews*, dieters who took chromium lost an average of only 1.2 pounds more than placebo-takers. So why am I recommending the nutrient?

Important scientific evidence: In 1999, I published a study in *Diabetes, Obesity and Metabolism* on 20 overweight women who were restricting calories and exercising regularly. For two months, the women took a placebo. In another two-month period, they took 600 micrograms (mcg) of chromium daily. They lost the same amount of weight on the supplement and the placebo. *But…*

When they took the placebo, they lost 92% of their weight as muscle and 8% as fat. When they took chromium, they lost 84% as fat and 16% as muscle. That is a crucial difference.

Pound for pound, muscle burns 60% more calories than fat. When you lose muscle during weight loss, you gain your weight back…as fat! And because you now have a fatter body, you're likely to gain back even more weight

---

Better Lunch Choices

In a survey of nearly 6,000 adults, those who ate at least one sandwich daily got considerably more calories and sodium than those who didn't eat sandwiches.

Why: Typical sandwich ingredients, such as bread, cheese and processed meat, tend to be high in calories and sodium. For adults over age 50, one sandwich had about half of the daily recommended dietary allowance of sodium.

Better options: Sandwiches made with healthier ingredients, such as fresh meat and vegetables, or salad…fruit…or low-sodium tuna.

Rhonda Sebastian, MA, nutritionist, Beltsville Human Nutrition Research Center, Maryland.

---

than you lost. That's exactly what happens to 90% of people who lose weight—they shed the pounds only to gain them back again (and then some). Chromium can help you not only firm your body during weight loss but also stop or at least reduce weight regain.

Suggested dosage: 200 mcg, three times a day, while dieting. After you've reached your weight-loss goal, switch to 200 mcg once a day. I have taken chromium daily for at least 15 years.

Important: It is best to take chromium separately from meals and other supplements, which can interfere with its absorption.

Secret Weight-Loss Weapon

What if there were a food that had an incredible power to help you lose weight or avoid gaining weight? You'd try it, right? Well, a new study shows exactly what that food is. It's beans and other legumes! To see what new benefits these nutrient-packed foods might have, researchers tracked adults who ate a daily serving (three-quarters cup) of beans, lentils, peas or chickpeas.

Result: They felt 31% fuller after meals than those who didn't eat legumes.

If you're trying to lose weight: Add legumes to your daily diet.

Cyril Kendall, PhD, nutrition researcher, University of Toronto, Canada.

Help from Medicare

Medicare offers free weight-loss counseling, but fewer than 1% of Medicare's 50 million beneficiaries use it—even though 30% of seniors are obese and eligible for counseling.

Problem: Many of the most knowledgeable providers, such as weight-loss specialists, are not allowed to participate, because Medicare reimburses only primary-care providers, nurse practitioners and physician assistants working in doctors' offices.

Also: Medicare requires that counseling be given during a separate appointment, not when patients come in for other services. For information, go to *Medicare.gov*.

Roundup of experts on senior obesity and Medicare requirements, reported at *MedPageToday.com*.

4 Super-Healthy Super-Easy Desserts

Emily von Euw, raw-food recipe creator and the author of *Rawsome Vegan Baking*. She lives in Vancouver, British Columbia, Canada. *ThisRawsomeVeganLife.com*

If you're looking for a new dessert that's healthful, the first ingredient you'll want to reduce is added sugar. But to do even better, the best trick is to add at least one superstar nutrient.

For something that's truly delicious and chock-full of amazing health benefits, try one of these four easy-to-make desserts—each with a superstar nutrient that's known for specific health benefits...

Chia Vanilla Pudding

Superstar nutrient: Chia seeds. Yes, these are the same seeds that cause Chia Pets to sprout, and these tiny black seeds are packed with cholesterol-lowering fiber—nearly 10 g per ounce. Chia seeds are also a good source of calcium.

And it gets even better. A Canadian study found that regular consumption of chia seeds helps lower blood sugar levels—an important bonus for people with diabetes.

How to prepare: In a blender, combine ¼ cup each of almonds and dates with ¾ cup of water until the mixture is smooth and creamy like pudding. Stir in 2 tablespoons of chia seeds, 1 teaspoon of vanilla extract, ½ teaspoon of ground cinnamon and ¼ cup of raisins and refrigerate for an hour, allowing the seeds to absorb the liquid. Water makes the seeds soft and gel-like—it will remind you of tapioca pudding. Sprinkle with toppings such as chopped nuts or fresh berries. Makes two to four servings.

Strawberry Sorbet

Superstar nutrient: Strawberries. These vitamin C–rich gems may help fight cancer. In one recent study, they slowed the growth of precancerous esophageal lesions. The fiber in strawberries is also believed to slash colorectal cancer risk.

If you don't like strawberries: Try raspberries—they're also delicious!

How to prepare: Blend 1 cup of frozen strawberries (or raspberries) with 1 tablespoon of maple syrup until it's the consistency of a creamy sorbet. (Add a pinch of cardamom, which promotes digestion, or crushed mint leaves, for an extra taste treat.) Makes one serving.

Coconut Delights

Superstar nutrient: Coconut oil. Long considered taboo due to its saturated fat, coconut oil is now gaining momentum as a healthful food when consumed in moderation, thanks to its high levels of medium-chain triglycerides, easily digested fats that deliver long-lasting energy and are rarely stored as fat.

How to prepare: Measure out 1¼ cups of shredded coconut. Place half the coconut in a food processor, and process until it reaches a chunky consistency (this may take several minutes). Add in the remaining coconut shreds and 1 tablespoon of melted coconut oil. Process this until the ingredients are well mixed. Mold the mixture into the shape of golf balls, flatten and then refrigerate for an hour until firmly set. Next, mix 4 tablespoons each of melted cacao butter and cacao powder with 2 tablespoons of your favorite liquid sweetener such as coconut nectar or maple syrup until smooth. When the balls are firmly set, dip them in the cacao mixture and allow to set again in the fridge for 30 to 60 minutes. Makes six large Coconut Delights.

Jewel Fruit Tart

Superstar nutrient: Almond butter. Similar to peanut butter in its main health benefits, almond butter offers protein for muscle maintenance and is rich in heart-healthy monounsaturated fats. But almond butter outdoes peanut butter as a source of calcium, potassium, iron and magnesium—all necessary for healthy bones.

How to prepare: To make the crust, pulse 2 cups of walnuts in a food processor until they become a rough flour. Add 2 cups of raisins, and process until a dough forms. Press the dough into a tart or pie tin, and refrigerate for two hours. For the filling, blend ½ cup of almond butter and ¼ cup each of melted coconut oil and maple syrup with ½ teaspoon of cinnamon until it's a smooth consistency (add water if needed). Gently spread the filling into the bottom of the chilled crust, and let harden in the fridge for 30 to 60 minutes.

Top off the tart with three to four cups of berries. Makes six to eight servings.

4 Spices That Could Save Your Life

Bill Gottlieb, CHC, editor of *Healing Spices: How to Use 50 Everyday and Exotic Spices to Boost Health and Beat Disease*, founder and president of Good For You Health Coaching, and author of 14 health books that have sold more than 2 million copies. *BillGottliebHealth.com*

Certain spices have been touted as good for our health. For example, cinnamon helps regulate blood sugar...ginger eases indigestion...and garlic can lower high blood pressure.

What most people don't realize: Several other commonly used spices are just as healthful (if not more so). *Here are four "secret" super-spices with healing powers...*

Black Pepper

Black pepper is rich in piperine, the pungent compound that triggers a sneeze when it hits the nerve endings inside your nose. Hundreds of studies show that piperine also triggers healing—energizing and protecting nearly every organ and system in your body. *Two standout benefits...*

• **Cancer.** Cellular and animal research demonstrates that piperine fights cancer. In a test of 55 natural compounds, piperine scored number one in killing triple-negative breast cancer, the most virulent type. In another study, it killed aggressive HER2 breast cancer cells—and even stopped the deadly HER2 gene from activating. Other research shows that piperine can slow, stop or kill prostate, colorectal, lung, cervical, liver and stomach cancers. Piperine also slows angiogenesis, the growth of new blood vessels that feed tumors. It even enhances the effectiveness of radiation and chemotherapy.

• **Arthritis and gout.** Piperine is anti-inflammatory—and studies show that it can stop destructive inflammation in cartilage cells (loss of cartilage is the cause of osteoarthritis) and reduce inflammation associated with gout. It also reverses the symptoms of arthritis in lab animals.

How to use: For the highest level of piperine, buy whole black peppercorns and grind as needed. (Green and white peppercorns are not as rich in piperine, and once the peppercorn is ground, piperine begins to decrease.) Add freshly ground black pepper liberally and often—in cooking and at the table. Try to add freshly ground pepper at the end of cooking because the benefits break down the longer the spice is heated.

Also helpful: Studies show that just smelling black pepper (in the form of black pepper oil) can cut nicotine cravings in smokers and strengthen "postural stability" in older people (thereby helping to prevent falls). Put a drop of oil on a tissue, and inhale for two minutes, two to three times a day. Black pepper oil is available at *Amazon.com* and other online retailers.

Oregano

Two major components of oregano—thymol and carvacrol—have been proven to have healing powers…

• **Heart disease and stroke.** In a study published in *Journal of International Medical Research*, people with high LDL (bad) cholesterol were divided into two groups—one group ingested oregano extract with every meal and one group didn't. Three months later, the oregano group had greater decreases in LDL, lower levels of C-reactive protein (a biomarker of artery-damaging inflammation) and greater increases in arterial blood flow.

In other studies, researchers found that oregano is more powerful than any other spice in stopping the oxidation of LDL—the breakdown of cholesterol by unstable molecules called free radicals that drives the formation of arterial plaque. Oregano also stops the activation of cytokines, components of the immune system that attack oxidized cho-

lesterol, sparking the inflammation that worsens heart disease.

• **Infections.** Oregano is antimicrobial. It can kill the parasite giardia more effectively than tinidazole, a prescription antiparasitic drug. It decimates *Candida albicans*, a yeast that can multiply in the intestinal tract and trigger a range of health problems, such as arthritis and depression. And it can neutralize *Staphylococcus aureus*, a common hospital-acquired infection.

How to use: You can buy oregano fresh or dried. I recommend using the dried form because it concentrates the therapeutic compounds. It often is used in salad dressings, marinades, chili and in Italian and Greek dishes. For optimum benefits, try to use at least one teaspoon of dried oregano daily.

Also helpful: During the winter, consider using oregano oil in supplement form to prevent colds and flu. Follow the directions on the label.

Basil

Basil is a traditional medicine in Ayurveda, the more than 5,000-year-old natural healing system from India, where it's used to treat diabetes, digestive disorders, skin problems and infections. The variety native to India is holy basil, and there are at least 30 more varieties worldwide. All of them contain basil's four main healing components—the antioxidants orientin and vicenin and the volatile oils eugenol and apigenin—that can help regulate blood sugar.

• **Type 2 diabetes.** In one study, people with type 2 diabetes who included more basil in their diets saw an average drop of 21 mg/dL in fasting blood sugar and a 15.8 mg/dL drop in postmeal blood sugar. In a similar, smaller study, three people with type 2 diabetes had remarkable decreases in fasting blood sugar levels when they added basil to their diets three times a day for five weeks—from 250 to 110 mg/dL, from 200 to 80 mg/dL, and from 230 to 90 mg/dL (99.9 mg/dL and lower is normal…100 to 125.9 mg/dL is prediabetes…126 mg/dL and higher is diabetes).

How to use: Dried basil has a larger concentration of the health-giving volatile oils than fresh. I recommend one-quarter to one-half teaspoon daily. Use dried basil in full-flavored sauces. Fresh basil still is rich in health-giving compounds. An easy way to enjoy fresh basil is to toss a handful of leaves into your favorite hot pasta and dress with extra-virgin olive oil.

Sage

The botanical name for sage—*Salvia officinalis*—comes from the Latin *salvare*, meaning "to save" or "to cure." *And sage lives up to its name...*

•**Memory problems.** One hour after people took a supplement of sage oil, they had better memory, more focused attention and more alertness, reported researchers in *Journal of Psychopharmacology.* In another study, people who smelled sage had a stronger memory and were in a better mood.

•**Anxiety.** In a study published in *Neuropsychopharmacology,* people who took a supplement of dried sage leaf were less anxious and felt calmer and more content than when they took a placebo.

Why it works: Sage may block the action of cholinesterase, an enzyme that destroys acetylcholine, a brain chemical that plays a role in memory, attention and alertness. Sage also might improve the functioning of cholinergic receptors on brain cells that receive acetylcholine.

How to use sage: Because of its robust flavor, sage is best used in hearty dishes such as pot roast, meat loaf and stuffing. It also goes well with squash, sweet potatoes and apples.

However: The amounts that improve mental and emotional functioning aren't easy to get with diet, so you may want to take a sage leaf supplement. I often recommend the herbal extract from Herb Pharm because it's made from the whole leaf that has been grown organically. Follow the directions on the label.

Should You Stop Eating Spinach?

Is spinach super nutritious...or does it alter a woman's calcium levels?

Both. Spinach contains oxalic acid, a natural compound in plant foods that interferes with calcium absorption. Oxalic acid is broken down in cooking, so eating steamed or sautéed spinach will keep it from interfering with calcium absorption. Spinach is incredibly nutritious, high in iron, folate and vitamin C, but if you're worried about your calcium, you may want to cut back on eating it raw and cook it instead.

Note: Talk to your doctor if you have gout or kidney stones, since oxalate-rich foods could worsen those conditions.

Janet Bond Brill, PhD, RD, nutrition, health and fitness expert and a fellow of the Academy of Nutrition and Dietetics. DrJanet.com

Got This? Don't Eat That

Michael T. Murray, ND, naturopathic physician and leading authority on natural medicine. Dr. Murray serves on the Board of Regents of Bastyr University in Kenmore, Washington, and has written more than 30 books. DoctorMurray.com

Let's say you've got arthritis...heartburn...heart disease...or some other common health problem.

You follow all your doctor's suggestions, but you still don't feel better. It could be that you're not getting the right medication or other treatment, but there's an even stronger possibility.

What often gets overlooked: Your diet. Far too many people sabotage their treatment—and actually make their health problems worse—by eating the wrong foods. Meanwhile, you could be helping yourself by eating certain foods that ease whatever is ailing you.

Common health problems that foods can worsen—or help...

Arthritis

Both osteoarthritis and rheumatoid arthritis involve inflammation that causes joint pain and/or swelling.

What hurts: Refined carbohydrates (sugar, white bread, white rice and most pasta). They cause a spike in glucose (blood sugar) that leads to inflammation.

What helps: Raw, fresh ginger. It's a potent inhibitor of prostaglandin and thromboxanes, inflammatory compounds involved in arthritis. And unlike anti-inflammatory medications, ginger doesn't cause an upset stomach. Be sure to use fresh ginger—it's better than powdered because it contains higher levels of active ingredients. For pain relief, you need to eat only about 10 g (about a quarter-inch slice) of raw, fresh ginger a day.

Smart idea: You can add raw ginger to any fresh fruit or vegetable juice with the help of a juice extractor. Ginger mixes well with carrot, apple, pear or pineapple juice. You also can grate fresh ginger and add it to any hot tea.

Cardiac Arrhythmias

Everyone notices occasional changes in the way the heart beats at certain times—during exercise, for example. But persistent irregularities could be a sign of arrhythmias, potentially dangerous problems with the heart's electrical system. The heart can skip beats or beat too slowly or too quickly—all of which can signal heart disease.

What hurts: Too much caffeine. Whether it's in coffee, tea or chocolate, caffeine stimulates the heart to beat more quickly, which triggers arrhythmias in some people.

What helps: Berries. All types of berries, including cherries, blackberries, raspberries and blueberries, are rich in procyanidins, plant pigments that reduce arrhythmias and improve blood flow through the coronary arteries. Aim for one cup of fresh berries daily (frozen are fine, too).

Also helpful: Concentrated extracts made from hawthorn. This herb contains the same heart-healthy compounds as berries. In Germany, it is commonly used to treat arrhythmias and congestive heart failure. If you have heart problems, a hawthorn extract containing 10% procyanidins (100 mg to 200 mg three times daily) is often recommended. Hawthorn can interact with heart medications and other drugs, so check with your doctor before trying it.

Heartburn

Also known as gastroesophageal reflux disease (GERD), heartburn is usually caused by the upward surge of digestive juices from the stomach into the esophagus. People who suffer from frequent heartburn can get some relief with lifestyle changes, such as not overeating and staying upright for a few hours after eating. But most people with heartburn don't pay enough attention to their diets.

What hurts: Alcohol and coffee are widely known to trigger heartburn. Many people, however, don't consider the effects of chocolate, fried foods and carbonated drinks, which also may weaken the esophageal sphincter (the muscle that prevents acids from entering

You're Cooking Chicken Wrong!

Forty percent of people undercook chicken.

Best: Always use a meat thermometer—slicing through the meat is not a good guide to whether chicken is properly cooked to 165°F.

Also: Do not wash chicken before cooking it—washing uncooked chicken can spread bacteria around the kitchen.

And: Wash your hands for at least 20 seconds before handling anything else after you touch raw chicken. Use a separate cutting board exclusively for chicken, and clean that board in the dishwasher.

Christine Bruhn, PhD, director, Center for Consumer Research, University of California at Davis.

the esophagus) or increase the intra-abdominal pressure that pushes acids upward.

What helps: Fresh (not bottled) lemon juice—two to four ounces daily in water, tea or apple or carrot juices. Lemon contains D-limonene, an oil-based compound that helps prevent heartburn. Also, use the peel if you can. It's an especially good source of D-limonene.

Eye Disease

Age-related macular degeneration (AMD) is a leading cause of vision loss, but it (as well as cataracts) can often be prevented—or the effects minimized—by eating carefully.

What hurts: Animal fat and processed foods. A study of 261 adults with AMD found that people who ate a lot of these foods were twice as likely to have a worsening of their eye disease compared with those who ate less of the foods. Animal fat also increases risk for high cholesterol, which has been linked to increased risk for cataracts.

What helps: Cold-water fish. The omega-3 fatty acids in fish can help prevent AMD and cataracts—or, if you already have one of these conditions, help prevent it from getting worse. Try to eat three to four weekly servings of cold-water fish, such as salmon or sardines.

Also helpful: Tomatoes, watermelon and other red fruits and vegetables (such as red peppers) that are high in lycopene. Green vegetables are also protective. Foods such as spinach and kale are high in lutein and other plant pigments that concentrate in the retina to help prevent eye disease.

Rosacea

Some 16 million Americans have rosacea, a chronic skin condition that causes bright-red facial flushing for at least 10 minutes per episode, along with bumps and pustules.

What hurts: Hot foods. "Hot" can mean temperature (a hot bowl of soup or a steaming cup of coffee or tea) or spicy (such as chili powder, cayenne or curry). Alcohol also tends to increase flushes.

What helps: If you have rosacea, ask your doctor to test you for *H. pylori*, the bacterium that causes most stomach ulcers and has been linked to rosacea. If you test positive, drink cabbage juice (eight to 12 ounces daily). It's not the tastiest juice, but it inhibits the growth of H. pylori. Make your own cabbage juice in a juicer (add some apples and/or carrots to improve the taste). If you have thyroid problems, check with your doctor—fresh cabbage may interfere with thyroid function.

How to Make Frozen Veggies as Good as Fresh

Linda Gassenheimer, award-winning author of several cookbooks, most recently, *No-Fuss Diabetes Desserts and Simply Smoothies: Fresh, Fast & Diabetes-Friendly Snacks & Complete Meals*. She writes the syndicated newspaper column "Dinner in Minutes." *DinnerInMinutes.com*

A s cold weather approaches, the fresh produce you want can be difficult to find or very expensive. Frozen vegetables can be a scrumptious alternative—and a terrific time-saver. Think of all the time it takes to wash and cut up veggies!

Bonus: Vegetables grown for freezing are picked at their peak and flash-frozen, preserving much of their nutrient value.

Here, delicious recipes that bring out the very best in frozen veggies...

Indian Spiced Carrots

Frozen sliced or crinkle-cut carrots are available in most markets. Adding Indian spices adds zing. Spices lose their flavor and color over time. If yours are more than six months old, it's time for new bottles.

1 Tablespoon canola oil
2 teaspoons ground cumin
2 teaspoons ground coriander
2 teaspoons mild curry powder
1 pound sliced frozen carrots (about 4 cups)

1 Tablespoon grated fresh ginger
½ cup water
½ cup light coconut milk
Salt and freshly ground black pepper, to taste
4 Tablespoons chopped cilantro

Heat oil in a large, nonstick skillet over medium-high heat. Add the cumin, coriander and curry powder. Cook about 30 seconds. Add the carrots, ginger and water. Cover with a lid, and cook five minutes. Remove the lid. If any liquid remains, cook uncovered until it has evaporated.

Remove from the heat. Add the coconut milk and salt and pepper to taste. Sprinkle the chopped cilantro on top. Serves four.

Roasted Baby Brussels Sprouts and Bacon

Look for baby Brussels sprouts. The roasted sprouts will be crisp on the outside and tender inside—and the bacon adds a delectable smoky taste. If you don't like bacon, you can sprinkle a little smoked paprika over them.

1 Tablespoon olive oil
1 pound frozen small Brussels sprouts (about 4 cups)
Salt and freshly ground black pepper
4 bacon slices, diced into ½-inch pieces

Preheat the oven to 400°F. Line a baking sheet with foil. Add the oil, and roll the Brussels sprouts in the oil making sure all sides are covered. Sprinkle with salt and pepper to taste, and toss well. Spread them in one layer on the sheet. Place the diced bacon over the Brussels sprouts. Roast 20 minutes. Remove from oven, and turn sprouts over. Roast another 10 minutes. Serves four.

Thai Green Beans

Look for thin, whole green beans. Toasted sesame oil has a rich sesame flavor, but regular sesame oil can be used.

2 Tablespoons crunchy peanut butter
1 Tablespoon low-sodium soy sauce
2 Tablespoons toasted sesame oil

2 teaspoons grated fresh ginger (optional)
1 pound frozen whole green beans (about 4 ½ cups)
Freshly ground black pepper, to taste
2 Tablespoons peanuts, chopped

Mix the peanut butter, soy sauce, 1 tablespoon of the toasted sesame oil and ginger together. Heat the second tablespoon of toasted sesame oil in a large, nonstick skillet over medium-high heat. Add the green beans. Sauté for five minutes. Add the peanut butter mixture, and stir to combine with the beans. Add black pepper to taste. Sprinkle peanuts on top. Serves four.

Hot Pepper Succotash

Hot pepper jelly adds zip to this American staple gleaned from the Native Americans who grew corn and beans side by side in the fields and cooked them together and called it succotash. Any type of hot pepper jelly can be used.

⅔ cup fat-free, low-sodium chicken broth
2 Tablespoons canola oil
3 cups frozen corn kernels
3 cups frozen baby lima beans
5 Tablespoons jalapeño pepper jelly
3 scallions, thinly sliced
Salt

Warm the broth and oil in a large, nonstick skillet over high heat. Add the corn and lima beans, and sauté for five minutes. Reduce heat to medium-high, and add the jelly. Stir until the jelly melts and coats the vegetables. Add scallions and salt to taste. Serves four.

Creamy Spinach

Frozen chopped onion can be found in most markets. If it is not available, use fresh chopped onion and add it to the spinach while it is defrosting in the microwave.

1 10-ounce package frozen chopped spinach
1 Tablespoon olive oil
1 cup frozen chopped onion
¼ cup light cream
¼ teaspoon ground nutmeg
Salt and freshly ground black pepper

Place the spinach in a microwave-safe bowl, cover and microwave on high for five minutes to defrost. (Or ahead of time, remove the spinach from the package, and place in a bowl in the fridge for 24 hours or on the counter top for several hours.)

Heat the olive oil in a medium-sized skillet over medium-high heat. Add the spinach and onion. Sauté for five minutes. Remove from the heat, and add the cream. Mix well. Add nutmeg and salt and pepper to taste. Stir to combine into the spinach. Makes two large servings or four small servings.

Better Way to Get Protein

Healthy adults whose protein intake was spread evenly throughout the day had 25% higher levels of muscle growth and repair than those who ate most of their daily protein with dinner—a typical eating pattern. The recommended dietary allowance (RDA) for protein is at least 46 g daily for women and 56 g for men. (If you have kidney disease, ask your doctor for advice on protein intake.)

Douglas Paddon-Jones, PhD, professor of nutrition, The University of Texas Medical Branch at Galveston.

The 3 Supplements Everyone Should Take

Alan R. Gaby, MD, contributing medical editor for *Townsend Letter*. He is author of the comprehensive textbook Nutritional Medicine, widely used by natural practitioners as a reference manual. *DoctorGaby.com*

Vitamin supplements have taken a beating lately. And plenty of people who use them to help ensure their good health are now left wondering whether these pills should be dumped in the trash.

But before you do that, there's another side to the vitamin question that you should know—most of the negative findings are mis-

reported and/or the studies are flawed. After decades of research (backed by more than 26,000 medical journal articles and 19 years of clinical practice treating thousands of patients), I am confident that supplements can and often do work. The question is, which supplements?

What Everyone Needs

In an ideal world, we'd get all our nutrients from foods—there's a powerful synergistic effect when vitamins and minerals are found in foods. But the reality is, most people don't get enough of these crucial nutrients. That's why certain individual supplements can help.

Even if you take a standard, over-the-counter multivitamin, such as Centrum or One A Day, you may benefit from the following supplements because most multis don't contain enough of these nutrients.

Exception: If you use a high-potency multivitamin (it has megadoses of nutrients and is usually labeled "high potency"), you're most likely getting enough of the necessary nutrients and probably don't need to add the supplements below. But you may still need these additional supplements if you have any of the health conditions described in this article.

Three Key Supplements

Supplements everyone should consider taking...*

•**B-complex.** The B vitamins—thiamine, riboflavin, niacin and several others—are a must for the body's production of energy. They also play a key role in the health of the brain and nervous system.

But when foods are refined—for example, when kernels of whole wheat are stripped of their outer covering of fibrous bran and inner core of wheat germ and turned into white

*Be sure to check with a nutrition-savvy health practitioner before taking any supplements. To find one near you, consult the American Holistic Medical Association, *HolisticMedicine. org*, or the American Association of Naturopathic Physicians, *Naturopathic.org*.

flour, as commonly occurs in American manufacturing practices—B vitamins are lost.

New scientific evidence: A study of 104 middle-aged and older adults, published this summer, showed that taking three B vitamins (folic acid, B-6 and B-12) lowered levels of the amino acid homocysteine in people with very high levels (such elevations are linked to heart disease) and improved several measurements of mental functioning, such as memory.

Typical dose of B vitamins: Look for a B-complex supplement that contains at least 20 mg of most of the B vitamins, including B-6, thiamine and niacin…and at least 50 micrograms (mcg) each of B-12 and biotin.

• **Magnesium.** Without this mineral, your body couldn't produce energy, build bones, regulate blood sugar or even move a muscle. But most Americans don't get enough of this mineral in their diets.

Magnesium is used by nutritionally oriented clinicians to treat many health problems, including insomnia, chronic muscle pain, headache, heart disease, diabetes, osteoporosis and hearing loss. Overall, magnesium is the most beneficial supplement I have seen in my patients.

Typical dose of magnesium: 200 mg, twice a day. A capsule or a chewable or liquid form is preferable to a tablet, because it is more easily absorbed. But all types of magnesium—including magnesium oxide, magnesium citrate and magnesium aspartate—are equally effective for most conditions. If you develop diarrhea, reduce the dose until diarrhea eases.

• **Vitamin C.** This vitamin is an antioxidant—a nutrient that protects you from oxidation, a kind of inner rust that destroys cells. A low level of oxidation is normal, but it's increased by many factors—such as stress and chronic disease.

Recent finding: A review of 13 studies involving nearly 4,000 people with colorectal adenoma (a benign tumor that can turn into colon cancer) found that people with

---

Pregnancy Danger

Low vitamin D increases risk for dangerous pregnancy disorder. Pregnant women who had blood levels of vitamin D lower than 50 nanomoles per liter had 40% higher risk for severe preeclampsia, a potentially fatal condition characterized by high blood pressure and excess protein in the urine.

If you are pregnant: Talk to your healthcare provider about whether you need to take additional vitamin D.

Study of 3,703 blood samples from pregnant women by researchers at University of Pittsburgh Graduate School of Public Health, published in *Epidemiology*.

---

the highest levels of vitamin C were 22% less likely to develop colon cancer.

Typical dose of Vitamin C: 100 mg to 500 mg daily, for general nutritional support. If you have a family history of colon cancer (for example, in a first-degree relative, such as a parent or sibling), consider taking 1,000 mg, three times daily.

"Add-on" Supplements You May Need…

Certain people may need additional suppprove their health. *Two key "add-on" supplements…*

• **Fish oil.** A large body of scientific research shows that fish oil can help prevent and treat heart disease.

Typical dose: About 1 g daily for people who want to reduce heart disease risk…and 2 g to 6 g daily for people diagnosed with the condition. People with coronary heart disease need 360 mg to 1,080 mg daily of eicosapentaenoic acid (EPA) and 240 mg to 720 mg of docosahexaenoic acid (DHA). Talk to a health practitioner before taking fish oil—it may increase bleeding risk.

• **Vitamin D.** Vitamin D deficiency is common, and it can increase risk for bone loss (osteoporosis), falls in older people (frailty), the flu, autoimmune diseases (such as rheumatoid arthritis, lupus and multiple sclerosis) and even cancer. Ask your doctor for advice on the best dose for you, and use vitamin D-3 (the type derived from sunlight and animal sources).

Juice for Healing Power

Michael T. Murray, ND, naturopathic physician and leading authority on natural medicine. Dr. Murray has written more than 30 books, including the newly revised and updated *The Complete Book of Juicing: Your Delicious Guide to Youthful Vitality.* DoctorMurray.com

Juice has gotten a bad rap. We're often advised to eat whole fruits and vegetables—for the fiber and because they are lower in calories than an "equal" amount of juice. But for the many Americans who don't eat the recommended three to five servings of vegetables and two to three servings of fruit daily, juice can be a lifesaver—literally. Juice is loaded with nutrients that protect against heart disease, cancer, diabetes, arthritis, Alzheimer's and other chronic conditions.

We can pack in a day's worth of fruits and vegetables in just 12 to 16 ounces of juice. *How to do it right…*

• **Opt for fresh juice, not packaged.** Packaged juices, whether in a can, bottle, carton or frozen, are lower in nutrients. And packaged juices have been pasteurized, which destroys health-giving compounds.

Example: Fresh apple juice contains ellagic acid, an anticancer nutrient that shields chromosomes from damage and blocks the tumor-causing action of many pollutants. In contrast, commercial apple juice contains almost no ellagic acid.

• **Use a quality juicer.** If you juice once or twice a week, try a high-speed centrifugal juicer. They're relatively inexpensive, starting at $100 or so. (Examples: Juice Fountain Duo or Juice Fountain Elite, both from Breville.)

If you juice more frequently, consider investing in a "slow juicer" ($300 and up) that typically operates at 80 revolutions per minute (RPM), compared with the 1,000 to 24,000 RPM of a centrifugal model. (I use The Hurom Juicer.) A slow juicer expels significantly more juice and better preserves delicate nutrients. And because the damaged compounds produced by a centrifugal juicer taste a little bitter, a slow juicer provides better-tasting juice.

Follow this basic juice recipe: Use four unpeeled carrots and two unpeeled, cored apples cut into wedges as a base for creating other juice blends by adding such things as a handful of kale, spinach, radishes and/or beets. Ideally, use organic fruits and vegetables. If not, be sure to wash them thoroughly.

• **Keep blood sugar balanced.** Fruit and vegetable juices can deliver too much natural sugar, spiking blood sugar levels, a risk factor for heart disease, diabetes and other chronic conditions.

What you need to know: The metabolic impact of the sugar in a particular food can be measured using the glycemic index (GI)—how quickly a carbohydrate turns into glucose (blood sugar). But a more accurate way to measure this impact is with the glycemic load (GL)—a relatively new calculation that uses the GI but also takes into account the amount of carbohydrate in a specific food. Beets, for example, have a high GI but a low GL—their carbohydrate is digested quickly, but there's not a lot of it. Charts providing the GI and the GL are available on the Internet. I like those at *Mendosa.com.*

Bottom line: Limit the intake of higher-GL juices such as orange, cherry, pineapple and mango. You can use them to add flavor to lower-GL choices such as kale, spinach, celery and beets.

Breakfast Before or After a Workout?

If you feel super hungry during your morning workout before breakfast, here's what to do…

While vigorous exercise after a full meal might cause you to feel nauseated or bloated, you can certainly grab a banana, a handful of trail mix or a granola bar to eat before your walk. Or you can eat part of your breakfast before you walk and enjoy the rest afterward.

Some people think they'll burn more body fat if they avoid eating before working out, but that's not true. You will lose body fat if you use more calories than you consume by the end of the day.

Nancy Clark, RD, sports nutritionist in private practice in Boston, and the author of Nancy Clark's Sports Nutrition Guidebook. NancyClarkRD.com

You Can Exercise Less and Be Just as Healthy

Barry A. Franklin, PhD, director of Preventive Cardiology and Cardiac Rehabilitation at William Beaumont Hospital in Royal Oak, Michigan. He is co-author, with Joseph C. Piscatella, of 109 Things You Can Do to Prevent, Halt & Reverse Heart Disease.

D o you struggle to fit the recommended amount of exercise into your busy schedule?

Well, what if we told you that the amount of exercise needed to reap health benefits might be less than you think? Maybe you could free up some of your workout time for other activities that are important to you and beneficial to your health—like playing with your kids or grandkids, volunteering for a favorite charity or cooking healthful meals.

The Latest in Exercise Research

A recent study published in the *Journal of the American College of Cardiology* found that people lived longest when they ran, on average, for 30 minutes or more, five days a week. Surprisingly, that research also showed that people who jogged at an easy pace for as little as five to 10 minutes a day had virtu-

ally the same survival benefits as those who pushed themselves harder or longer.

Also surprising: A study recently done at Oregon State University found that one- and two-minute bouts of activity that add up to 30 minutes or more per day, such as pacing while talking on the telephone, doing housework or doing sit-ups during TV commercials, may reduce blood pressure and cholesterol and improve health as effectively as a structured exercise program.

How to Exercise Smarter, Not Harder

Here are four strategies to help you exercise more efficiently…

•**Recognize that some exercise is always better than none.** Even though exercise guidelines from the Centers for Disease Control and Prevention (CDC) call for at least 150 minutes of moderate exercise each week, you'll do well even at lower levels.

A Lancet study found that people who walked for just 15 minutes a day had a 14% reduction in death over an average of eight years. Good daily exercises include not only walking but working in the yard, swimming, riding a bike, etc.

If you're among the multitudes of Americans who have been sedentary in recent years, you'll actually gain the most. Simply making the transition from horrible fitness to below average can reduce your overall risk for premature death by 20% to 40%.

•**Go for a run instead of a walk.** The intensity, or associated energy cost, of running is greater than walking. Therefore, running (or walking up a grade or incline) is better for the heart than walking—and it's easier to work into a busy day because you can get equal benefits in less time.

For cardiovascular health, a five-minute run (5.5 mph to 8 mph) is equal to a 15-minute walk (2 mph to 3.5 mph)…and a 25-minute run equals a 105-minute walk.

A 2014 study of runners found that their risk of dying from heart disease was 45% lower than nonrunners over a 15-year follow-up.

In fact, running can add, on average, three extra years to your life.

Caution: If you take running seriously, you still should limit your daily workouts to 60 minutes or less, no more than five days a week. (See below for the dangers of overdoing it.) People with heart symptoms or severely compromised heart function should avoid running. If you have joint problems, check with your doctor.

• **Ease into running.** Don't launch into a running program until you're used to exercise. Make it progressive. Start by walking slowly—say, at about 2 mph. Gradually increase it to 3 mph...then to 3.5 mph, etc. After two or three months, if you are symptom-free during fast walking, you can start to run (slowly at first).

• **Aim for the "upper-middle."** I do not recommend high-intensity workouts for most adults. Strive to exercise at a level you would rate between "fairly light" and "somewhat hard."

How to tell: Check your breathing. It will be slightly labored when you're at a good level of exertion. Nevertheless, you should still be able to carry on a conversation.

Important: Get your doctor's OK before starting vigorous exercise—and don't ignore potential warning symptoms. It's normal to be somewhat winded or to have a little leg discomfort. However, you should never feel dizzy, experience chest pain or have extreme shortness of breath. If you have any of these symptoms, stop exercise immediately, and see your doctor before resuming activity.

Watch out: Many hard-core runners love marathons, triathlons and other competitive events. Be careful. The emotional rush from competition increases levels of epinephrine and other "stress" hormones. These hormones, combined with hard exertion, can transiently increase heart risks.

Of course, this doesn't mean that you shouldn't enjoy a daily run...or a few long ones—just don't overdo it!

Make Exercise Safer and Much More Comfortable

Colin Milner, CEO of the International Council on Active Aging, a Vancouver, British Columbia–based organization dedicated to improving fitness and quality-of-life issues in older adults.

Let's face it. Exercise sometimes hurts. So when we fear that our bodies might rebel, we're tempted to put off exercise or even skip it.

That's a shame because it doesn't make sense to deprive ourselves of exercise—it's hands-down the most powerful health protector there is. So what's the solution?

By choosing the right workout aids, you can dramatically ease the discomfort of key exercise routines. *Here's what works best for...*

Stretching

Who among us isn't just a little—or a lot—stiff and achy at times? Stretching is perhaps the best exercise you can do to loosen up those tight, inflexible muscles. It will help limber you up and improve your range of motion—both of which make it easier to do day-to-day activities such as grabbing groceries off a high shelf.

But if you're not very flexible to begin with, stretching is likely to cause some discomfort.

What helps: Gaiam Multi-Grip Stretch Strap ($12.98, *Gaiam.com*). With multiple handholds along the strap, this product allows you to ease into your stretches with greater control than you could on your own or if you relied on a regular strap without handholds.

Walking

Walking is the easiest, most approachable workout there is. But if you've got pain due to arthritis, back problems or a hip or other joint replacement...or balance problems, even walking can be difficult.

Adding walking poles helps reduce impact on your joints, normalize your gait and improve your balance. The addition of poles also helps to boost your cardio endurance and increase your caloric burn—with poles, your heart rate will be 10% to 15% higher compared with traditional walking, and you'll burn about 400 calories per hour versus 280 calories.

What helps: ACTIVATOR Poles ($99.99 per pair, *UrbanPoling.com*). These aren't just any old walking poles. They feature bell-shaped, rubber tips for added grip and reduced vibration. With a doctor's prescription, this product may be covered by insurance.

Also: For people with peripheral neuropathy, a type of nerve damage that leads to numbness, tingling and/or weakness in the feet and other limbs, it can be tough to rely on walking as a form of exercise.

What helps: WalkJoy ($3,495 per pair, *WalkJoy.com*). This device is attached with straps worn below the knees. Sensors in the device signal healthy nerves around the knees (which are unaffected by peripheral neuropathy), letting your brain know that one foot has hit the ground and it's time to lift the toes of the opposite foot for another step.

WalkJoy is FDA-approved and available by prescription.

Swimming

Swimming is a great low-impact, whole-body exercise for people who are watching their weight, building cardio strength or looking for relief from arthritis pain.

For the average recreational swimmer, however, efficient breathing can be challenging. Many swimmers feel like they're struggling for air...or their necks tire or become painful from constantly twisting and lifting.

What helps: Finis Swimmer's Snorkel ($35.99, *FinisInc.com*). Unlike many snorkels, which are designed for scuba divers, this product was created specifically for swimmers. Its adjustable head bracket lets you wear it with a swim cap and/or goggles while allowing you to keep your head in a fixed position so that you don't have to remove your mouth from the water to breathe.

Cycling

Riding a bicycle is another great low-impact exercise. It has been shown to improve muscle strength and promote lung and heart health. The problem is, traditional bike saddles (on both stationary and road bikes) place a lot of pressure on the perineum (the area between the genitals and the anus). This contributes to pain and erectile dysfunction in men and numbness in women.

What helps: ISM Cruise Saddle ($99.95, *ISMseat.com*). This is a noseless saddle, which directly supports your "sits" bones (at the base of the buttocks) while easing pressure on the perineum. Research has found that no-nose saddles reduce numbness in women.

Simple Solution to Stop The Dangers from Too Much Sitting

Taking a five-minute walk every hour counters the negative effects of sitting at a desk or on a couch for long hours. Extended sitting is bad for blood pressure and cholesterol and contributes to obesity. Researchers believe the increase in muscle activity aids blood flow, which improves arterial function and could even prolong life span.

Study by researchers at Indiana University School of Public Health, Bloomington, published in *Medicine & Science in Sports & Exercise.*

Get in Shape for Free

Charles B. Inlander, consumer advocate and health-care consultant based in Fogelsville, Pennsylvania. He was the founding president of the nonprofit People's Medical Society, a consumer advocacy organization credited with key improvements in the quality of US health care, and is the author or coauthor of more than 20 consumer-health books.

Up until two years ago, my wife and I paid more than $900 in annual membership fees—year after year—

to belong to a gym. Today, we go to the same gym and have a membership to more than 11,000 fitness centers across the country… without paying a dime out of pocket. That's because our Medicare supplemental health insurance carrier offers the SilverSneakers (SilverSneakers.com) fitness program as a bonus. But you don't have to be age 65 or older to access free fitness programs. Hundreds of health insurance companies (plans vary by state) offer similar no-charge fitness center memberships for any of their policyholders or through employer-sponsored plans. *Here's my advice on finding free fitness programs in your area…*

•**Just ask!** In order to get your business, or your employer's, most health insurers now offer fitness memberships and other services that are included in the regular monthly premium price. So call your insurer, or ask your employer, to find out if your insurer offers free fitness center memberships or other fitness options.

Insider tip: If you have a medical condition, such as diabetes, Parkinson's disease or arthritis, your insurer or employer may offer, or provide access to, free fitness programs aimed specifically at your condition. Ask when you call.

•**Look locally.** You may be surprised to learn that there are many free exercise and fitness programs right around the corner from you. Most community senior centers offer free classes. If you belong to your local YMCA/YWCA, Jewish Community Center or similar organization, there are usually several fitness classes offered at no extra charge. Many community swimming pools, both indoor and outdoor, now offer free lap sessions for any resident or through what is now known as "Silver Splash" programs for older adults.

Insider tip: Don't forget about your community hospital. In many areas, hospitals now offer free fitness programs and fitness lectures focused on specific health-related topics, such as cancer recovery/prevention and cardiac rehab.

•**Get creative.** Of course, you can also set up your own fitness program at little or no cost. Walking is probably the easiest, most beneficial form of exercise to do economically. You can organize a walking group with friends or neighbors and use some great smartphone applications to create a fun exercise program that will keep you engaged.

What I use: Runtastic (available for iPhones and Android models) automatically logs in your miles, calories burned and more (check your phone's app store for fitness, walking, running or personal-trainer apps). Since many apps are free, you can try them out with little risk. There are also some excellent websites to help you set up a home workout program or walking regimen.

One of my favorites: Boston's Beth Israel Deaconess Medical Center has a comprehensive, consumer-friendly website to help you set up your own walking program (*BIDMC. org/walking*).

CoolSculpting: The Shortcut to the Perfect Body

Neil S. Sadick, MD, clinical professor of dermatology at Weill Cornell Medical College in New York City and a cosmetic dermatologist in private practice at Sadick Dermatology. *SadickDermatology.com*

You've struggled through endless sit-ups, strained through strength training, sweated through spinning, and your diet regimen is impeccable. But your love handles and fat rolls persist. If you are committed to a healthy lifestyle, but frustration with lingering fat is tempting you toward liposuction or plastic surgery, chill out. There's a much safer and noninvasive way to eliminate those annoying stomach- and back-fat bulges—with lasting results and minimal risks. Forget plastic surgery for what a gym workout won't fix. This body-sculpting technique may be the key to claiming the trimmer figure you've been striving for.

Get That Sleek Physique

Demand for cosmetic-enhancement procedures has increased by 250% in the past two decades, but as people increasingly aspire to look Mah-velous, they are also becoming savvier. Instead of risky cosmetic surgery, folks are increasingly opting for nonsurgical body-sculpting techniques, according to Neil S. Sadick, MD, clinical professor of dermatology at Weill Cornell Medical College in New York City.

Among the few nonsurgical body-sculpting techniques available, cryolipolysis, a technique that freezes fat away, has been around the longest—five years—and so more is known about its effectiveness and safety than other, newer techniques, such those that use ultrasound or radiofrequency waves to melt away fat. Cryolipolysis is also a rapid procedure—taking one to two hour-long sessions—and side effects are minimal. Plus, a small survey of cosmetic dermatologists and their patients, recently conducted by a team of researchers from the University of British Columbia and University of Southern California's Keck School of Medicine, showed that the procedure not only dissolves fat and has some effect on cellulite, but also tightens and improves skin texture.

Skin texture and tightness were rated as moderately to significantly improved in 93% of patients who had work done on their abdomens, arms and back. For patients who had work done on their thighs, skin texture was rated as moderately-to-significantly improved in 73%. And 82% of patients reported a moderate to significant improvement in skin tightening. But cryolipolysis's effect on cellulite was so-so—55% of patients and 36% of dermatologists said they noticed a moderate-to-significant improvement.

Just Cool It

Cryolipolysis targets fat cells (adipocytes), which are more sensitive to cooling than other cells of the skin and nearby tissue. Get adipocytes cold enough, and they will ultimately be destroyed. The procedure, which is FDA-approved and marketed as Cool-Sculpting, involves placing cooling panels on the area to be worked on, said Dr. Sadick. Suction pulls the area into a well between the cooling panels and freezes the fat in its grip without damaging the skin or surrounding tissue. After being frozen, the fat cells crystallize, break down and pass into the bloodstream and are eliminated just like other body waste.

The technique takes one to two hours, depending on the area being worked on. No anesthesia, needles or pain medication is needed, although some people feel pulling, tugging or tingling and, rarely, cramping during the procedure. No prep or recovery restrictions are required either. Redness of the skin can last for a few minutes to a few hours immediately after the procedure. Common side effects–such as bruising and numbness of the area—usually disappear within two weeks.

But, although you can resume normal activities immediately after the procedure, don't expect to see the slimmer, trimmer you the minute you run home to gaze in a mirror. It takes about four weeks for the fat to begin to wear away…and six months until complete results are seen.

Although most patients need only one session to achieve the desired results, some may need two or occasionally three. Most patients are happy with the results and come back for a touch up about four to six months after the procedure, Dr. Sadick said. And so long as you maintain a healthy diet and exercise program, studies so far show that results are permanent, said Dr. Sadick.

Is It for You?

Cryolipolysis is meant for body contouring and not major weight reduction or bulk fat removal. It is commonly used on the abdomen, love handles, lower back and buttocks, and thighs and arms—and newer applicators, CoolSmooth and CoolFit, are designed to specifically treat the inner and outer thighs. The best candidates are people who are near or at their ideal weight, exercise regularly, eat a healthy diet and are willing to do their part to maintain the results of cryolipolysis with smart lifestyle choices, said Dr. Sadick.

For those interested in exploring this fat-reduction option, the best place to find a cosmetic dermatologist in your area who specializes in cryolipolysis is through the American Society for Dermatologic Surgery. The average cost for a cryolipolysis procedure is $1,500. Remember, since it is considered a cosmetic procedure, it mostly likely won't be covered by your medical insurance plan.

The Quick, Powerful Workout You're Probably Not Getting

Wayne L. Westcott, PhD, professor of exercise science at Quincy College in Quincy, Massachusetts, and a strength-training consultant for the American Council on Exercise and the American Senior Fitness Association. He is also coauthor of several books, including Strength Training Past 50.

Until recently, fitness gurus have advised people to "take the stairs" mainly as a substitute for do-nothing elevator rides.

Now: Stair-climbing is becoming increasingly popular as a workout that's readily accessible (stairs are everywhere)...often climate-controlled (indoor stairs)...and free.

It burns more calories than walking...strengthens every muscle in the legs...and is good for your bones as well as your cardiovascular system. It may even extend your life span.

Compelling research: A study found that participants who averaged eight flights of stairs a day had a death rate over a 16-year period that was about one-third lower than those who didn't exercise—and more than 20% lower than that of people who merely walked.

A Concentrated Climb

Walking is mainly a horizontal movement, with an assist from forward momentum. Stair-climbing is a vertical exercise. Your body weight is lifted straight up, against gravity. Climbing stairs also involves more muscles—in the calves, buttocks and the fronts and backs of the thighs—than walking. Even the arms get a workout. Canadian researchers found that it required double the exertion of walking on level ground—and 50% more than walking up an incline.

As a weight-loss tool, stair-climbing is hard to beat. An hour of climbing (for a 160-pound person) will burn about 650 calories. That compares with 400 calories an hour for a 15-minute-mile "power walk"...and 204 calories for a leisurely stroll.

It's Easy to Start

Inconvenience is one of the biggest barriers to exercise. It sometimes feels like a hassle to change into workout clothes and drive to a health club...or even exercise at home. But you can always find a set of stairs—in your neighborhood, at work, at the mall or at home.

You don't need fancy workout gear to climb stairs (uncarpeted stairs are preferred). Because it doesn't involve side-to-side movements, you don't necessarily need to invest in specialized shoes. You can do it in any pair of athletic shoes or even work shoes, as long as they don't have high heels.

How to Climb

When getting started, begin with a single flight of stairs. When that feels easy, take additional flights or increase the intensity by going a little faster. Work up to five minutes, then slowly increase that to 10, 15 and 20 minutes, if possible, three times a week. *Other tips...*

• **Keep your upper body straight.** There's a natural tendency to lean forward when you climb stairs, particularly because a forward-leaning position feels easier. Remind yourself to stand straight when you're climbing and descending. It will give your legs a better workout...strengthen your abdominal and other core muscles...and help improve your balance.

• **Swing your arms.** You don't need an exaggerated swing, but keep your arms moving—it helps with balance and provides exercise for your arms and shoulders. You'll often see stair-climbers with their hands or arms on the rails. It's OK to use the rails if you need the support, but it reduces the intensity of the exercise. It also causes the stooped posture that you want to avoid.

• **One step at a time.** Unless you're a competitive stair-climber, you'll probably do best by taking just one step at a time. Ascending stairs is a concentric exercise that increases muscle power...it's also the part of the workout that gives most of the cardiovascular benefit.

Coming down the stairs is an eccentric (also called "negative") movement that puts more stress on the muscles and increases strength.

Important: Descend the stairs slowly, and keep "jolts" to a minimum. It sounds counter-intuitive, but the descents cause more muscle soreness than the climbs.

You can take two steps at a time on the ascent—if your balance is good and you're bored with single-step plodding. The faster pace will increase the intensity of your workout, particularly when you give your arms a more exaggerated swing. To minimize jolts and maximize safety, however, stick to single steps on the descent.

To End Your Workout

The "Figure 4" stretch is a great way to conclude a stair-climbing workout. It stretches the calves, hamstrings, gluteals, low back and upper back.

What to do: While sitting on the floor with your right leg straight, bend your left leg so that your left foot touches your right thigh. Slowly 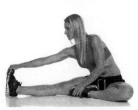 reach your right hand toward your right foot. Then grasp your foot, ankle or lower leg, and hold for 20 seconds. Repeat on the other side.

Caution: Stair-climbing should be avoided if you have serious arthritis or other joint problems. It's less jarring than jogging, but it's still a weight-bearing exercise that can stress the joints. People with joint issues might do better with supported exercises, such as cycling, rowing or swimming.

Before taking up stair-climbing as a form of exercise, check with your doctor if you're middle-aged or older, have arthritis, a history of heart or lung disease or if you've been mainly sedentary and aren't confident of your muscle strength—or your sense of balance.

Stair-Stepping Without a Staircase

If you want to climb stairs without using a staircase, consider buying a commercial "stepper," such as those from StairMaster. Some have components that work the arms as well as the legs. Stair-steppers, however, don't provide the benefit of actual stair-climbing, which uses more muscles because of the descents. These machines can be costly (at least $2,500 for a new one but much less for a used one on Craigslist or eBay). They typically hold up for years of hard use.

Caution: I don't recommend "mini-steppers" that sell for as little as $60. They have hydraulics, bands or other systems that cause the steps to go up and down, but the equipment usually breaks quickly.

When to Lift Weights

Don't lift weights before cardio exercise. People who did upper-body exercises before cycling had a 35% decline in endurance.

Possible reason: Working the shoulders, arms, chest and back may also tire the legs as lactate and other fatigue-related substances move through the bloodstream.

Study by researchers at Nottingham Trent University, Nottingham, England, published in *Medicine & Science in Sports & Exercise.*

The One-Minute Workout Miracle

Jonathan Little, PhD, exercise physiologist and assistant professor in the School of Health and Exercise Sciences at University of British Columbia-Okanagan, Kelowna.

Even if you enjoy aerobic workouts, you probably wish that they took less time. *Good news:* New research shows that you can get all of the metabolic and cardiovascular benefits of aerobic exercise in about 60 minutes a week.

The secret is high-intensity interval training (HIIT) where you exercise intensely for one minute and leisurely for another minute, working up to a total of 20 minutes three times a week. *How it works...*

New Thinking

For years, the American College of Sports Medicine has advised Americans to walk, bike or get other forms of moderate-intensity aerobic exercise for at least 30 minutes, five days a week. That's two-and-a-half hours—minimum.

HIIT can be a refreshing change. You do the same activities (walking, biking, stairclimbing, etc.), but you do them hard—ideally at 80% to 90% of your estimated maximal heart rate. On a 1-to-10 scale, you'll rate the exertion between 7 and 8 (compared with about 5 for conventional aerobic workouts).

Here's the good part. After just 30 to 60 seconds of pushing yourself, you take a break. During the recovery phase, you keep moving, but at a leisurely pace—a slow walk, slow pedaling on the bike, etc. You rest for the same length of time that you exercised—between 30 and 60 seconds. Then you push yourself again. Each on-off cycle is one interval.

Exercise scientists used to think that HIIT was helpful mainly for athletes or very fit adults who wanted to take their fitness to an even higher level. But new studies suggest that this technique can be equally effective—and, in most cases, equally safe—for just about everyone who is in reasonably good health.

Important Benefits

For our recent study, we recruited 41 "regular" people who typically engaged in aerobic activities only two or fewer times a week. After they completed preliminary tests and questionnaires, they completed a single workout that involved HIIT (one minute on, one minute off, for a total of 20 minutes), conventional high-intensity aerobic exercise (20 minutes)...or conventional moderate-intensity aerobic exercise (40 minutes). Each participant did all three workouts, in a randomized order, separated by about one week.

At the end of the study, 24 of the participants said that they preferred HIIT, compared with just 13 who preferred conventional, moderate-intensity aerobic workouts. The remaining four people preferred the conventional high-intensity aerobic workout.

This is an important finding because people who enjoy exercise are more likely to keep doing it. Just as important, the study showed that nonathletes are able to do HIIT. Mixing the high-intensity "challenges" with frequent rest breaks boosted their confidence.

Other benefits...

•**Higher metabolism.** You actually burn fewer calories during an HIIT session than you would during a standard aerobic workout. But HIIT elevates your basal metabolic rate for up to 24 hours after the workout. You burn more calories post-exercise than you normally would.

Researchers at McMaster University in Hamilton, Canada, studied participants who followed a 20-week program of conventional aerobics and others who followed a 15-week HIIT program. The first group burned 48% more calories per session than the HIIT group, but the HIIT group burned 900% more fat over the 15 weeks than the first group burned in 20 weeks.

•**Cardiovascular health.** A number of studies have looked at the effects of HIIT in patients with heart disease. They found that participants had better outcomes—improved blood lipids, less insulin resistance, more elastic blood vessels, etc.—than those who did traditional workouts.

•**Improved fitness.** The body's ability to use oxygen is among the best measures of cardiovascular health and longevity. People who do these workouts have improved peak oxygen uptake after as little as two weeks.

Important warning: There's some evidence that the resting component makes HIIT safer than traditional aerobic workouts for people with heart disease or other chronic conditions. But any form of vigorous exercise can be risky for those with health problems. Get the OK from your doctor before trying it.

A Typical Workout

To do an HIIT workout, you first need to pick your activity. It could be walking, biking, swimming, jogging, stair-climbing or any other form of aerobic exercise. *After that...*

•**Warm up.** Take three to five minutes just to get ready—with slow walking, easy pedaling, etc.

•**Do a "speed" session.** If you're new to HIIT, I recommend limiting your initial speed sessions to 30 seconds each. You can increase the time each time you work out. Your goal will be 60 seconds.

As discussed above, you want an exertion level that you would rate as a 7 or 8 out of 10. If you're not sure if you're pushing hard enough, use the talk test—you should have just enough wind to blurt out a short word or two. If you can speak an entire sentence, increase the exertion.

•**Now take a break.** The recovery phase will last just as long as the exertion phase. If you exercised for 30 seconds, rest for 30 seconds. As noted above, "rest" doesn't mean doing nothing. You'll keep doing the activity, but at an easy pace—say, between 15% and 20% of your maximum ability (1 or 2 on a 0-to-10 scale).

•**Immediately start the next interval.** After resting, repeat the speed part of the exercise. Do it for 30 seconds...recover for 30 seconds...and so on.

•**Increase the intervals.** I advise people who are new to HIIT to complete a total of four intervals. If that feels like too much, you can do just one or two, increasing the number when you feel ready. In our studies with nonathletes, we started with four intervals during the first session. We added one interval during each subsequent session until they reached a total of 10. We found that most people adjusted quickly.

•**Three times a week.** Because these workouts are more intense than a conventional, moderate-intensity workout, you don't want to do them every day. Your muscles need time to recover. Every other day is optimal.

•**Be flexible.** The typical HIIT workout involves a 1:1 ratio—one minute of exertion followed by one minute of rest. But there's nothing magical about this ratio. For someone who has been sedentary for a long time, I might recommend a 30-to-60-second exertion phase followed by a two-minute or even a four-minute break. In general, the more intensely you exercise, the more rest you'll need. Your body will tell you what you need.

Cooldown Myth

A postworkout cooldown is usually not necessary. Cooldowns have long been advocated as a way to prevent muscle soreness.

But: A study found that exercisers who did a formal cooldown after a strenuous workout had the same amount or more muscle pain the next day as people who did not do a cooldown. The one benefit of a cooldown is that it prevents blood from pooling in the lower body and possibly causing dizziness, but to get that benefit, all that is needed is a few minutes of walking.

The New York Times.

Appendix 2
MEDICAL MISCONCEPTIONS THAT HARM YOUR HEALTH

Do You Really Need a Hysterectomy?

Daniel M. Morgan, MD, associate professor, department of obstetrics and gynecology, University of Michigan Medical School, Ann Arbor. His study appeared in the *American Journal of Obstetrics and Gynecology.*

One of every three women will have an operation to remove her uterus before she turns 60 years old. Something is wrong with that statistic. Shedding a uterus should not be a rite of passage, like sporting silver hair or joining AARP. Doctors may tell you that the operation is no biggie, but removing a body part is always a big deal. Hysterectomies involve anesthesia, often an abdominal incision and, like all surgery, the risk that something will go wrong.

If you've been told that hysterectomy is the best option to clear up a uterine problem such as endometriosis (a painful condition whereby uterine tissue grows outside of the uterus), fibroids (noncancerous growths) or abnormal bleeding—or if you know someone who was advised to have a hysterectomy—hold on. Although there are times when having a hysterectomy is the right move, such as when cancer is a threat, some procedures are unnecessary, according to researchers from University of Michigan. In fact, a lot of women are getting hysterectomies for no good reason at all. What's more, alternative treatments to hysterectomy don't look like they are being tried as often as they should be.

Hold On to Your Uterus

The University of Michigan team looked through the medical records of 52 Michigan hospitals to evaluate how many of the hysterectomies done in the first 10 months of 2013 were actually appropriate. After weeding out women who had medically valid reasons for heading straight to surgery, such as those with cancer or a life-threatening hemorrhage, the researchers ended up with a study population of about 3,400 women. For each of these, the researchers looked for documentation that other medical treatments had been either tried or at least recommended before the woman's hysterectomy. These other treatments included drug or hormone therapy, endometrial ablation (therapeutic removal of cells that line the uterus) and various other uterus-sparing surgical procedures.

The results: About two-thirds of the women considered or tried at least one other treatment before having a hysterectomy, but most still had hysterectomies done for conditions for which uterus-sparing procedures were available. Most alarming is that nearly one in every five women had her uterus surgically removed for no clear reason. This was particularly seen among the younger women—the rate of needless hysterectomies was 38% in women younger than 40 compared with 8% in women older than 50.

Why would a woman have a hysterectomy for seemingly no medically valid reason? The researchers only went by what they could find in the patients' medical records and did not interview any of the patients or their physicians. Their educated guess is that many of the younger women were having hysterectomies to correct abnormal bleeding caused by ovulatory dysfunction. But ovulatory dysfunction is usually a hormonal problem and should be first treated with hormones or other medicines—not a scalpel—according to the American Congress of Obstetricians and Gynecologists. So if young women really are getting hysterectomies to solve bleeding problems, many of the doctors recommending and performing the procedures may be out of line. (But another study will to be done to investigate if this is really so.)

Know Your Options

Before agreeing to a hysterectomy, make sure it is the best and most appropriate treatment for what ails you. Make sure that the doctor fully explains your diagnosis, how the problem can be treated, and the risks and benefits of each and every treatment option. Then, with your doctor, make a list of options to try in order of preference so if the most preferred doesn't work, another option or two can be tried before resorting to a hysterectomy.

Is Your Medication Dose Wrong for You?

Heather Whitley, PharmD, associate professor in the Auburn University Harrison School of Pharmacy in Auburn, Alabama. She is also associate affiliate professor at The Institute for Rural Health Research at the University of Alabama, Tuscaloosa, and the lead author of *"Sex-Based Differences in Drug Activity,"* which appeared in the journal *American Family Physician*.

I f you are a man and take a sleeping pill in the middle of the night, you may fall asleep quickly and wake up feeling refreshed. If you're a woman and take the same pill, you may fall asleep just as fast but find that you are slogging through the morning with a drug-powered hangover.

Just a fluke? Absolutely not.

An under-recognized problem: While scientists have long suspected that men and women don't respond in the same ways to certain drugs, a growing body of research shows that these differences are more significant than previously thought.

Why this matters: You may be taking a drug—or be prescribed one in the future—in a dose that's not right for you...or in a class that is not the most effective for your condition. *What you need to know...*

How Gender Slipped Under the Radar

Since 1992, when the sedative *zolpidem* (Ambien) was first introduced in the US, the recommended maximum dose for men and women has been the same—10 mg.

A startling finding: Recently, evidence came to light that women who took the same dose of zolpidem as men had blood levels that were 45% higher. The "standard" dose, in other words, was essentially an overdose for women.

Meanwhile, zolpidem has also been implicated in cases of so-called "sleep driving," in which people who have taken the drug drive their cars while not fully awake.

Now the FDA has stepped in and cut the recommended dose of zolpidem for women in half, to 5 mg. The daily dose for the extended-release version is up to 12.5 mg for men and 6.25 mg for women.

But it's not just sleeping pills that affect men and women differently. Entire classes of medications—such as beta-blockers, opioid painkillers and heart medications—have sex-specific effects.

Why haven't we heard more about this?

Until the early 1990s, women of childbearing age were excluded from most drug-based research. The majority of drugs were tested only in men. Based on these results, doctors assumed that any research that cleared a medication as being safe and effective for men would also apply to women—but they didn't really know.

Today, medications are routinely tested in roughly equal numbers of men and women—but there are still hundreds, maybe thousands, of drugs on the market whose outcomes have never been analyzed based on gender. What's more, data do not always separate outcomes based on age, ethnicity and other factors. So the recommended dose may not be the optimal amount for certain people.

Which Drugs Are Suspect?

You'd expect that a small woman would require a lower dose of medication than a large man. But size is only one difference.

Because women have a higher percentage of body fat, on average, drugs that are lipophilic—that is, accumulate in fatty tissue—cause longer-lasting effects in women than in men.

315

On top of that, women tend to metabolize (break down) some medications more slowly than men, so women can be more likely to accumulate higher-than-expected concentrations of those drugs in their bodies.

A woman's digestive process is also generally slower than a man's, which means that women may have to wait for a longer time after meals in order to take some medications "on an empty stomach."

Trust your gut: If you start taking a new medication and your instincts tell you that something's wrong, pay attention. You may need a different drug or dose.

The research on sex-based drug effects is still in the early stages. There are probably hundreds, if not thousands, of drugs that affect men and women differently.

Among the drugs that women should use with caution...

Sedatives

Benzodiazepine sedatives, such as *diazepam* (Valium), accumulate in fat and have longer-lasting effects in women. Women may find themselves feeling drowsy the next day...less alert than usual...and having slower reaction times. (Zolpidem, the medication discussed earlier, has similar effects.)

My advice: If you are a woman taking one of these medications for anxiety, back spasms or any other condition, ask your physician, "Could I take a lower dose because I'm a woman?"

Blood Pressure Drugs

Beta-blockers, such as *metoprolol* (Lopressor), *atenolol* (Tenormin) and *propranolol* (Inderal), have stronger effects on women. For example, women who take them tend to have a greater drop in blood pressure and heart rate than men, particularly during exercise.

My advice: All patients should be started on the lowest possible dose, then gradually adjusted (titrated) every few weeks until the desired effects are achieved.

Let your doctor know if you're experiencing dizziness, fatigue or other symptoms—this could signal that you're taking a dose that's too high for you.

Calcium channel blockers, including *amlodipine* (Norvasc) and *felodipine* (Plendil), are among the most commonly used drugs for high blood pressure. One potential side effect of these drugs is edema (fluid accumulation in the body)—and women tend to experience more of this edema than men.

My advice: Rather than taking a diuretic to manage edema, women (and men) who have this side effect might do better without a calcium channel blocker at all.

They can frequently switch to an ACE inhibitor such as *lisinopril* (Zestril), which also provides blood pressure–lowering effects—and does not cause edema. Alternatively, adding an ACE inhibitor to the calcium channel blocker can reverse edema.

Painkillers

Opiate analgesics, such as morphine, *oxycodone* (OxyContin) and *hydromorphone* (Dilaudid), have a greater analgesic effect in women.

In fact, women usually get pain relief from a 30% to 40% lower dose than that required for men. Women who do not take the lower dose are also more likely than men to experience side effects, including unwanted sedation.

My advice: Tell your doctor that you want the lowest effective dose. It can always be increased if you need more relief.

Heart Medication

Low-dose aspirin is routinely recommended to prevent heart attacks and/or strokes. This benefit has been shown to occur in both men and women who have already had a heart attack or stroke but is less clear-cut in those who have not. Clinical studies have found that low-dose aspirin helps prevent stroke in healthy women ages 55 to 79 and heart attack in healthy men ages 45 to 79. Preventive low-dose aspirin may be especially beneficial for men and women with cardiovascular risk factors, such as high blood pressure, high cholesterol, diabetes, family history or smoking.

My advice: Men and women should discuss with their doctors whether they need low-dose (81-mg) aspirin to prevent a heart attack or stroke, especially since even small doses of aspirin increase the risk for gastric bleeding. Unlike some other drugs in which side effects are amplified for women, low-dose aspirin is less likely to cause gastric bleeding in women than in men.

Medical Tests That Can Cause More Harm Than Good

Reid B. Blackwelder, MD, FAAFP, president of the American Academy of Family Physicians. He is also a practicing family physician in Johnson City, Tennessee, and professor of family medicine at Quillen College of Medicine at East Tennessee State University, also in Johnson City.

Are you getting cookie-cutter medical care? Too many people are—and one glaring example of this is the number of tests and procedures that are being prescribed regardless of the individual's specific health situation.

In fact, there's more and more evidence that many of the tests that are given so routinely are causing more harm than good.

Here are some popular tests that are often not necessary...*

CT Scans For Low-Back Pain

If your low back is giving you fits, your doctor may order an X-ray or even a more detailed test such as a CT scan to see what's going on.

Problem: Americans are receiving doses of radiation from X-rays and CT scans (not

*The tests in this article are evaluated at *ChoosingWisely.org*, a Web site that advises patients and doctors on a wide range of tests and procedures. Developed by more than 50 medical specialty societies, such as the American Academy of Family Physicians and the American College of Surgeons, the information is based on the most current scientific evidence. Remember to check with your doctor for advice that's tailored to your specific needs.

to mention spending enormous amounts of money) to diagnose a problem that will likely go away on its own in a few weeks. In some cases, an incidental finding that's not even related to the pain leads to unnecessary back surgery.

New thinking...

• **Unless you are experiencing worsening nerve damage** (such as loss of bladder or bowel control or loss of sensation or muscle power in your legs) or have cancer (which could possibly spread to the back), you probably don't need an imaging test within the first six weeks of your back pain.

Also: There is no medical or legal reason to get X-rays as a "baseline" for work-related back injuries.

Bone-Density Tests

For years, physicians have been routinely recommending bone-density tests using dual-energy X-ray absorptiometry (DXA). The test estimates the amount of bone in the hip and spine, which is a marker for osteoporosis. Until recently, women have often been advised to have a "baseline" DXA screening at menopause...then periodically after that.

Problem: Being labeled with "preosteoporosis" (commonly known as osteopenia) can start you on a medical journey of repeated DXA testing and use of medications that may be harmful. For example, osteoporosis drugs known as *bisphosphonates—risedronate* (Actonel), *ibandronate* (Boniva) and *alendronate* (Fosamax)—have been shown, in rare cases, to cause an unusual fracture of the thigh bone when one of these medications is taken for longer than five years.

And evidence shows that this test is not always a reliable predictor of fractures even in high-risk patients who are already receiving drug therapy for osteoporosis.

New thinking...

• **Unless you are a woman age 65 or older or a man age 70 or older**—or you have a special risk factor for osteoporosis, such as family history, smoking or alcohol abuse or use of corticosteroid drugs—you probably don't need DXA screening.

•**If your DXA test results show that you have normal bone mass,** you don't need to be tested again for up to 10 years, provided you don't break a bone or show other signs of osteoporosis, such as losing more than an inch in height.

Carotid Artery Imaging

Your carotid arteries carry blood from your heart through the neck to your brain. If those arteries become narrowed from a buildup of plaque (a condition known as carotid artery stenosis, or CAS), your blood flow is slowed and your risk for stroke increases. Doctors can use ultrasound, magnetic resonance angiography (MRA) or computed tomography angiography (CTA) scans to check for plaque in these arteries.

Problem: If testing does show a blockage, you may be advised to take medication that won't necessarily improve your life expectancy. You may even be urged to undergo surgery (endarterectomy) to clear the artery. However, this is a difficult and complex operation that in rare cases leads to stroke, heart attack or even death.

New thinking…

•**Unless you are experiencing symptoms, such as stroke,** transient ischemic attack (a so-called "mini-stroke") or unexplained dizziness, you probably do not need to be screened for CAS. Evidence shows that the harms of screening (and subsequent treatment) in people without symptoms usually outweigh the benefits.

If you do undergo screening for CAS, surgery is generally not recommended unless you have more than 70% blockage in one or both of your carotid arteries and you have had a stroke or ministroke in the previous six months.

EKG and Stress Test

During your routine physical, your doctor may have ordered an electrocardiogram (EKG or ECG) to measure your heart's electrical activity and/or a cardiac stress test to check the same functions but under condi-tions where you are "stressed" via exercise or medication.

Problem: Unnecessary stress testing can lead to false-positive tests—indicating that something is wrong when you are actually healthy. This can mean more follow-up tests, including CT scans or coronary angiography, both of which expose you to radiation. And in rare cases, an angiography actually leads to a heart attack in people who have the test. Sometimes, after a "bad" EKG or stress test, a doctor may also prescribe unnecessary heart medication.

New thinking…

•**If you don't have any heart-related symptoms (such as chest pain or short-ness of breath),** the evidence shows that an annual EKG or other cardiac screening is unlikely to prevent a heart attack, catch a hidden heart problem or otherwise make you any healthier than you already are.

•**If you are getting noncardiac thoracic surgery (for example, on the lungs, esoph-agus or other organs in the chest),** you do not need to have stress testing before the operation unless you have a history of heart problems. In healthy patients, testing rarely changes how they are treated, so it's gener-ally not necessary.

Are You Getting the Most from Your Blood Tests? Even Doctors May Miss Signs of Health Problems

James B. LaValle, RPh, CCN, clinical pharmacist, nutritionist and founder of LaValle Metabolic Institute, an integrated-care practice in Cincinnati. He is the author of *Your Blood Never Lies: How to Read a Blood Test for a Longer, Healthier Life. JimLaValle.com*

Unless your doctor tells you there's a problem, you may not give much thought to the blood tests that you receive periodically.

But standard blood tests and certain other blood tests that you may request from your doctor can offer valuable—even lifesaving—clues about your health, including explanations for such vexing conditions as short-term memory loss and fatigue.

What you may not realize: If your doctor says that your test results are "normal," this is not the same as "optimal" or even "good."

For example, a total cholesterol reading of 200 mg/dL is considered normal, even though the risk of developing heart disease is sometimes higher at this level than it would be if your numbers were lower. Always ask your doctor what your target should be.

Blood test results that you should definitely make note of—and certain tests you may want to request...*

• **Low potassium.** Low potassium (hypokalemia) is worrisome because it can cause fatigue, constipation and general weakness, along with heart palpitations.

Causes: An imbalance of the hormone insulin often causes low potassium. It also can be due to problems with the adrenal glands or a loss of fluids from vomiting and/or diarrhea. A magnesium deficiency or a high-sodium diet can lead to low potassium, too. It is also a common side effect of certain medications, including diuretics, such as hydrochlorothiazide...laxatives...and some asthma drugs, such as albuterol.

Normal potassium: 3.6 mEq/L to 5.2 mEq/L.

Optimal potassium: 4.5 mEq/L to 5.2 mEq/L.

What to do: If your potassium is not optimal, your doctor will probably recommend that you eat more potassium-rich foods, such as fruits (bananas, oranges, cantaloupe)...vegetables (tomatoes, sweet potatoes)...and whole grains (quinoa, buckwheat). You'll also be advised to reduce your sodium intake to less than 2,300 mg daily—high sodium depletes potassium from the body. Additional-

*These blood tests typically are covered by health insurance.

ly, you may be advised to take a magnesium and potassium supplement.

Also: Keep your stress level low. Chronic stress can lead to a high level of the hormone cortisol—this can overwhelm the adrenal glands and lead to low potassium.

• **"Normal" glucose.** Most people know that high blood glucose (126 mg/dL or above) is a warning sign of diabetes. But you may not be aware that slight increases in blood sugar—even when it is still within the so-called normal range—also put you at greater risk.

Surprising: Among 46,000 people who were tracked for 10 years, for every one-point rise in fasting blood glucose over 84 mg/dL, the risk of developing diabetes increased by about 6%. Vascular and kidney damage may begin when glucose reaches 90 mg/dL—a level that's within the normal range.

Causes: High blood glucose usually occurs when the body's cells become resistant to the hormone insulin and/or when the pancreas doesn't produce enough insulin. Obesity and genetic factors are among the main causes.

Normal glucose: 65 mg/dL to 99 mg/dL.

Optimal glucose: 70 mg/dL to 84 mg/dL.

What to do: If your fasting glucose isn't optimal or if tests show that it's rising, try to get the numbers down with regular exercise, weight loss and a healthier diet.

Powerful spice: Add one-quarter teaspoon of cinnamon to your food each day. People who take this small dose can lower their blood glucose by 18% to 29%.

Alternative: A standardized cinnamon extract in capsule form (125 mg to 250 mg, two to three times daily).

• **High homocysteine.** Most doctors recommend a homocysteine test only for patients with existing heart problems. Everyone should get it. High homocysteine may damage arteries and increase the risk for heart disease and stroke.

Causes: Homocysteine rises if you don't get enough B-complex vitamins or if you're unable to properly metabolize methionine, an amino acid that's mainly found in meat, fish and dairy. Vegetarians tend to have higher homocysteine levels. Other causes include a lack of exercise, chronic stress, smoking and too much caffeine.

Normal homocysteine: Less than 15 umol/L.

Optimal homocysteine: 8 umol/L or below.

What to do: If your homocysteine level isn't optimal, take a daily B-complex vitamin supplement that has at least 50 mg of vitamin B-6.

Also helpful: A fish oil supplement to reduce inflammation and protect the arteries. Take 1,000 mg, two to three times daily.*

• **Low DHEA.** This is a hormone that's used by the body to manufacture both testosterone and estrogen. It's also an antioxidant that supports the immune system and increases insulin sensitivity and the body's ability to metabolize fats. DHEA is not usually measured in standard blood tests, but all adults should request that their levels be tested.

Low DHEA is a common cause of fatigue, weight gain, depression and decreased libido in men and women of all ages. Over time, it can damage the hippocampus, the "memory center" of the brain.

Causes: It's normal for DHEA to slightly decrease with age. Larger deficiencies can indicate an autoimmune disease (such as rheumatoid arthritis) or chronic stress.

Normal DHEA: Levels of this hormone peak in one's late 20s. Normal levels vary widely with age and gender.

Optimal DHEA: The high end of the normal range is optimal—it reflects a reserve of DHEA.

Examples: 200 mcg/dL to 270 mcg/dL for men…and 120 mcg/dL to 180 mcg/dL for women.

What to do: If your DHEA level isn't optimal, managing emotional stress is critical. Get at least eight hours of sleep every night…exercise aerobically for about 30 minutes, three to four times a week…and practice relaxation techniques, such as yoga and meditation.

Also helpful: A daily supplement (25 mg to 50 mg) of DHEA. If you take this supplement, do so only under a doctor's supervision—you'll need regular blood tests to ensure that your DHEA level doesn't get too high.

• **High LDL-P (LDL particle number).** Traditional cholesterol tests look only at triglycerides and total LDL and HDL cholesterol. I advise patients to get a fractionated cholesterol test for a more detailed picture.

Important: Patients with a large number of small LDL particles have an elevated risk for a heart attack even if their overall LDL level is normal. The greater the number of these cholesterol particles, the more likely they are to lodge in the lining of blood vessels and eventually trigger a heart attack.

Causes: Genetics is partly responsible for high LDL and LDL-P. A poor reading can be due to metabolic syndrome, a group of factors that includes abdominal obesity, elevated triglycerides and high blood pressure. A diet high in animal fats and processed foods also can cause an increase in LDL-P.

Normal LDL-P: Less than 1,300 nmol/L. Optimal LDL-P: Below 1,000 nmol/L on an NMR lipoprofile (this test is the most accurate).

What to do: If your LDL-P level is not optimal (and you have not had a coronary event), I recommend exercise…weight loss… blood pressure and blood sugar management…more antioxidant-rich foods such as vegetables, berries and legumes…and three to five cups of green tea daily—it's a potent antioxidant that minimizes the oxidation of cholesterol molecules, which is important for reducing heart attacks.

Also: Daily supplements of bergamot extract, which has been shown to change the size of cholesterol particles (Earl Grey tea, which is flavored with oil of bergamot, provides a less potent dose)…and aged garlic extract, which has a beneficial effect on multiple cardiovascular risk factors. If these steps do not sufficiently improve your LDL-P level,

---

*Check with your doctor before using fish oil, especially if you take a blood thinner—fish oil can interact with it and certain other medications.

talk to your doctor about taking a statin and/or niacin.

Guard Against Radiation Danger

Leo Galland, MD, director of the Foundation for Integrated Medicine in New York City. He has held faculty positions at Rockefeller University, Albert Einstein College of Medicine of Yeshiva University and Stony Brook University.

Let's say your doctor has advised you to get an X-ray or a CT scan. You're likely to book the appointment without giving it much thought. But before you do so, it's worth asking whether you really need the test.

A growing threat: In the 1980s, about 15% of a typical person's lifetime exposure to radiation came from medical tests. Now these tests account for about half of one's lifetime exposure. Why the increase? Doctors are now prescribing more imaging tests, and newer tests, such as computed tomography (CT) scans, produce more radiation than those available in the past.* This is true even though some CT scans now have lower radiation levels than when they were first introduced.

A Double-Edged Sword

There's no question that imaging tests save lives. They can reveal hidden problems and have greatly improved doctors' ability to diagnose and treat serious diseases. But the use of CT scans, to give just one example, has increased 20-fold in the last 25 years. Fortunately, the cancer risk from a single scan—or even a few scans—is negligible.

The real risk: Research shows that repeated CT scans over a lifetime could increase one's risk of developing cancer by 2.7% to 12%. Cancers that have been linked to medi-

*X-rays, computed tomography (CT) and positron emissions tomography (PET) scans produce damaging radiation...ultrasounds and magnetic resonance imaging (MRI) scans do not.

cal radiation include leukemia and malignancies of the breast, thyroid and bladder.

Should You Worry?

Everyone is exposed to small amounts of radiation. Cosmic rays, radon gas and radioactive minerals in the soil are among the most common sources. Typically, the amount of radiation from these "background" sources adds up to only about 3 millisieverts (mSv), a standard unit of measurement, a year—not enough to worry about.

However, imaging tests exponentially add to your lifetime exposure.

Examples: About 1.5 mSv from a spinal X-ray...6 mSv from a pelvic CT scan...and about 20 mSv from a whole-body positron emission tomography (PET)/CT scan to detect cancer.

Questions to Ask

Before agreeing to a test, ask your doctor why it's needed and if the results will possibly change your diagnosis or treatment (if not, you don't need the test). If an imaging test is crucial, you can ask whether there's a radiation-free alternative, such as ultrasound, or whether a lower-radiation test is available—say, an X-ray instead of a CT scan. Also be sure that the medical facility where you will receive the imaging test has been accredited by the American College of Radiology (ACR). To check a facility's accreditation status, go to the ACR website, *ACR.org*.

Also helpful: Keep a log of any radiation-based tests that you get. You can refer to your radiation history whenever you and your doctor are considering a medical test that will expose you to radiation.

Supplements to Consider

Emerging evidence suggests that radioprotective supplements can help reduce the risks of radiation exposure. The research isn't conclusive (and is primarily extrapolated from findings related to radiation from nuclear accidents), but lab studies have found that some supplements may help protect you from the dangers of radiation exposure, including that from medical tests. *Examples…*

•**Ginkgo extract.** After the nuclear meltdown at Chernobyl, scientists studied a number of natural products to see what could help reduce radiation damage in first responders. They found that a ginkgo extract, known as Egb 761, reduced the damaging effects of radiation on chromosomes—and the benefits persisted for several months after workers stopped taking it. Other studies have found similar results.

My advice: Take Egb 761 for a week after having a CT scan or other imaging tests. It's available at health-food stores and from online retailers such as *Amazon.com*.

Typical dose: 120 mg daily.

Good product: Tebonin.

Possible side effect: Egb 761 can increase bleeding when it's combined with aspirin or other blood-thinning drugs, such as *warfarin* (Coumadin). Ask your doctor if it's safe for you to use.

•**Hesperidin.** This flavonoid (a type of antioxidant) is found in fruits, especially citrus. It is also available as a dietary supplement.

An animal study published in *The British Journal of Radiology* found that hesperidin taken before radiation exposure reduced blood-cell damage. In human tests, results were similar—it reduced radiation-induced damage by about one-third.

My advice: Take 250 mg of hesperidin about one hour before testing. It's unlikely to cause side effects.

Radiation Doses

Depending on the type of imaging test you receive, the radiation dose can vary widely. *For example…*

•**Bone densitometry (DEXA)** requires an approximate radiation dose of 0.001 millisieverts (mSv).

•**Mammography** requires an approximate radiation dose of 0.4 mSv.

•**X-ray of the spine** requires an approximate radiation dose of 1.5 mSv.

•**Computed tomography (CT)** of the head requires an approximate radiation dose of 2 mSv.

•**CT of the chest** requires an approximate radiation dose of 7 mSv.

•**X-ray of the lower gastrointestinal tract** requires an approximate radiation dose of 8 mSv.

•**CT of the abdomen and pelvis** requires an approximate radiation dose of 10 mSv.

•**Coronary CT angiography (CTA)** requires an approximate radiation dose of 12 mSv.

Source: Radiological Society of North America, *Radiology Info.org*.

Don't Let What Happened to Joan Rivers Happen to You

David Sherer, MD, anesthesiologist and former physician-director of risk management for a major HMO in the metropolitan Washington, DC, area. He is author, with Maryann Karinch, of *Dr. David Sherer's Hospital Survival Guide. DrDavidSherer.com*

Ever since Joan Rivers died after a routine surgical procedure at an outpatient center in Manhattan, people have been wondering if they're better off having surgery in a hospital.

The reality is that the vast majority of outpatient procedures go off without a hitch. But you can reduce your risk by getting involved before the procedure. *Important steps…*

Check Your Physical Status

Ask your doctor about your "physical status classification." The American Society of Anesthesiologists uses a numerical scale to assess a patient's surgical risks. Patients with higher physical status (PS) scores (four or five) because of health problems should have procedures done in hospitals because their risk for complications is higher.

Example: A patient who needs a knee replacement also might have poorly controlled diabetes, kidney insufficiency and nerve damage. His/her PS might be rated as four—too high to safely have a major procedure at an outpatient center.

In general, patients with PS scores of one through three—with one being generally healthy and three indicating that they have serious diseases that aren't life-threatening—are good candidates for outpatient procedures.

Pick Your Surgeon Carefully

Don't assume that every surgeon in an outpatient center has the same experience—or the same credentials.

Suppose that you're planning to get Botox or Restylane injections. These are not as simple as most people think. For the best results—and the lowest risk for complications—you should have the procedure done by a physician who is board-certified in plastic and reconstructive surgery.

Caution: In many states, many procedures can be done by any physician who has undergone minimal training in these procedures, such as a weekend course or three-day seminar. These doctors might be board-certified in something but not necessarily in the field that concerns you.

Also important: The amount of experience. Studies have clearly shown that doctors who do a lot of procedures have better results, with fewer complications, than those who do them less often.

Example: If I were planning to have LASIK eye surgery, I wouldn't feel comfortable seeing a surgeon who had done the procedure 50 times. I would want someone whose total cases numbered in the hundreds or even thousands.

Insist on Pain Control

Most people assume that their surgeons will do everything possible to minimize postoperative pain. Not true. Some doctors are reluctant to order strong painkillers on an ongoing basis because they worry that the patient will become addicted. Or they mainly use narcotics (opioids, such as codeine and morphine) that dull pain but can cause unpleasant and sometimes dangerous side effects, including impaired breathing, constipation, itching, nausea and vomiting.

Poorly controlled pain is among the most serious postoperative complications. It impairs immunity and increases the risk for infection…slows healing times…and can increase the risk for blood clots when patients hurt too much to move normally.

My advice: Tell your surgeon that you're terrified of pain. Ask what he/she plans to use to relieve your pain—and emphasize that you would like to avoid narcotics if at all possible.

Also, ask about *bupivacaine* (Exparel), a nonnarcotic anesthetic that was recently approved by the FDA. The active ingredient is encapsulated in liposomal (fat-based) particles and slowly released over 72 hours. When injected into the surgical area, it relieves pain as effectively as narcotics with fewer side effects.

Beware of Supplements

Tell your doctor about everything that you're taking. Surgeons and anesthesiologists routinely ask patients about medications that they're using. They don't always think to ask about supplements.

This is a dangerous oversight because many supplements—along with garden-variety over-the-counter medications such as aspirin—can interact with the drugs that are used during and after surgery.

Examples: Garlic supplements increase the risk for excessive bleeding, particularly when they're combined with aspirin. The herbs ephedra and kava can interfere with anesthetics.

Patients who are taking natural remedies—including vitamin E, echinacea, ginseng, valerian and St. John's wort—should ask their doctors if they need to quit taking them. You may need to stop two weeks or more before the procedure. Aspirin should be discontinued two to three days before.

Plan for the Worst

Even routine procedures sometimes go south. Most outpatient surgical centers are equipped with crash carts (used for cardiac emergencies) and other equipment and drugs for handling serious complications—but some don't have these on hand.

Ask the surgeon if a crash cart will be available. *Also ask…*

• **Is there *dantrolene* (Dantrium)?** It can reverse a rare but deadly complication from anesthesia known as malignant hyperthermia. The drug is always stocked in hospitals, but an outpatient center might not have it.

• **Is there *succinylcholine* (Anectine, Quelicin)?** It's a fast-acting paralytic agent that assists doctors in quickly intubating patients who can't breathe—one of the most dangerous complications of anesthesia. It has been reported that Joan Rivers might have lived if this drug had been available.

Don't Put Up with Nausea

It is estimated that 30% of all postsurgical patients will experience nausea, retching or vomiting. These are among the most common surgical complications.

My advice: Tell your anesthesiologist/surgeon if you've suffered from surgery-related nausea in the past. He/she can administer *granisetron* (Kytril) or *ondansetron* (Zofran), which helps prevent nausea in most patients.

Get Moving

Try to get moving as soon as you can. Surgeons used to recommend lengthy bed rest for postsurgical patients. They now know that it's better to move around as soon as possible to prevent constipation, urinary retention and muscle weakness, among other common complications.

As soon as you're able, get up and walk (with your doctor's permission, of course). If you can't stand right away, at least move in bed. Stretch your legs. Move your arms. Roll over, sit up, etc. Any kind of physical movement increases blood flow and improves recovery times. It also improves the movement of your lungs, which can help prevent postsurgical pneumonia.

---

4 Secrets to Avoiding a Misdiagnosis

Trisha Torrey, Baldwinsville, New York–based patient advocacy consultant, also known as "Every Patient's Advocate," *EveryPatientsAdvocate.com*, and the author of *You Bet Your Life! Ten Mistakes That Every Patient Makes*. She is also the founder and director of the Alliance of Professional Health Advocates and lectures across the country on the best ways to navigate the health-care system.

Ten years ago, I noticed a golf ball–sized lump on my torso. My family doctor sent me to a surgeon, who removed the lump and sent it to a lab for testing.

A few weeks later, I got the news from my doctor: "You have a very rare type of lymphoma." I froze with fear. The second blow came when an oncologist told me that if I didn't start chemotherapy right away, I'd be dead within months.

But I didn't feel sick, and my intuition told me that something was off with the diagnosis. So I sought a second opinion from another oncologist, who reviewed my case and had the biopsy analyzed again. As it turned out, I didn't have cancer. The lump was simply an inflamed bundle of fat cells. I didn't need chemo, and 10 years later I'm fine.

So how do you make sure that you or a loved one never experiences a misdiagnosis nightmare? It happens a lot. Twelve million Americans are misdiagnosed each year.

For the past decade, I have dedicated my life to helping people become smarter patients and, in the process, avoid misdiagnoses. Some of what I've learned may sound a little unconventional, but I know from my experience and that of other patients that the steps below work. *How to avoid a misdiagnosis…*

Secret #1: Track your symptoms. You probably know to write down your questions before seeing a doctor, but I suggest that you first spend at least a little time tracking your symptoms. Medical symptoms can be vague, inconsistent and wax and wane unexpectedly, so patients often don't give their doctors enough facts to ensure a correct diagnosis. Without such details, it's easy for physicians to jump on the most obvious—though sometimes incorrect—diagnosis.

What to do: If you're not dealing with an emergency, keep a diary of your symptoms before you see your doctor. Include a clear description of all your symptoms and when they started. Also, be sure to include any triggers—anything that makes the symptoms worse…or better.

Of course, don't let your symptom tracking become an excuse to delay going to the doctor. Even if your appointment is the next day or so, you can use that time to organize your notes on what you've observed so far. And once you've tracked your symptoms, you'll be better prepared to write down your questions for the doctor.

Secret #2: Make a list of possible diagnoses. If you've got an unexplained symptom, most doctors tell you to avoid the Internet. You will just confuse yourself, they reason. I disagree. If you've got a weird symptom, you want to know what may be causing it so you can ask the doctor intelligent questions.

When doing research online, just make sure you don't jump to conclusions. And skip Web sites that are sponsored by pharmaceutical companies or businesses trying to sell you something. Also, disregard comments and forums populated by non–health professionals. Up-to-date and reliable health information is available at such sites as *Medline Plus.gov*…*HealthFinder.gov*…and *UptoDate.com* (it's used by many doctors around the world—click on "Patients and Caregivers").

In my own situation, using the Internet helped me to realize that cancer wasn't the only possible diagnosis, and it compelled me to ask many more questions.

Important: Don't try to diagnose yourself…and don't talk yourself out of going to the doctor.

Secret #3: Ask this crucial question. Your doctor has just given you a diagnosis. Now what? Rather than launching into a discussion about the best treatments for the diagnosis you've just received—as most often occurs—I suggest that you stop and ask the doctor, "What else could it be?"

Specifically, ask the doctor for the "differential diagnosis"—that is, the conditions he/she ruled out. Then ask how he ruled them out. Listen carefully—if there are any gaps in the case he makes for your diagnosis, they are likely to come up at this time. After this explanation, ask about anything you don't understand. Be concise and stay focused. If you start to ramble, your doctor won't stay engaged.

Secret #4: Don't be afraid of your doctor. There are ways to get what you need and ask your questions without offending anyone.

What you need to know: A good, ethical doctor won't be upset by your desire for additional medical opinions. Getting more than one opinion is crucial, especially if your doctor has recommended any invasive type of treatment such as chemotherapy, surgery or a long-term drug prescription.

Ask for your own medical records and take them to additional opinion appointments. Your goal is to find at least two doctors who give you the same diagnosis, maximizing your odds of getting a correct one. Let new doctors draw their own conclusions about your diagnosis rather than sharing previous opinions they can simply agree with.

If your online research doesn't jibe with what your doctor has told you, don't be confrontational. Instead, ask questions like, "I recently read about this [diagnosis or treatment]. Can you tell me why you ruled that out?" This acknowledges your doctor's extensive education and experience but puts him on notice that you've done your homework and need to know more.

Drugs That Work Against Each Other

David Lee, PharmD, PhD, assistant professor in the College of Pharmacy at Oregon State University in Portland. Dr. Lee is also a coauthor of a recent paper on therapeutic competition that was published in the journal *PLoS ONE*.

Most people who have a chronic health problem such as osteoarthritis, high blood pressure or diabetes are accustomed to taking medication to help control their symptoms.

But if you have more than one chronic condition—and take medication for each of them—you could be setting yourself up for other problems.

The risk that often goes undetected: Taking medication prescribed for one disease may actually worsen another health problem. This situation, known as "therapeutic competition," has received surprisingly little attention from the medical profession.

Are You At Risk?

Therapeutic competition can occur at any time in a person's life. But the risk increases with age—the older we get, the more likely we are to have chronic medical conditions and use more medications. Because our bodies metabolize medication less efficiently as we age, we're also more likely to develop side effects that can worsen other health problems.

Modern medicine has not done very much to help the situation. For one thing, polypharmacy—the use of multiple medications—has become more common than ever before.

For people with more than one chronic medical condition, frequent conflicts occur if you have…

High Blood Pressure

If you also have chronic obstructive pulmonary disease (COPD), drugs that you take to ease your breathing, such as the beta-adrenergic agonist *albuterol* (Proventil) or a corticosteroid, may raise your blood pressure.

If you are also being treated for depression, an antidepressant such as *venlafaxine* (Effexor) or *duloxetine* (Cymbalta) could push your blood pressure higher. COX-2 inhibitors such as *celecoxib* (Celebrex), commonly used for osteoarthritis, also may increase blood pressure.

Diabetes

Corticosteroids taken for COPD can raise blood sugar levels, worsening diabetes. If you have an enlarged prostate and take an alpha-blocker such as *tamsulosin* (Flomax) or a beta-blocker such as *atenolol* (Tenormin) for high blood pressure, the drug can mask symptoms of low blood sugar, such as shakiness.

COPD

If you also have high blood pressure or angina and take a non-selective beta-blocker such as *propranolol* (Inderal), the drug could worsen lung symptoms.

Heart Disease

COPD drugs, including albuterol…tricyclic antidepressants such as *imipramine* (Tofranil), taken for depression…and COX-2 inhibitors for osteoarthritis also can make heart disease worse.

Atrial Fibrillation

Osteoporosis drugs, including bisphosphonates such as *alendronate* (Fosamax)…and Alzheimer's drugs, including cholinesterase inhibitors such as *donepezil* (Aricept), may worsen atrial fibrillation.

Osteoporosis

Corticosteroids used to treat COPD often lead to significant bone loss. Glitazones taken for diabetes and proton pump inhibitors such as *omeprazole* (Prilosec), commonly prescribed for gastroesophageal reflux disease (GERD), can accelerate bone loss.

GERD or Peptic Ulcers

Warfarin (Coumadin) or *clopidogrel* (Plavix), often prescribed for atrial fibrillation or heart disease, as well as nonsteroidal anti-inflammatory drugs (NSAIDs), can cause bleeding that worsens GERD and ulcers. Bisphosphonates taken for osteoporosis may aggravate esophageal damage that commonly occurs with GERD and ulcers.

How to Protect Yourself

If you have more than one chronic condition and take two or more medications to treat them, it is crucial that you watch for signs of therapeutic competition, such as new symptoms that are unexplained or begin soon after a new medication is started. Any new health condition actually may be an adverse effect of medication.

Important steps to avoid therapeutic competition...

•**Try to cut back on the drugs you take.** The less medication you're on, the less likely one of your drugs will adversely affect another condition. Ask your doctor whether it's advisable to reduce the overall number of prescriptions you take. A drug you have been taking for years may no longer be necessary. You may also be able to make lifestyle changes—such as getting more exercise—that will allow you to cut back on blood pressure or diabetes medication.

•**Get the right medication.** If it seems that a drug is worsening another condition, ask your doctor about less harmful alternatives. Some medications are more selective—that is, their effects on the body are more focused on the target illness, making unintended consequences for other conditions less of a danger.

Example: Nonselective beta-blockers, such as propranolol, often worsen COPD symptoms, but medications with more selective action, such as *metoprolol* (Lopressor), are usually just as effective for the heart problem they're prescribed for without adversely affecting your lungs.

Get a Yearly Medication Check

If you suffer from multiple ailments, you need to tell all your doctors about the medications you take. Also, talk to your pharmacist each time you pick up a new prescription to make sure your drugs aren't working against each other.

To ensure that no drug-related problems develop: Once a year, have a pharmacist (ask one at your drugstore) review all your medications. This service includes a discussion of side effects, interactions and alternatives. For many people, Medicare Part D and some private health plans will pay for this service. If not, it usually costs less than $100.

Thyroid Supplements Contain Potentially Dangerous Levels of Hormones

Study titled "Thyroxine and triiodothyronine content in commercially available thyroid health supplements," published in *Thyroid.*

Tired and sluggish? Gaining weight? Maybe you've seen ads for certain dietary supplements that purport to rev up metabolism and increase energy by providing vitamins, minerals and herbs that "support the thyroid." But if you're tempted to try them, hold on!

Reason: A shocking study has uncovered the fact that many such "thyroid-boosting" supplements contain dangerous ingredients that can have very serious side effects, especially for the heart—so it's outrageous that they're being sold over the counter to unwary consumers. *Here's what you need to watch out for...*

Shocker of an Analysis

Doctors have reported seeing a number of patients who are hyperthyroid, meaning that they have excessively high levels of thyroid hormone in their blood—despite the fact that their thyroid glands seem to be functioning perfectly normally. Some such patients have acknowledged taking nutritional supplements marketed to boost thyroid function or promote weight loss.

To investigate the connection, researchers purchased 10 different over-the-counter supplements (readily available in retail stores and online) that claimed to improve "thyroid health"…provide "thyroid support"…or act as "thyroid supplements." Five of the products were labeled as herbal supplements. The other five were labeled as containing "raw thyroid" tissue, concentrate or powder from bovine sources—meaning from cow thyroid glands.

In the lab, the researchers analyzed the supplements to see whether they contained actual thyroid hormones—specifically, thyroxine (also called T4) and triiodothyronine (T3), the two hormones that our thyroid glands naturally produce. Every product was tested three times…and to reduce any possible bias, the lab workers conducting the analyses were unaware of the identities of the products they were testing.

What they discovered: Nine of the 10 supplements tested contained at least one of the thyroid hormones…and five of the 10 contained both. Of the five so-called herbal products (which you would expect to contain only herbs), all contained T3 and two also contained T4—even though the package labels did not mention anything about animal thyroid products and even though an animal source is the only way that T3 and T4 could have wound up in the supplements.

The products contained varying amounts of the thyroid hormones, but even the smallest dose is clinically significant because it can interfere with the endocrine system's delicate feedback system that carefully regulates the levels of various hormones that interact with each other.

Big concern: Judging by the doses listed on labels, some products contained thyroid hormone amounts even greater (in one case, more than six times greater) than prescrip-

tion drugs used to treat diagnosed cases of underactive thyroid.

What's the Harm?

What's the big deal about taking these thyroid hormones if our bodies naturally produce them anyway? Plenty. A functioning endocrine system is finely tuned to secrete just the right amount of hormones to maintain homeostasis, or a state of balance. Too much thyroid hormone can lead to atrial fibrillation, a heart-rhythm disorder in which the heart beats chaotically, increasing the risk for stroke and heart failure…congestive heart failure, in which the heart can't circulate enough blood to meet all of the body's needs…osteoporosis…anxiety and insomnia. That's why people who take prescription medication to regulate their thyroid levels are carefully monitored by their doctors.

Bottom line: If you think your thyroid isn't working as it should—because you feel sluggish, you're always cold when others around you are not, or you're gaining weight for no apparent reason—do not simply dose yourself with so-called thyroid-boosting supplements. They can be dangerous and can even trigger thyroid disease in healthy people. Instead, see your doctor for a proper

---

Diet Pill Labels Are Misleading

A recent study by the FDA found that nine of 21 diet pill products marketed as all-natural contained beta-methylphenethylamine, an amphetamine-like compound that has not been tested on humans.

And: All the products' labels claimed that they included a natural ingredient taken from a bushy plant in Texas and Mexico called *Acacia rigidula*…but researchers could not find the substance in tests of the plant.

Study of 21 diet pills by scientists at the US Food and Drug Administration, Washington, DC, published in *Journal of Pharmaceutical and Biomedical Analysis*.

diagnosis—and if you already took any thyroid-boosting supplements, share this information with your doctor. A blood test can reveal whether your thyroid hormone levels are off. If they are, your doctor can help you get them back on track safely...and if they aren't, you and your doctor can start figuring out what's really causing your symptoms.

Rapid-Weight-Loss Diets: Proceed with Caution

Frank Lammert, PhD, professor of medicine, Saarland University Medical Center, Homburg, Germany. His study was published in *Clinical Gastroenterology and Hepatology*.

Rapid-weight-loss diets can be tempting quick fixes. You know the circumstances. You want to quickly lose a few pounds to look great in a suit or dress that you plan to wear to a reunion...or you aim to fit into a slinky gown for a wedding reception...or to look your hunky best for a vacation cruise.

You know that rapid-weight-loss and crash diets are self-sabotaging because they can mess with your metabolism and hormones, but there's another painful reason why you should steer clear of rapid-weight-loss dieting—gallstones.

The biggest risk factor for gallstones is carrying too much weight, especially around the middle, but rapid weight loss can also bring on gallstone formation. Recent research is providing insight into how gallstones can be prevented naturally in dieters, although some dieters might not like what these researchers have to say.

The Gall of It

About half a million Americans have their gallbladders removed each year because of gallstones. Gallstones are formed by different substances. Those that most commonly form in people who are overweight or who go on rapid-weight-loss diets are made from excess cholesterol in bile (also called gall), which is produced by the liver and stored in the gallbladder. (Bile is used as a digestive enzyme in the small intestine.) The stones can range in size from grains of sand to golf balls.

Gallstones may cause no symptoms or health problems at all—but if a stone gets stuck in a bile duct of the gallbladder, it can cause severe pain (it's often compared with the pain of childbirth) and other complications, such as jaundice (yellowing of skin and eyes). Symptoms include sudden, rapidly worsening pain in the upper right or middle part of the abdomen or pain between the shoulder blades or under the right shoulder. The pain can last for minutes or hours and then pass. (Seek immediate attention if the pain becomes so severe that you can't sit still or if jaundice develops.)

Preventing Gallstones

A recent study by German and Danish researchers led by Frank Lammert, PhD, professor of medicine at Saarland University Medical Center in Homburg, Germany, identified two ways to prevent gallstones during weight loss. One way is preventive treatment with *ursodiol* (Actigall, Urso), a prescription drug used to prevent gallstones and dissolve existing ones in patients who need but either can't have or don't want gallbladder surgery. The other way, which may sound counterintuitive, is to follow a diet higher in fat—although this isn't how many "lose-weight-fast" dieters want to eat.

In two small published studies that the team looked at, gallstones developed in 38% and 67% of patients on very-low-fat diets and none on higher-fat diets. Overall, the research team (which analyzed 13 published clinical trials on the topic of gallstones and weight loss) found that patients whose weight-loss diets contained between 19% and 30% fat had fewer gallstones than those whose diets contained between 3% and 5% fat. The reason? Scientists theorize that a meal that is higher in fat stimulates the gallbladder to move bile between the liver and intestines at a fast enough pace to prevent gallstone formation.

Weight Loss: How Much and How Fast?

To minimize risk of developing gallstones during weight loss, losing 1.5 kg (about 3.3 pounds) a week was best. This might make some dieters impatient, but remember that slow and steady calorie control is the best way to lose weight and keep it off.

For people considering weight-loss surgery, be aware that rapid weight loss of more than 25% of body weight immediately after surgery is associated with an increased risk of gallstones. Patients planning weight-loss surgery should talk to their doctors about taking ursodiol as a preventive measure. Ursodiol is actually a synthetic version of a bile acid that is already naturally found in the body, but, as with all drugs, side effects can sometimes occur. The most common are stomach upset, diarrhea, dizziness, back pain, hair loss and cough. Rare allergic reaction also can occur.

Because gallstones can form in as short a time as four weeks, ursodiol should be started within a few days after surgery. It can be stopped three to six months later. (Gallstone formation levels off about six months after the surgery.) Eating a higher proportion of fat is also helpful.

Of course, losing those extra pounds benefits health, but keep your doctor in the loop and consider working with a nutritionist or physician specializing in weight loss (such as an endocrinologist or bariatric physician) to help ensure that your weight-loss plan is effective and that you're not putting yourself at risk for an attack of gallstones.

What's Really in That Generic Drug?

Jack E. Fincham, PhD, RPh, professor of pharmacy administration at Presbyterian College School of Pharmacy in Clinton, South Carolina.

Generics cost 80% less, on average, than brand-name drugs. They contain the same active ingredients and supposedly do the same job. What's not to like? A lot, it turns out. In June, two large manufacturers of the generic version of the heart drug Toprol-XL issued a recall because the drug wasn't dissolving properly—a problem that was identified when patients taking the drug started complaining of chest pain and other heart symptoms.

This isn't an isolated incident. Generic drugs may be similar to their brand-name counterparts, but they are not identical. *What you need to know about generic drugs...*

Doubts About Quality

For years, major medical groups such as the American Heart Association (AHA) have expressed concerns that generics may cause more side effects than brand-name drugs—and the AHA as well as many other such groups advise always getting a doctor's approval before using a generic drug.

Generics account for about 80% of all prescriptions in the US and save Americans billions of dollars a year, but some experts worry that patients, in some cases, are trading quality for economy—and may be taking serious risks.

Sobering statistics: A survey of more than 500 doctors found that nearly 50% worried about the overall quality of generics...and more than 25% said that they would hesitate

---

See Your Doctor in the Morning

Doctors are more likely to prescribe antibiotics later in the day. About 5% more patients receive unnecessary antibiotics for respiratory infections toward the end of a doctor's day than at the beginning.

Theory: Doctors experience a "wear down" through the day, which makes them more likely to prescribe antibiotics.

Analysis of data from more than 21,000 doctor visits by researchers at Brigham and Women's Hospital, Boston, published in *JAMA Internal Medicine*.

to prescribe these drugs for themselves or their families.

The Face-Off

Key differences between generic and brand-name drugs...

• **Bioequivalence.** You would think that the amount of a drug that's absorbed by the body would be the same in generic and brand-name versions. This isn't always the case.

According to FDA guidelines, generics are required to reach maximum blood concentrations that are between 80% and 125% of the levels achieved by brand-name drugs. Suppose that you switch to a generic that delivers medication at the low end of the range. You may find your symptoms aren't as well-controlled as they used to be. If the drug is at the high end, you'll be more likely to have side effects.

• **Timed-release.** Medications that release their active ingredients slowly are among the trickiest to copy. Even when the active ingredient is the same in two versions of the same drug, how it is released in the body might be different.

• **Fillers.** The active ingredients in generic and brand-name drugs are the same, but the extra ingredients—such as binding agents, preservatives and pill coatings—may be different. These ingredients are supposed to be inert. But new research suggests that they may affect how drugs dissolve or how they're absorbed by the body.

• **Testing.** The same investigational drug studies that are needed for FDA approval of brand-name drugs are not required for all generic drugs. For example, the FDA requires only a very small number of people (sometimes just 20) for its bioequivalence studies.

How to Protect Yourself

There's no reason to swear off generic drugs. The cost savings can be tremendous, and most generics provide the same benefits—with no greater risk for side effects—as brand-names. But you have to choose them carefully. *My advice...*

• **Be wary of timed-release medications.** Also called extended-release, they are used for conditions such as pain, depression and asthma that require long-term control...or for convenience. They're usually designated with abbreviations such as ER (extended release), LA (long acting) or LTR (long-term release).

Problems with the timed-released components are more of an issue with generics than with brand-name drugs. This doesn't mean you should avoid generics. What matters is the predictability of the timed-release drug. If your symptoms are well-controlled by a generic version, stick with the same drug—preferably one that's made by the same manufacturer (see below). You're more likely to have problems when you first switch from a brand-name drug to a generic substitute.

• **Take exactly the same drug.** Pharmacies use generic products from multiple manufacturers. Different drug companies use different manufacturing techniques as well as different ingredients. Even if you think you're taking the same drug, there may be subtle variations in such areas as effectiveness and side effects each time the prescription is filled. You can avoid these

---

When NSAIDs Are Deadly...

Painkillers may be linked to blood clots. A meta-analysis of six studies of venous thromboembolism—a type of clot that includes deep vein thrombosis and pulmonary embolism—showed an 80% higher clot risk in people who use naproxen, ibuprofen and other nonsteroidal anti-inflammatory drugs (NSAIDs) compared with nonusers. For patients known to have increased risk for venous thromboembolism because of genetic factors or extended immobility, acetaminophen may be a safer pain reliever. Talk to your doctor.

Patompong Ungprasert, MD, instructor in the department of rheumatology at Mayo Clinic, Rochester, Minnesota, and leader of an analysis published online in Rheumatology.

variations by making sure that your prescription comes from the same company.

What to do: Check the prescription bottle for the manufacturer of the drug you take. If it's not there, your pharmacist can tell you. Also, ask him/her if it's possible to use a single company for each refill.

This is crucial if the drug has a narrow therapeutic index (NTI)—a fine line between an effective dose and a toxic dose.

Examples: Some blood-thinning drugs (such as warfarin)…drugs used for seizures (such as phenytoin)…and antipsychotic drugs (such as lithium).

• **Track results.** Be suspicious if a drug that you've been taking for months or years suddenly seems less effective or seems to be causing new side effects. It's possible that your condition has changed—or you could be receiving a drug made by a different manufacturer.

Important: If you start using a new pharmacy, let the pharmacist know the manufacturers of all your medications. Also, ask your doctor to give you copies of all your test results. Track your numbers—for cholesterol and blood sugar, for example. If you notice a change, tell your doctor right away. It's possible that you just need a dosing adjustment. It's also possible that a generic isn't the best choice for you.

• **Switch drugs.** If you're not getting the best results from a new generic medication, don't assume that you need a different drug. You might simply need to switch to the brand-name version.

What to do: Ask your doctor to prescribe the brand-name drug for a few months. If you notice an improvement in your symptoms and test results, it might be worth sticking with it even if it costs more. Or if you are not happy with the results of your generic but would rather avoid the high cost of a brand-name, ask your pharmacist to recommend another generic.

Is the Cheaper Store-Brand Supplement Really As Good?

Edgar Dworsky, creator of the consumer advocate websites *ConsumerWorld.org* and *MousePrint.org.* Formerly, he served as consumer education consultant for the Federal Trade Commission and was a Massachusetts assistant attorney general.

Store-brand vitamins and supplements can save you money, but they may not be as perfect a match to national brands as you often are led to believe.

Examples…

• **Walgreens One Daily Women's 50+ Multivitamin** (about $13) may seem like a good substitute for Centrum Silver Women 50+ Multivitamin/Multimineral Supplement (about $16). But the Walgreens supplement contains only 23 specific vitamins, minerals and nutrients, while Centrum has 31, including boron and potassium, which are not in the Walgreens version, and higher daily doses of vitamins A, C and E. Which is better? That may depend on an individual shopper's nutritional needs. But what's clear is that the Walgreens version isn't an exact substitute for the national brand.

• **CVS Advanced Eye Health softgel tablets** (about $17) say on the label that they're "comparable" to the AREDS 2 study formula softgels popularized by Bausch & Lomb PreserVision (about $35). The Bausch & Lomb product contains all six ingredients that were used in that study by the National Institutes of Health, which resulted in slower progression of age-related macular degeneration, a very serious eye condition that could lead to partial blindness. The CVS product contains only two of the six ingredients—lutein and zeaxanthin—while leaving out all of the study's proven vitamins and minerals (vitamin C, vitamin E, copper and zinc).

Bottom line: Compare ingredients carefully.

Beware of Medical Apps

A study published in *The Journal of the American Medical Association Dermatology* by researchers from University of Pittsburgh Medical Center looked at four apps that claimed to diagnose melanoma. Three misread actual melanomas as "unconcerning" 30% of the time. Another study looked at all cancer-related apps and found that almost half did not contain scientifically validated data. The only apps that now require FDA approval are those that meet the definition of a medical device—for example, a mobile app that can be used as an electrocardiography machine.

Analysis by IMS Institute for Healthcare Informatics, based in Danbury, Connecticut.

Appendix 3
OPTIMUM AGING

What You Know About Aging Is Wrong!

Marc E. Agronin, MD, adult and geriatric psychiatrist who is medical director for mental health and clinical research at Miami Jewish Health Systems and affiliate associate professor of psychiatry and neurology at University of Miami Miller School of Medicine, both in Florida. He is a contributor to *The Wall Street Journal* experts blog at *Blogs.WSJ.com/experts.*

O ld age is often portrayed as a time of loneliness, depression and significant cognitive decline. But most research shows that the opposite is true for most people.

Among the common myths about getting older...

***Myth #1*: Depression hits.** No one loves the physical changes of age, let alone the likelihood of dealing with age-related illnesses.

But the emotional prospects are better than you think. The rates of major depression, for example, actually go down with age. A recent study that tracked participants for about 10 years found that their feelings of well-being increased until they reached their 70s. The feelings plateaued at that point but still didn't fall.

People who develop serious medical problems or experience traumatic life events (such as the death of a spouse) obviously will be more likely to suffer from depression than those who have an easier path. But even in the face of adversity, older people are resilient—they've accumulated enough wisdom to help them through hard times.

***Myth #2*: You'll be lonely.** One of the inevitabilities of aging is the loss of friends and family members. Older people do spend more time alone. But that's not the same as feeling lonely or isolated.

A number of studies have shown that the quality of relationships improves with age. You may have fewer close friends in your 70s than you did in your 50s, but you'll probably find that the connections have matured and become richer and more fulfilling.

Remember your earlier relationships—how often were they tumultuous and emotionally fraught? Studies have shown that older adults tend to be more positive about their relationships and less likely to experience social tensions.

***Myth #3*: Your mind slips.** Yes, it will, in some ways—but the typical "slips" that most people experience will be offset by improvements in other mental areas.

Take memory and the ability to concentrate. Both start to decline by middle age. You won't be as quick at math, and your verbal skills won't be quite as sharp. You'll retain the ability to learn, but new information will take longer to sink in.

At the same time, you'll notice improvements in other mental abilities. You'll have a lot of accrued knowledge, along with an edge in reasoning and creative thinking. You won't keep up with the youngsters on cognitive tests, but you may perform better in real-world situations.

To keep your mind active, take up painting or other hobbies. Read challenging novels. Learn another language, or learn to play a musical instrument. People who stretch themselves mentally can improve memory and cognitive skills and possibly slow the rate of subsequent declines.

Myth #4: **No more sex**. In surveys, older adults often report more sexual satisfaction than is reported by their younger counterparts. They might have sex less often, but they tend to enjoy it more.

A national survey of sexual attitudes, published in *The New England Journal of Medicine*, found that, on average, the frequency of sexual activity declines only slightly from the 50s to the 70s.

And the sexual attitudes among seniors are sufficiently frisky to make their grandchildren blush. About 50% of people ages 57 to 75 reported engaging in oral sex. More than half of men and about 25% of women masturbated.

Good health (and an available partner) are among the best predictors of a robust sex life. Sex-specific disorders—such as erectile dysfunction in men and vaginal dryness in women—now can be overcome with a variety of aids and treatments. Even when sexual activity does decline (or disappear), older adults enjoy cuddling and other intimacies.

Myth #5: **Falls are normal**. Falls are never a normal part of aging…and they're not merely accidents. Anyone who is unsteady on his/her feet has a health problem that needs to be addressed. It could be osteoporosis, reduced muscle strength, impaired vision, disturbed sleep or side effects from medications.

Warning: Falls are the main cause of more than 90% of hip fractures and a leading cause of emergency room visits and deaths.

People who get any kind of exercise—a daily walk, working around the house, digging in the garden—are much less likely to fall or to suffer serious injuries should they have a misstep.

Important: A good night's sleep. We've found that people who don't sleep well tend to have more disorientation and balance problems, particularly if they happen to be taking sleep medications that contain the antihistamine diphenhydramine.

It Takes a Virtual Village

Susan McWhinney-Morse, founder of Beacon Hill Village, reported by Karen Larson, editor of *Bottom Line/Personal. BottomLinePublications.com*

Back in 1999, Susan McWhinney-Morse faced a dilemma. She loved her Boston town house but was worried that she'd have to struggle to obtain needed support.

Her solution: She helped launch a nonprofit group that would provide her—and other retirees in her area who wished to remain in their homes—with help and social activities. Today that nonprofit group, Beacon Hill Village, has nearly 400 members. What's more, it has inspired approximately 150 similar "virtual villages" around the country, with roughly 120 more in the planning stages.

These virtual villages do not typically provide actual day-to-day support to members, just guidance about where and how to obtain support. They vet local service providers—from plumbers to home health aids. (Some of these providers offer discounts to group members.) They connect members in need of assistance with fellow members or local volunteers who are willing to help. And they typically have someone on staff who can advise members about the ins and outs of senior services. Virtual villages also sponsor get-togethers and outings. Membership fees typically are $300 to $500 a year, though a few villages charge as much as $1,000.

The Village to Village Network website (*VTVNetwork.org*) can help you locate groups in your area. If there is no group nearby, click the "Start a Village" link on the site to learn more.

Antiaging: Hope or Hoax?

S. Jay Olshansky, PhD, research associate at the Center on Aging at The University of Chicago and professor, School of Public Health, University of Illinois at Chicago.

Antiaging experts are popping up like flowers in springtime, promising to help people look and feel their best. Many of them are, in fact, doctors, whether MDs, NDs or some other type. You probably have some of these doctors where you live.

But doesn't the very phrase "antiaging" set off alarm bells? We're all aging. Every day, we're a day older. So, what are all these antiaging docs really able to do? And how do we avoid all the hucksters?

For some answers, we spoke with S. Jay Olshansky, PhD, research associate at the Center on Aging at The University of Chicago. He's spent 28 years studying aging...and he doesn't sell a cure for it. *His information may surprise you...*

Not an Exact Science

The first thing to know is that the American Board of Medical Specialties (ABMS) does not recognize antiaging as a specialty, so there is no such thing as becoming "board-certified" in the area. A group of doctors did, however, organize their own association in 1992—the American Academy of Anti-Aging Medicine. According to its site, the Academy offers certification to anyone with an MD, DO, DPM (Doctor of Podiatric Medicine) or MBBS (Bachelor of Medicine/Bachelor of Science) degree who passes a written and an oral exam and meets some other modest requirements. About 24,000 people have signed up. But since ABMS doesn't recognize the Academy or its certification, personally it's not enough of a credential to satisfy me that a doctor is an expert in the subject of aging.

Dr. Olshansky suggested that an antiaging doctor's certification, though, is less important than the particular type of treatments that he or she recommends. *So let's take a look at a few of the most common treatments that are offered...*

Common Antiaging Treatments

Dr. Olshansky said that part of the typical antiaging regimen is based on prescribing three types of hormones—synthetic human growth hormone (HGH), dehydroepiandrosterone (DHEA) and bioidentical estrogen. Though opinions on these hormones vary widely among experts, in Dr. Olshansky's view, none of them has been scientifically proven to be effective in making people grow younger or live longer. *Specifically...*

• **HGH might help you boost skin elasticity,** mental acuity and muscle mass (but not strength) in the short term, but its potential side effects include carpal tunnel syndrome, aching muscles and joints, and—most worrisome—heart disease, diabetes and possibly speeding up the rate at which cells turn cancerous, said Dr. Olshansky.

• **DHEA is said to improve bone density,** mental concentration and memory, but there's no scientific evidence backing up those claims—plus, studies show that this hormone can reduce HDL "good" cholesterol, cause acne and increase facial hair in women, said Dr. Olshansky.

• **Bioidentical estrogen is recommended by some antiaging doctors to women because it's been shown to relieve menopausal symptoms such as hot flashes,** dry skin, reduced libido and other problems. However, there is no scientific proof that bioidentical estrogen is any safer than synthetic estrogen, which has been linked to a number of diseases, including breast cancer, said Dr. Olshansky.

True Antiaging Treatments

We would all like one magic cure-all, but Dr. Olshansky told me that when it comes to maintaining energy, mental sharpness, strong bones, flexibility, clear skin and more as you age, the only tried-and-true methods are the same ones that you've been hearing about since you were a little kid. *Here are the three keys...*

- **Exercise.** Cardio plus weight training provides the same benefits as injecting yourself with HGH, but without its exorbitant cost ($12,000 a year or more) and dangerous side effects, and the benefits are immediate.

- **Diet.** Choose foods dense in vitamins, minerals and amino acids—these (of course) include low-fat protein and colorful fruits and vegetables.

- **Medical monitoring.** Dr. Olshansky said that everyone over age 50 should get regular checkups and tests for general health by an MD. If you want or need care above what your general practitioner can provide, talk to a specialist, too. An endocrinologist is generally best equipped to address hormone imbalances, and a geriatrician can coordinate treatment of age-related diseases.

What the Future Holds

Exercise, diet and medical monitoring (along with follow-up) can slow down the manifestations of aging a little or at least make you feel younger, said Dr. Olshansky. In the future, we might actually be able to slow down aging itself.

Scientists are studying genes to learn how we might turn certain ones "on" or "off" to prevent or delay health problems and live longer. Caloric restriction is also showing possibility for prolonging vigor, and research continues on how stem cells may someday allow repair of damaged tissue in older people and others. It is an exciting frontier...but it is a frontier, so don't believe everything you hear out there, even from doctors.

More Evidence That Hormone Therapy Might Not Help Women's Hearts

Henry Boardman, MD, cardiovascular medicine department, University of Oxford, England.

Suzanne Steinbaum, MD, director, women and heart disease, Lenox Hill Hospital, New York City.

Taraneh Shirazian, MD, assistant professor, obstetrics, gynecology and reproductive sciences, Icahn School of Medicine at Mount Sinai, New York City.

Cochrane Library, news release.

There's yet another study looking at the potential dangers of hormone replacement therapy for menopausal symptoms, and this one supports the notion that the treatment may not help women's hearts.

The research, a review of collected data on the issue, found that hormone replacement therapy (HRT) does not protect most postmenopausal women against heart disease and may even increase their risk of stroke.

Also, the findings suggest that the harms and benefits of hormone therapy may vary depending on a woman's age when she started the therapy, explained study lead author Henry Boardman, MD, of the cardiovascular medicine department at the University of Oxford in England.

"This 'Timing Hypothesis' may be the critical key to the use of HRT," agreed one expert, Suzanne Steinbaum, MD, director of women and heart disease at Lenox Hill Hospital in New York City.

"For certain women who fit the criteria, being on HRT early in menopause may be beneficial, and the fear of taking it may be unfounded," said Dr. Steinbaum, who was not involved in the new study.

The findings were published in the journal *Cochrane Library*.

Background

A woman's natural supply of estrogen diminishes after menopause, and HRT has been widely used to control menopausal symptoms. HRT has also been used to help prevent heart disease in postmenopausal women, the researchers noted.

However, results from the Women's Health Initiative study released in 2002 found that long-term use of HRT boosted a woman's odds for breast cancer as well as strokes. Those findings caused a steep drop-off in the number of women using HRT.

New Study

In the new study, Dr. Boardman and colleagues analyzed data from a variety of studies involving more than 40,000 women worldwide. The women used HRT for periods between seven months to over 10 years.

Overall, the results showed no evidence that the therapy reduces the risk of death from any cause, death from heart disease, or nonfatal heart attack or angina in healthy women or those with heart disease.

In fact, hormone therapy was associated with a slightly increased risk of stroke, the researchers found.

Timing seemed to matter, however. There was some evidence that women who began hormone treatment within the first 10 years of menopause appeared to have a small amount of protection against death and heart attack, and no increased risk of stroke. However, these women did appear to have an increased risk of blood clots.

Implications

"The evidence we have provides some support for the so-called 'timing hypothesis,' but we should bear in mind the size of this effect," said Dr. Boardman.

"When we looked at the results according to the age of women, or by how long since their menopause that they started treatment, we found that if 1,000 women under 60 years old started hormone therapy we would expect six fewer deaths, eight fewer cases of heart disease and five extra blood clots over about seven years, compared to 1,000 similar women who did not start hormone therapy," Dr. Boardman added.

So the study findings "need to be carefully considered," he said.

"This is a complicated health issue, where the same treatment offers benefits in some women, but harms in others."

Expert Commentary

Dr. Steinbaum agreed that women may need to make the decision to take HRT on a case-by-case basis, in consultation with their physician.

"Hormone replacement therapy for postmenopausal women has been controversial," she said. "This new study published in the *Cochrane Library*, looking at over 40,000 women, added to the confusion, but also helped to establish potential guidelines."

Taraneh Shirazian, MD, is an assistant professor of obstetrics, gynecology and reproductive sciences at the Icahn School of Medicine at Mount Sinai, in New York City. She said that, as of now, HRT "use is recommended for the shortest period of time for symptom control due to the risks of blood clots, stroke and slight increase in breast and ovarian cancer risk."

"This study suggests that if used further from menopause, the cardiac benefit is not obtained and that the risks of blood clots and stroke increase," Dr. Shirazian added. "It is important to consider starting age of HRT, other medical conditions, and family history of breast/ovary cancer when considering the use of HRT in individual women."

For more information about hormone replacement therapy, visit the website of the American Academy of Family Physicians, *familydoctor.org*. Search "hormone replacement therapy."

HRT Linked to Ovarian Cancer

Hormone replacement therapy (HRT) is linked to ovarian cancer risk. In a recent analysis of more than 21,000 postmenopausal women, those who used either oral or patch HRT to ease menopause symptoms, even for the commonly recommended limit of less than five years, were 20% more likely to develop ovarian cancer than those who never used HRT.

If you are considering HRT: Talk to your doctor about your cancer risk.

Valerie Beral, DBE, MD, director, Cancer Epidemiology Unit, University of Oxford, UK.

Neroli Oil Soothes Menopausal Symptoms

Study titled "Effects of Inhalation of Essential Oil of *Citrus aurantium L. var. amara* on Menopausal Symptoms, Stress, and Estrogen in Postmenopausal Women: A Randomized Controlled Trail," published in *Evidence-Based Complementary and Alternative Medicine.*

Are menopausal symptoms—the hot flashes, night sweats, insomnia and moodiness among all else—cramping your style…stressing your relationships…in short, ruining your life? Sure, hormone replacement therapy (HRT) is an option, but maybe its risks, such as blood clots, gallstones, breast cancer and stroke, have nixed that idea for you.

There's another great way that's helping women wind down and recharge.

No, it's not another supplement, mind trick or exercise routine. It's aromatherapy using a lusciously exotic scent—neroli oil.

Sniff Test

Neroli oil is extracted from the blossoms of the bitter orange tree and is rich in limonene, a compound that has antianxiety and muscle-relaxing effects. Neroli oil vapor, when inhaled, is known to relieve anxiety, stress and depression, reduce high blood pressure and stimulate an underactive libido. Because symptoms such as mood swings and underactive libido are so common in menopause, a group of Korean researchers decided to sci-

entifically test whether neroli oil had an effect on those and other menopausal symptoms.

Here's what they did. The team recruited 63 healthy menopausal women and divided them into three groups. One group received several vials of a 0.1% concentration of neroli essential oil in scentless sweet almond oil… the other, a 0.5% concentration (in scentless sweet almond oil)…and the third group received plain scentless sweet almond oil (a placebo).

The women sat in a comfortable position every morning and evening for five days and inhaled the oil vapor for five minutes at each sitting. To inhale the scent, the women simply poured a small vial of oil on a fragrance pad and held the pad about 12 inches from their noses while they breathed normally.

Before and after the five-day treatment period, each woman was given special questionnaires that rated and scored their quality of life and levels of stress and sexual desire. Blood pressure and pulse were also checked, and blood tests were done to measure cortisol (a stress hormone) and estrogen levels.

The results: Compared with the placebo group, women inhaling neroli felt better and had fewer hot flashes. After the five days of daily aromatherapy, their quality-of-life scores improved by an average of 28% in the women smelling 0.1% neroli oil and 20% in the women smelling 0.5% neroli oil compared with an average 7% improvement in women smelling the placebo oil.

Sexual desire also got a lift in the women who inhaled neroli oil, most especially if they were inhaling the 0.5% concentration. It improved by an average 113% in women using the higher concentration and 27% in women using the 0.1% concentration. Meanwhile, sexual desire took a 50% dive in women using the placebo oil.

How to Benefit from Neroli Oil

Some pure essential oils, such as clove and cinnamon, come with strong precautions because they can irritate the skin or lungs. Neroli oil is much milder. Still, no undiluted essential oil should be daubed on the skin straight out of the bottle—remember, this is concentrated stuff. A few drops should be placed in a scentless "carrier oil," such as sweet almond oil or jojoba oil.

To approximate your own 0.5% concentration of neroli oil, the ratio should be four drops of the essential oil per ounce of carrier oil. (A good aromatherapy oil will come with its own dropper.)

Don't want to fuss with mixing essential oils and carriers? Another simple way to enjoy aromatherapy is to place up to five drops of an essential oil in a pot of hot water and, keeping a safe distance of about a foot away, breathe the steam. Or consider purchasing an aromatherapy diffuser and vaporizer. They come in different styles and have different user directions that come with the packaging. These gadgets either warm an essential oil or mix it with steam to create a scented vapor. They cost anywhere from a few bucks to about $60 and can be easily found in department stores or online through Amazon. com and other sellers.

No side effects were seen in the study, so why not take a few minutes a day to stop and smell the neroli to manage The Change?

Menopausal Vaginal Dryness? Pueraria Mirifica Can Help

Laurie Steelsmith, ND, LAc, licensed naturopathic physician and acupuncturist with a private practice in Honolulu. Dr. Steelsmith is coauthor, with her husband Alex Steelsmith, of *Great Sex, Naturally: Every Woman's Guide to Enhancing Her Sexuality Through the Secrets of Natural Medicine*. DrLaurieSteelsmith.com

For most women, the change of life is a scourge. And one set of symptoms is particularly troubling for women and their partners—vaginal dryness. There's a natural substance that will help you keep celebrating your sexuality. It's an herb available in capsule or cream form that acts like natural estrogen to prevent and repair the damage done by estrogen depletion.

Better Hot Flash Defense

Hot flashes? Don't sweat it. That's the conclusion of research involving about 200 menopausal women.

Study details: Women who have the highest levels of "self-compassion"—that is, the ability to go easy on one's self in difficult or embarrassing situations—find hot flashes and night sweats to be less disruptive than do women who are self-critical.

If you suffer from hot flashes: Try gently telling yourself that this will pass, or make a physical gesture such as placing your hand over your heart.

Lydia Brown, MA, doctoral researcher, The University of Melbourne, Australia.

The herb is called *Pueraria mirifica*. Native to Thailand, it is a tuberous root rich in phytoestrogens, making it a good option for women who want relief but don't want the risks of hormone-based remedies, says naturopathic doctor and sexual health expert Laurie Steelsmith, ND, LAc, coauthor of the book *Great Sex, Naturally*. And a recent experimental study bore this out. It tested a cream formulation of Pueraria mirifica in postmenopausal macaque monkeys and showed that the herb was just as effective as conjugated estrogen cream in repairing vaginal tissue that becomes thin and dry because of estrogen depletion. (The researchers used macaques because they naturally experience menopause and their reproductive organs and hormones are similar to those of humans.)

Restorative Effects

In this study, one group of macaques received a vaginal application of 0.1% Pueraria mirifica cream and another received a 1.0% application daily for one month. A third group received a daily application of conjugated equine estrogen cream, which is used in humans in oral and topical estrogen-based hormone therapy. Vaginal cells were collected from the macaques in a way similar to that of a Pap smear and studied on a weekly basis for three months that spanned pretreatment, treatment and posttreatment periods.

The results: Healthy cell growth lining the vaginal wall increased two-fold beginning at day seven of the treatment period for macaques treated with either 1.0% Pueraria mirifica cream or conjugated equine estrogen cream. (The weaker 0.1% cream also spurred cell growth but not as robustly, and it took a much longer time to kick in). Vaginal pH became more normalized, too. These restorative effects lasted as long as the macaques continued to receive treatment and reverted when treatment was stopped. The researchers also noted that the effects of the cream were comparable to the effects seen in other studies of capsule formulations of Pueraria mirifica.

Is It Right for You?

Dr. Steelsmith, who was not involved in this study, told us that she thought the study was well-done and provided reassurance for women who want a natural option to vaginal estrogen creams. However, although a cream formulation was experimentally used in macaques in the study, Dr. Steelsmith has concerns about over-the-counter cream formulations for vaginal use. They may be irritating or cause allergic reactions, she said. Rather than prescribing a marketed product, she said she would have a cream specially compounded if she were to prescribe it to a patient.

She prescribes Pueraria mirifica in capsule form at a dosage of 100 milligrams (mg) to 200 mg per day. The brand she prefers to prescribe is Nature's Answer Pueraria mirifica Estro Balance with DIM. DIM, which stands for diindolylmethane, is a phytonutrient found in cruciferous vegetables such as broccoli, brussels sprouts, cauliflower, cabbage and kale. It promotes favorable estrogen metabolism in the liver, and so boosts Pueraria mirifica's restorative effects.

The herb is not without potential side effects. For one, its estrogenic effects can cause breast enlargement in some women—which may or may not be an unwelcome effect. In fact, capsule and cream formulations are sold for that very purpose.

More importantly, women who have had or are at risk for estrogen-related cancers, including ovarian, endometrial and breast cancer, should not use Pueraria mirifica for the same reason they should not use other estrogenic supplements or drugs. "In addition, it's definitely not for women who have chronic breast cysts, heavy menstrual bleeding, a history of chronic liver disease, diabetes, migraines, systemic lupus or a history of blood clots," said Dr. Steelsmith. Herbal formulations of the herb can also interact with certain drugs, such as Luvox, Inderal and Clozaril to name a few.

Although formulations of Pueraria mirifica are available without prescription, Dr. Steelsmith stressed that it is wise to consult with a licensed naturopath first. Pueraria mirifica's strong estrogenic effect in the right amount can be beneficial, but too much can contribute to disease, she said.

Weight-Loss Surgery Improves Incontinence

Weight-loss surgery improves urinary incontinence. Of the obese women in a weight-loss program who had urinary incontinence prior to surgery, about two-thirds reported that their incontinence symptoms had improved or disappeared after weight-loss surgery. Other studies have shown that weight loss reduces incontinence because less weight is pressing on the bladder.

Study of 1,565 women by researchers at University of California San Francisco School of Medicine.

Have a Cup of Chamomile for a Long Life

Chamomile may do more than calm your nerves. This popular tea and herbal remedy was linked to a 33% lower risk for death in women, but it had no similar effect on men, according to a recent study of nearly 1,700 adults age 65 and older.

Chamomile's beneficial effects may be due to its antioxidant and anti-inflammatory properties, combined with its ability to help reduce anxiety and depression. Women may benefit from drinking chamomile tea daily (but avoid it if you're allergic to ragweed).

Bret Howrey, PhD, assistant professor of family medicine, The University of Texas Medical Branch at Galveston.

Too Late for Estrogen?

Even if you went through menopause years ago, you haven't missed the "window" for starting estrogen. It is generally considered safest to begin estrogen therapy within 10 years after menopause, but this is not a rigid rule.

Some women may decide years after menopause that they would like to begin estrogen (to curb hot flashes or night sweats, for example), and this calls for personalized decision-making that weighs the benefits versus the risks for the individual patient. Estrogen has been found to raise risk for blood clots, stroke and breast cancer (especially when taken with progestin). Some women who are not candidates for the pill form of estrogen may still be able to take a low-dose skin patch, gel or spray.

JoAnn E. Manson, MD, DrPH, professor of medicine and women's health, Harvard Medical School, Boston.

Brain Harm from Early Menopause

Menopause at age 40 or younger may hurt your brain, reports Joanne Ryan, PhD. Premature menopause increased the risk for poor verbal memory by 56% and poor visual memory by 39%.

Likely link: Estrogen levels, which affect brain function, decline at menopause. Low-

dose hormone therapy may benefit women undergoing premature menopause. Talk to your doctor about the pros and cons.

Joanne Ryan, PhD, postdoctoral research fellow in neuropsychiatry at Inserm U1061, Montpellier, France, and leader of a study of 4,868 women, published in *BJOG: An International Journal of Obstetrics & Gynaecology*.

Nerve Block Injection Helps Reduce Hot Flashes

David R. Walega, MD, associate professor of anesthesiology, Feinberg School of Medicine of Northwestern University, Chicago. His study was published in *Menopause*.

It's like an inner inferno suddenly erupts, leaving you drenched in sweat and red in the face from heat and embarrassment. No wonder women who suffer from menopausal hot flashes—and that includes about 80% of us at some point in our lives—are desperate for relief. The treatment options leave a lot to be desired, however. Hormone therapy helps but has been linked to increased risk for breast cancer and heart disease...oral medications that reduce hot flashes (gabapentin, clonidine) can have intolerable side effects...and botanical therapies such as black cohosh and phytoestrogens haven't proved to be very effective.

A real breakthrough: A treatment usually used to control nerve pain or heavy sweating helps reduce hot flashes, too—and the effects of a single treatment last for six months or more, according to a recent study.

A Single Shot Does the Trick

To understand the study, you need a little physiology lesson. The stellate ganglion is a collection of nerves located in front of the vertebrae at the base of the neck, connecting to the arms and face. These nerves are part of the sympathetic nervous system that activates our fight-or-flight response when we're stressed, so they're not involved with sensation or movement. When a tiny amount of local anesthetic is injected into this bundle of nerves, a procedure called a stellate ganglion block, it temporarily inactivates the nerves. Doctors typically administer the injection to relieve nerve pain in the head, neck, chest or arm…ease angina…or help control very excessive sweating in those same areas.

Some earlier studies suggested that stellate ganglion blocks also reduced vasomotor symptoms (hot flashes, night sweats) in women—so researchers put it to the gold-standard test by doing a randomized, placebo-controlled study. Participants included 40 women who experienced an average of 10 hot flashes daily, with most hot flashes rating as moderate to very severe. (Side note: We're not talking about 10 quick little surges of mild warmth. A moderate hot flash lasts up to 15 minutes and involves sweating, clammy skin, dry mouth, tense muscles, racing heart and/or heat in part or all of the body. A severe hot flash lasts up to 20 minutes, feels like a "raging furnace" and is accompanied by weakness, headache, extreme perspiration, anxiety and/or panic attacks. A very severe hot flash is a "boiling eruption" that lasts up to 45 minutes and is characterized by rolling perspiration, heart irregularities, dizziness, nausea, cramps and difficulty breathing!)

Study procedure: Half of the women were randomly assigned to receive the actual stellate ganglion injection. The other half got a placebo—a sham procedure in which a bit of saline was injected beneath the skin close to, but not actually into, the stellate ganglion. All injections were done using an imaging technique called fluoroscopic guidance (like an X-ray "movie") so that the needle went precisely where it was supposed to go. Only the anesthesiologist giving the injections knew which patients got the real block and which ones got the sham.

For the first three months after the procedure, the women's self-reported symptoms were reduced by about the same amount in both groups—despite the fact that the skin tests showed actual reductions only in the block group—suggesting that a strong placebo effect was at work in the sham group. However, that placebo effect seemed to wear off over time. Compared to the start of the study, the frequency of self-reported moderate-to-very-severe hot flashes occurring in the four to six months after the procedure fell by 52% in the block group but by only 4% in the sham group…while the intensity fell by 38% in the block group but only 8% in the sham group.

How does the procedure work? That's not fully understood, but it could be that the block induces changes in blood flow to regions of the brain that regulate body temperature…and/or that it modulates norepinephrine or nerve growth factor, neurotransmitters that seem to change before and during a hot flash.

The women in this study continued to show benefit from the stellate ganglion block throughout the six-month study. Additional research is needed to determine just how long the effects of a single injection last—they might last even longer than six months.

If you are interested in trying this treatment: Ask your doctor to refer you to an anesthesiologist who is experienced at doing stellate ganglion blocks. You certainly don't want just anybody injecting your neck, given the many critical nerves and blood vessels there—possible risks include seizure, collapsed lung, nerve damage and temporary numbness or weakness from the neck down. However, injuries are very rare when the procedure is done by a well-qualified practitioner. In this study, the only side effects of the treatment were temporary ones that lasted just a few hours—drooping eyelids, eye redness, warmth in the face, hoarseness—which are normal and expected with a stellate ganglion block.

Sex and Menopause

A study of menopausal women's sexual desire found that those with higher natural levels of testosterone tended to have stronger desire and to be more easily aroused. However, the researchers also found that sexual desire was more closely tied to the quality of the women's relationships and their mood than their testosterone levels.

John F. Randolph, Jr., MD, professor of obstetrics & gynecology and epidemiology, University of Michigan Schools of Medicine and Public Health, Ann Arbor.

Older Women Like Their Sex Lives

According to a recent study, older women are happy with their sex lives even though they have sex less often. Sexual frequency decreases with age, but two-thirds of older women say that they reach orgasm every time or almost every time they have intercourse.

Study of 806 women, mean age 67, by researchers at University of California-San Diego School of Medicine and Veterans Affairs San Diego Healthcare System, published in *American Journal of Medicine*.

Testosterone Cream for Women

Does testosterone cream help make sex more pleasurable for women?

Testosterone is known as the "male" hormone—but women's bodies produce some, too. A testosterone deficiency in women may lead to lack of interest in sex. Prescription testosterone cream, which is compounded by a pharmacist and applied to the clitoris in small amounts (0.05 mg to 1 mg) daily, can help improve sensation, desire and arousal. It also increases the size of the clitoris (which may be diminished in postmenopausal women), making it more accessible. The treatment may take a month or more to work.

Barbara Bartlik, MD, a sex therapist in private practice and assistant professor, Weill Cornell Medical College, New York City.

Estrogen for Wrinkles

Mark A. Stengler, NMD, naturopathic medical doctor and author of *The Natural Physician's Healing Therapies*, founder and medical director of the Stengler Center for Integrative Medicine in Encinitas, California, and adjunct associate clinical professor at the National College of Natural Medicine in Portland, Oregon. *MarkStengler.com*

Wrinkles are a natural part of aging. Still, many patients, especially women, ask me if there is a natural way to combat them. Fortunately, there is—with a cream containing specific formulations of bioidentical estrogen.

Let me explain how it works: As we age, hormone production declines. The drop in estrogen production reduces the amount of hyaluronic acid in the skin, a substance that helps the skin retain moisture. This reduction also decreases collagen (which supports the skin's structure) and elastin (a protein), which makes skin thinner and less elastic.

Studies have shown that maintaining levels of estrogen has an effect on the aging of skin. There are three main types of estrogen produced by the body—estradiol, estrone and estriol, which is the weakest of the three. No side effects are associated with using a small amount of estriol topically.

One study conducted by researchers at the University of Vienna of perimenopausal and postmenopausal women, published in *International Journal of Dermatology*, found that those who applied 0.3% topical estriol cream to the face and neck for six months experienced reduced signs of skin aging. Skin elasticity and firmness improved significantly as did wrinkle depth. The study also determined that the estrogen cream did not increase blood levels of any hormones but may have caused a minor side effect, breast tenderness.

My view: A topical estriol cream can reduce wrinkles in perimenopausal and postmenopausal women. It also can be safely used by women younger than perimenopausal age as well as by men, if they want to reduce wrinkles. Anyone interested in these creams must ask their holistic doctors or dermatologists about getting a prescription for them. To find a compounding pharmacy in your area, contact the International Academy of Compounding Pharmacists (800-927-4227, *Iacprx.org*).

People can take estriol for wrinkles indefinitely. Amounts do not need to be adjusted for potency as people age.

Cool Way to Firm Up Saggy Skin

Neil Sadick, MD, clinical professor of dermatology at Weill Cornell Medical College, and medical director of Sadick Dermatology and Sadick Research Group, all in New York City. He also is author of *The New Natural: Your Ultimate Guide to Cutting-Edge Age Reversa. SadickDermatology.com*

Are you sick of wrinkled, sagging skin, but apprehensive about getting a face-lift? You're right to worry about the pain, the anesthesia, not to mention the cost. And what if something goes wrong? There is an alternative…and it doesn't involve knives or needles.

The wrinkle-removing, nonsurgical technology is called Venus Freeze. The results aren't nearly as dramatic as those a face-lift might provide, but it is noninvasive and painless and costs significantly less than cosmetic surgery. The procedure uses radiofrequency energy and magnetic pulses to tighten sagging skin and smooth out wrinkles and cellulite on the face, neck, upper arms, belly, hips and/or thighs.

We spoke with Neil Sadick, MD, a clinical professor of dermatology at Weill Cornell Medical College in New York City. As one of the developers of Venus Freeze, Dr. Sadick has been using the treatment in his practice for several years and has performed it on nearly 1,000 patients to date. He told me, "A small number of people don't get the desired effect, but over 80% have significant improvement."

How it works. The Venus Freeze apparatus consists of a boxy energy-generating unit plus a handheld applicator that looks similar to a computer mouse. The energy it emits penetrates multiple layers of skin, uniformly heating the tissues to about 40°C (104°F). In response, the skin's fibers of collagen (protein-based connective tissue) immediately shorten and thicken, tightening the skin… and over the next several weeks, new collagen forms that provides additional support. Fat-cell volume also decreases, improving the appearance of cellulite. In addition, the treatment induces the release of growth factors needed for new blood vessel formations, thus promoting the flow of blood, nutrients and oxygen to the tissues.

Because Venus Freeze is fairly new, having been cleared by the FDA late in 2010, there isn't a lot of peer-reviewed research available yet (a fact that will no doubt give some people pause). However, one study recently published in *Journal of Dermatological Treatment* is promising—on a scale of one to 10, patients' average satisfaction level was eight and their average pain score was only 1.5.

In another study, this one conducted by Dr. Sadick, 31 patients (mostly middle-aged women) received 10 weekly or twice-weekly treatment sessions for facial wrinkles. None of the participants experienced pain, burns, skin damage or scarring. Three months later, when an independent dermatologist and a plastic surgeon analyzed before-and-after photos, 97% of patients received improved scores on a standard wrinkle scale.

According to Dr. Sadick, there are no long-term safety risks with Venus Freeze (though people who have concerns about any possible risks that might be associated with other radiofrequency and/or electromagnetic devices—cell phones, microwave ovens, overhead power lines—may not feel comfortable with this new technology). *If you are interested in trying it, here's what you'll want to know…*

•**What it can and cannot do.** Venus Freeze is worth considering if you have fine facial wrinkles or jowls yet don't have a tremendous amount of sagging skin, Dr. Sadick said. But if your complexion is already showing considerable signs of aging, the treatment isn't for you.

As for using Venus Freeze elsewhere on the body, don't count on it to dramatically whittle your waistline, eliminate underarm jiggles or slenderize thighs—it's no substitute for good old-fashioned weight loss and toning exercises or for liposuction. However, the technology can improve the appearance of mild-to-moderate cellulite and tighten loose skin in various areas. Dr. Sadick recommends Venus Freeze for people with saggy skin on their upper arms or thighs and for women whose bellies remain stretched out after childbirth.

• **What to expect during treatment.** During this office procedure, the practitioner holds the applicator against the skin and moves it in continuous circular or sweeping motions. Each area takes about 10 minutes to treat. No anesthesia is needed—patients generally feel a slight sensation of warmth, if anything, and can return to normal activities immediately afterward. Side effects consist primarily of slight swelling and/or redness that fade within an hour. There is minimal risk for burns, Dr. Sadick said.

Venus Freeze is available in many areas of the country. To find a provider near you, check VenusTreatments.com. Before you settle on a practitioner, Dr. Sadick suggests asking candidates the following questions…

• *"Who performs the treatment?"* You want a physician or physician assistant, not an aesthetician.

• *"How many patients have you treated with this technology?"* Opt for someone who has performed Venus Freeze on at least 25 patients, Dr. Sadick said.

• *"What does the treatment cost?"* This varies depending on your location and the area of the body being treated, but you can expect to pay several hundred dollars per session.

• *"How many sessions will I need?"* Dr. Sadick usually recommends five to seven weekly treatments initially, with a follow-up session for maintenance every three to six months thereafter. Be skeptical if anyone promises to transform your skin in a single session…or tries to rope you into committing to a dozen or more sessions.

Simple Ways to Look Younger

Eudene Harry, MD, medical director of Oasis Wellness & Rejuvenation Center in Orlando, Florida. She is the author of *Live Younger in 8 Simple Steps: A Practical Guide to Slowing Down the Aging Process from the Inside Out. LivingHealthyLookingYounger.com*

It's a fact of life that our skin becomes more wrinkled as we age. But you may be surprised to learn that our skin starts changing as early as age 30 for both women and men. Of course, you can "refresh" your appearance with Botox and skin fillers, but even "inexpensive" cosmetic procedures cost hundreds of dollars.

A better option: Healthful foods and effective skin-care products. Used properly, natural approaches can take years off your appearance.

Step 1: Tweak Your Diet

While you might think that skin-care products are the logical choice to smooth wrinkled skin, it's wise to first work from the "inside out" to give your skin the nutrients it needs to look its best.

Increasing laboratory evidence and positive reports from patients suggest that the following foods promote younger-looking skin…

• **High-sulfur foods.** Sulfur is known to be one of the "building blocks" of collagen, a protein that strengthens skin and gives it elasticity. Fortunately, sulfur is found in a number of foods.

My advice: At least once a day, eat sulfur-rich foods.

Good choices: Eggs, chives, legumes (such as black, white or kidney beans) and fish that is high in omega-3 fatty acids (such as salmon and sardines).

•**Grape juice or red wine.** These contain flavonoids known as proanthocyanidins and proteins called tenascins—both help make the skin smoother and more elastic.

My advice: Enjoy a daily glass of grape juice—or red wine if your doctor says daily alcohol consumption is appropriate for you. Both are high in proanthocyanidins.

In addition, a grape seed extract supplement (typical dose 200 mg once a day) is beneficial, but check first with your doctor if you take medication, especially a blood thinner—the supplement may interact with certain drugs.

•**Soy foods.** Tofu, soy milk and other foods derived from soy can make skin appear significantly younger. This is mainly due to genistein, an antioxidant in soy that slows skin aging and increases collagen. Genistein and other compounds are linked to increased skin elasticity and plumpness. These compounds give the skin a "glow" that makes it appear younger.

My advice: Have one or more daily servings of soy foods.

Good choices: Edamame (steamed soy beans) and miso (a fermented paste used in cooking). Check first with your doctor if you have breast cancer or kidney disease or take any medication. Soy may be harmful for some breast cancer and kidney disease patients…it may also interact with certain drugs, including blood thinners and some antidepressants.

Also: To help keep skin hydrated, drink eight eight-ounce glasses of water each day.

Step 2: Use The Right Skin-Care Products

Skin-care products can help smooth wrinkles and provide other benefits, but there are so many on the market that most people are confused about which to use. *Best choices for younger-looking skin…*

•**Topical vitamin C.** About 80% of the dermis (the second layer of skin) consists of that all-important protein collagen. Because collagen production declines with age, it's a good idea to promote collagen production any way you can.

That's where vitamin C enters the picture. The body uses vitamin C to produce collagen, but whatever is consumed orally doesn't reach adequate concentrations in the skin to boost collagen. That's why you need to apply it topically.

My advice: Use skin-care products (such as lotions and sunscreens) that have ascorbic acid (vitamin C)—the best form of the vitamin for absorption as well as collagen production and sun protection. Studies show that topical vitamin C can reduce the appearance of fine lines and wrinkles in as little as three months.

To save money: Buy powdered vitamin C at a health-food store, and mix in a small pinch each time you use a moisturizer/sunscreen that does not contain the vitamin.

•**Retinoic acid.** This is a form of vitamin A that is added to hundreds of over-the-counter (OTC) skin-care products. It is also available by prescription. Retinoic acid increases cellular turnover, the rate at which cells divide. This makes the skin appear brighter, smoother and plumper.

My advice: Use OTC retinol cream once daily. Apply it at night because it temporarily increases the skin's sensitivity to sun. Most products have a concentration of 1% or less. Prescription-strength retinoic acid usually is not necessary.

•**Moisturizer.** Everyone should use this as they age. Adding moisture to skin cells makes them expand, which improves skin volume and texture. Moisturizers protect the skin from environmental factors (heat, dryness and pollution) that undermine skin health.

My advice: Use moisturizer with sunscreen at least twice a day. I advise a vitamin C–enhanced moisturizer that includes green-tea extract. Both ingredients improve the skin's ability to absorb the moisturizer.

Compounds in green tea also reduce skin inflammation and sun-related skin damage. Soy moisturizers may provide similar benefits.

Also important: Exfoliation, an effective form of controlled trauma that stimulates the skin to produce more collagen. Every week or two, use a gentle facial scrub with fine grains and a soft facial brush. This practice also removes the dead skin cells that dull your complexion.

Sensitive skin sometimes cannot tolerate even a mild scrub. An ultrasonic brush, such as Clarisonic ($100 to $200 at department stores and online), with a hydrating cleanser is a good alternative.

A chemical peel once or twice a year is another good way to remove dead skin cells. OTC peels contain glycolic acid, lactic acid or salicylic acid, usually in a concentration of about 5% to 10%. Peels should also contain moisturizing ingredients to minimize irritation. If you're new to chemical peels, talk with your dermatologist before using one of these products, since they can irritate skin, especially sensitive skin.

---

6 Herbs That Slow Aging

Donald R. Yance, CN, MH, RH (AHG), clinical master herbalist and certified nutritionist. He is author of *Adaptogens in Medical Herbalism and Herbal Medicine, Healing & Cancer. DonnieYance.com*

You can't escape aging. But many Americans are aging prematurely. *Surprising fact:* The US ranks 42nd out of 191 countries in life expectancy, according to the Census Bureau and the National Center for Health Statistics.

The leading cause of this rapid, premature aging is chronic stress. Stress is any factor, positive or negative, that requires the body to make a response or change to adapt. It can be psychological stress, including the modern addiction to nonstop stimulation and speed. Or it can be physiological stress—such as eating a highly processed diet...sit-

ting for hours every day...absorbing toxins from food, water and air...and spending time in artificial light.

Chronic stress overwhelms the body's homeostasis, its inborn ability to adapt to stress and stay balanced, strong and healthy. The result?

Your hormonal and immune systems are weakened. Inflammation flares up, damaging cells. Daily energy decreases, fatigue increases and you can't manage life as effectively. You suffer from one or more illnesses, take several medications and find yourself in a downward spiral of worsening health. Even though you might live to be 75 or older, you're surviving, not thriving.

We can reduce stress by making lifestyle changes such as eating better and exercising. You also can help beat stress and slow aging with adaptogens. These powerful herbs balance and strengthen the hormonal and immune systems...give you more energy... and repair cellular damage—thereby boosting your body's ability to adapt to chronic stress.

Important: Adaptogens are generally safe, but always talk with your doctor before taking any supplement.

Here are six of the most powerful adaptogens...

• **Ashwagandha.** This adaptogen from Ayurveda (the ancient system of natural healing from India) can help with a wide range of conditions.

Main actions: It is energizing and improves sleep, and it can help with arthritis, anxiety, depression, dementia and respiratory disorders, such as asthma, bronchitis and emphysema.

Important benefit: It is uniquely useful for cancer—some researchers claim it can help kill cancer cells...reduce the toxicity of chemotherapy (and prevent resistance to chemotherapeutic drugs)...relieve cancer-caused fatigue...and prevent recurrence.

• **Eleuthero.** This is the most well-researched adaptogen (with more than 3,000 published studies). It often is called the "king" of adaptogens. (It was introduced in the US as "Siberian ginseng," but it is not a ginseng.)

Main actions: Along with providing energy and vitality, eleuthero protects the body against the ill effects of any kind of stress, such as extremes of heat or cold, excessive exercise and radiation. More than any other adaptogen, it helps normalize any type of physiological abnormality—including high or low blood pressure...and high or low blood sugar.

Important benefit: Eleuthero is a superb "ergogenic" (performance-enhancing) aid that can help anyone involved in sports improve strength and endurance and recover from injury.

• **Ginseng.** Used as a traditional medicine in Asia for more than 5,000 years and the subject of more than 500 scientific papers, ginseng has two primary species—*Panax ginseng* (Korean or Asian ginseng) and *Panax quinquefolius* (American ginseng).

Main actions: Ginseng is antifatigue and antiaging. It increases muscle strength and endurance and improves reaction times. It also strengthens the immune system and the heart and helps regulate blood sugar.

Important benefits: American ginseng can be beneficial for recovering from the common cold, pneumonia or bronchitis (particularly with a dry cough)...and chronic stress accompanied by depression or anxiety.

Korean or Asian ginseng is helpful for increasing physical performance, especially endurance and energy. It is effective for restoring adrenal function and neurological health such as learning and memory.

• **Rhaponticum.** This herb contains more anabolic (strengthening and muscle-building) compounds than any other plant. It is my number-one favorite herb for increasing stamina and strength.

Main actions: It normalizes the central nervous and cardiovascular systems...improves sleep, appetite and mood...and increases the ability to work and function under stressful conditions.

Important benefit: This herb is wonderful for anyone recovering from injury, trauma or surgery.

• **Rhodiola.** Rhodiola has gained popularity over the past few years as studies show that it rivals eleuthero and ginseng as an adaptogen. It is widely used by Russian athletes to increase energy.

Main actions: Rhodiola increases blood supply to the muscles and the brain, enhancing physical and mental performance, including memory. It normalizes the cardiovascular system and protects the heart from stress. It also strengthens immunity.

Red flag: Don't use rhodiola alone—it is extremely astringent and drying. It is best used along with other adaptogens in a formula.

• **Schisandra.** This herb has a long history of use as an adaptogen in China, Russia, Japan, Korea and Tibet. The fruit is commonly used, but the seed is more powerful.

Main actions: Schisandra can treat stress-induced fatigue...protect and detoxify the liver...treat insomnia, depression and vision problems...and enhance athletic performance.

Important benefit: This adaptogen may help night vision—one study showed it improved adaptation to darkness by 90%.

Combinations Are Best

Any one herb has limitations in its healing power. But a combination or formula of adaptogenic herbs overcomes those limitations—because the adaptogens act in concert, making them more powerful.

This concept of synergy—multiple herbs acting together are more effective than one herb acting alone—is key to the effectiveness of the herbal formulas of traditional Chinese medicine (TCM) and Ayurveda. Both these ancient forms of medicine often employ a dozen or more herbs in their formulas.

But it's not only the combination of herbs that makes them effective—it's also the quality of the herbs. There are many more poor-quality adaptogens on the market than high-quality (or even mediocre-quality).

My advice: Look for an herbalist or herbal company that knows all about the source and content of the herbs it uses.

Example: Herbalist & Alchemist, a company that grows most of the herbs used in its products.

Or find a product sold to health practitioners, who then sell it to their patients—this type of product is more likely to be high-quality.

Example: MediHerb, from Standard Process.

Herbal formulas from my company, Natura Health Products, also meet these criteria for high quality.

Say What? A Surprising Link to Hearing Loss for Women

Derek J. Handzo, DO, otolaryngology resident and Kathleen Yaremchuk, MD, chair of the department of otolaryngology–head and neck surgery at Henry Ford Hospital in Detroit. They are coauthors of a study on diabetes and hearing loss presented at a recent Triological Society Combined Sections Meeting.

Needing to turn up the volume on the TV or radio yet again…straining to catch a dinner companion's words in a crowded restaurant…having trouble identifying background noises. It's normal to notice an increase in such experiences as we get older.

But: A recent study has highlighted an important and often overlooked risk factor that can make age-related hearing loss among women much worse than usual—diabetes that was not well-controlled.

Researchers reviewed the medical charts of 990 women and men who, between 2000 and 2008, had had audiograms to test their ability to hear sounds at various frequencies…participants also were scored on speech recognition. Study participants were classified by age, gender and whether they had diabetes (and, if so, how well-controlled their blood glucose levels were).

Results: Among women ages 60 to 75, those whose diabetes was well-controlled were able to hear about equally as well as women who did not have diabetes—but those with poorly controlled diabetes had significantly worse hearing. (For men, there was no significant difference in hearing ability between those with and without diabetes, no matter how well-controlled the disease was, though this finding could have been influenced by the fact that men generally had worse hearing than women regardless of health status.)

Now hear this: Diabetes also increases the risk for heart disease, vision loss, kidney dysfunction, nerve problems and other serious ailments…so this new study gives women with diabetes yet one more important motivation for keeping blood glucose levels well under control with diet, exercise and/or medication.

If you have not been diagnosed with diabetes: If your hearing seems to be worsening, ask your doctor to check for diabetes—particularly if you have other possible warning signs, such as frequent urination, unusual thirst, slow wound healing, blurred vision and/or numbness in the hands and feet.

DIY Hearing Test

Why this test?* It can help identify hearing loss.

The prop you'll need: A perfectly quiet room.

What to do: Rub your right thumb and index finger together continuously to create a kind of "whisper" sound. Raise your right arm so that it's level with your ear and your arm is roughly forming a right angle. Continue rubbing your thumb and index finger

*This self-test is not a substitute for a thorough physical exam from your doctor. Use them only as a way to identify potential problem areas to discuss with your physician.

together. Can you still hear the sound? If not, move your hand toward your right ear, stopping when you can just hear the sound. Repeat on the left side.

Watch out: You should be able to hear this "finger rub" when your hand is six inches or more away from your ear.

Beware: If you need to be closer than six inches to hear the sound in either ear, you may have hearing loss. See an audiologist or otolaryngologist (ear, nose and throat specialist) for an evaluation.

While many people dismiss hearing loss as a mere inconvenience, it can have serious repercussions, such as getting into a car wreck because you can't hear the sound of a car approaching from the side.

David L. Katz, MD, MPH, internist and preventive medicine specialist. He is author of *Disease-Proof: The Remarkable Truth About What Makes Us Well.*

Don't Feel Ready for a Hearing Aid?

Barbara E. Weinstein, PhD, professor of audiology and head of the Audiology Program at The City University of New York Graduate Center. She is the author of the textbook *Geriatric Audiology.*

If you are reluctant (or can't afford) to use a hearing aid, there are dozens of personal sound amplification products (PSAPs), over-the-counter devices that can help you hear a little better but don't cost as much as hearing aids, which run up to $3,000 each.

Not Quite a Hearing Aid

Hearing aids are recommended for those who have been diagnosed with hearing loss by an audiologist. PSAPs, which come in many shapes and sizes, often resembling a Bluetooth headset, are meant to amplify sounds in situations where hearing is difficult, such as large gatherings or noisy restaurants.

In reality, it's not an either-or choice. Only 20% to 25% of people who could benefit from a hearing aid actually use one. PSAPs, with their lower price and availability on the Internet, in pharmacies and in stores such as RadioShack, can serve as "training wheels" for people who want to hear better but hesitate to shell out big bucks for a hearing aid.

Important: The hearing aids sold by audiologists are approved by the FDA as medical devices and must meet certain standards related, for example, to frequency ranges and distortion. PSAPs, on the other hand, are classified as electronic products. They aren't subject to FDA review, so you can't assume that they'll work for you. However, some PSAPs already rival the quality of "official" hearing aids and will keep getting better as technology improves.

Know What You Need

Before you look into PSAPs, get tested by an audiologist. About 14% of adults in their 50s, one-quarter in their 60s and more than one-third of those age 65 and older have some degree of age-related hearing loss. But do not assume that your hearing is normal—or that hearing loss is inevitable.

You may think that your hearing is becoming impaired because of your age when, in fact, it may be due to a medical issue, such as infection, abnormal bone growth, an inner-ear tumor or even earwax—all of which can be treated and sometimes reversed.

If your hearing loss is not related to a medical issue, a PSAP may be appropriate in the following situations…

• **You have trouble hearing the TV.** It is a common complaint but fairly easy to overcome. Inexpensive earbuds or a headset that merely amplifies the sound may be all that you need. Some products are wireless or have long cords that plug directly into the TV.

• **You have trouble hearing in quiet environments.** Speech can sound muffled or be entirely unintelligible if you have age-related hearing loss. Even if you can easily hear background sounds (such as music), you might struggle with the high-frequency sounds that are characteristic of speech.

If you plan to use a PSAP mainly at home or in other quiet settings (such as a museum or a hushed restaurant), look for a device that amplifies high frequencies more than low ones. You'll hear voices more clearly without being overwhelmed by the volume of sounds.

Warning: Some inexpensive products boost both high and low frequencies indiscriminately—avoid them. Your best choice will be a product that allows you to make adjustments and fine-tune it in different settings.

• **You have trouble hearing in noisy environments.** Even mild hearing loss can make it hard to hear voices over the din of clattering plates, a chattering crowd and background music. A simple amplifier won't work because it will make all of the sounds louder.

Better: A device that amplifies the sounds you want to hear while filtering out the rest. Look for a PSAP that has a directional microphone that will pick up speech while muting noise…noise cancellation to filter out low-frequency background sounds…volume control…and multiple channels that are suitable for different sound environments.

• **You're on the fence.** It's common for people to put off getting a hearing aid because of embarrassment or cost. (Hearing aids aren't covered by Medicare or most insurance plans.) You might be telling yourself, "Maybe I'll get one when I'm a lot older."

Important: Don't wait too long. The parts of the brain associated with hearing become less active when they aren't used. You need to hear sounds to keep this brain circuitry working and actively processing speech.

You might want to use a PSAP while you're making up your mind about hearing aids. Even if you get a PSAP that just boosts volume, it will keep the brain signals firing. In my opinion, it's reasonable to use one of these devices for a few months or even a few years. You can always buy a hearing aid later.

Great PSAP Models

Personal sound-amplification products you may want to consider…

• **For TV listening.** Sennheiser Wireless RS Headphones look like old-fashioned stereo headsets, but they let you turn up the sound. $100 to $600, *Sennheiser.com.*

• **For more volume in loud environments.** Able Planet Personal Sound 2500 AMP is packed with high-end electronics to reduce background noise while amplifying sounds you want to hear (such as voices). $900 a pair, $500 for one, *HearingHealth. AblePlanet.com.*

• **For more volume in both loud and quiet places.** The Bean Quiet Sound Amplifier by Etymotic provides amplification of soft speech without distorting sounds. $700 a pair, $375 for one, *QSABean.com.*

• **For more volume at a low cost.** Dozens of affordable products mainly increase volume without other features.

Example: Sonic SE4000X SuperEar Personal Sound Amplifier, a handheld amplifier you can attach to a pocket, belt, hat or purse strap. About $40, *SonicTechnology.com.*

All of the PSAP manufacturers listed here offer a money-back guarantee if the product is returned within 30 days.

Are These Common Pills Harming Your Hearing?

Sharon G. Curhan, MD, instructor in medicine at Harvard Medical School and a physician and clinical researcher at the Channing Division of Network Medicine at Brigham and Women's Hospital, both in Boston. She is the lead author of a study on analgesic use and hearing loss in women published in *American Journal of Epidemiology.*

Headaches, muscle aches, toothaches, menstrual cramps—whatever type of workaday pain you're prone to, chances are that you reach for an over-the-counter painkiller to deal with the discomfort.

After all, you've got plenty of readily available options, including *acetaminophen*

(Tylenol) plus the various nonsteroidal anti-inflammatory drugs (NSAIDs), such as *ibuprofen* (Advil, Motrin), *naproxen* (Aleve) and aspirin. In fact, such pain relievers are the most commonly used medications in the US.

But watch out: The pills that ease pain also may do damage to women's hearing, recent research shows.

Perhaps you heard about a similar finding in a previous study that focused solely on men? Well, given that women use nonprescription painkillers even more than men do, researchers thought it was important to determine whether these pills were risky for female ears, too.

So they analyzed data on 62,261 women who were 31 to 48 years old and who reported normal hearing at the start of the study. Periodically during the 14-year follow-up, all the women answered questions about their use of painkillers and 10,012 of them reported losing some of their hearing. *Here's what the research revealed about...*

• **Ibuprofen.** Compared with women who used ibuprofen less than once per week, the risk for hearing loss was 13% greater among those who regularly used it two to three days per week...21% greater for those using it four to five days per week...and 24% greater for those using it six or more days per week.

• **Acetaminophen.** Compared with women who took acetaminophen less than once per week, the risk for hearing loss among women who regularly took it two or more days per week ranged from 11% to 21%...and the risk tended to be higher with increasing use.

• **Aspirin.** Surprisingly, taking either low-dose or regular aspirin two or more days per week was not associated with an increased risk for hearing loss among women. This was unexpected, given that the earlier men's study did show such a connection.

• **Naproxen.** There was not enough information to determine whether other types of NSAIDs, such as naproxen, also were associated with increased risk for hearing loss.

How the drugs hurt our ears: Researchers theorize that frequent use of ibuprofen may reduce blood flow to the cochlea (the

spiral-shaped cavity of the inner ear), resulting in cell damage that diminishes the organ's function. Acetaminophen is thought to deplete factors (such as the antioxidant glutathione) in the cochlea that protect it from noise and other sources of damage.

Bottom line: Hearing problems become common as we age, affecting one-third of women in their 50s and almost two-thirds of women in their 60s. Yet even mild hearing loss can impair the ability to connect with others, adversely affect work and significantly reduce quality of life. That's why it is so important to identify and avoid preventable causes of hearing loss, such as excessive use of analgesic medications.

Realize, too, that more than your ears are at risk—because these drugs also can cause ulcers, gastrointestinal bleeding, increased blood pressure, kidney damage, liver damage and/or other serious problems. So if you often find yourself reaching for pain relievers, work with your doctor to identify the cause of your pain and discuss alternative ways to control discomfort. Also note that many cold and sinus medications combine analgesics with other ingredients, so check labels to make sure you're not ingesting painkillers more often than you realize.

Eating Fish Helps Hearing

According to a recent finding, women who consume at least two servings of fish a week had a 20% lower risk for hearing loss.

Reason: Blood-supply problems to the ears can cause hearing loss, and a higher intake of fish—rich in omega-3 fatty acids—may help to maintain blood flow.

Other ways to protect hearing: Exercise regularly, manage your weight, and avoid excessively loud noises—or wear protection if you can't.

Sharon E. Curhan, MD, instructor in medicine and a clinical researcher in epidemiology at Brigham and Women's Hospital, Boston, and leader of a study of 65,215 women, published in *American Journal of Clinical Nutrition*.

Wrinkle-Fill Injections Could Make You Go Blind

Study titled "Cosmetic facial fillers and severe vision loss," published in *JAMA Ophthalmology.*

Some people are willing to go to great lengths (and expense) to get rid of their wrinkles, if only temporarily...so they visit a dermatologist for cosmetic filler injections intended to restore a smoother, more youthful appearance to the skin. But there's a potentially devastating side effect of such wrinkle treatments—a side effect that doctors typically do not caution patients about. It is irreversible vision loss.

You read that right. Some people, in their quest to look younger, literally go blind on the spot, according to a recent report published in *JAMA Ophthalmology. Here's the story...*

Cosmetic Filler Cautionary Cases

Cosmetic fillers are sometimes called "liquid face-lifts" because a fluid—usually a product made with hyaluronic acid, collagen, the patient's own fat or some other material—is injected into the folds of the skin to smooth out wrinkles and creases. The effects generally last for a few months until the filler material is absorbed into the body. Filler injections are the second-most-common minimally invasive cosmetic procedure, after Botox injections, with nearly two million filler procedures performed per year in the US.

In a recent report, ophthalmologists in Los Angeles described the cases of three patients they saw who experienced vision loss after receiving filler injections...

An otherwise healthy woman in her 60s immediately lost all vision in her right eye after getting fat injections around her hairline. Her eye doctor was not able to reverse the blindness.

A woman in her 40s got a collagen injection to smooth out forehead creases. When she opened her eyes afterward, she couldn't see out of her right eye at all. After aggressive treatment by her ophthalmologist, she regained a slight ability to perceive light with that eye.

A man in his 30s noticed some loss in the visual field in his left eye the day after getting a hyaluronic acid filler injection in his forehead. Three weeks later, when there was no improvement, he went to the eye doctor... one year later, his vision was still impaired.

The Danger Explained

The ophthalmologists who reported these problems suspect that the injections can plunge the filler material into a crease or fold with such force that the filler winds up where it doesn't belong. It enters the bloodstream and gets into an artery that feeds the eye. Tiny bits of filler then block the retinal artery and/or become embedded in the retina, leading to potentially severe and seemingly irreversible vision loss.

Why are filler injections legal if they can have such devastating consequences? Well, the various types of fillers are FDA-approved for use in the lips and/or areas around the nasolabial folds (the creases that run from the nose to the corners of the mouth). Though the fillers are not specifically approved for use in the forehead, doctors are permitted to use approved drugs "off-label" (in ways other than those that are specifically approved)... even when the safety of such usage has not been established. In injecting cosmetic fillers into patients' foreheads, many doctors do just that.

Also, in some cases, product manufacturers may be misleading consumers into believing that it's OK to use the product anywhere on the face. For example, the website for the hyaluronic acid filler Restylane says that the product "can be used to add volume and fullness to the skin to correct moderate to severe facial wrinkles and folds, such as the lines from your nose to the corners of your mouth." Using the term "such as" implies that it's fine to use the material in other areas of the face besides the nasolabial folds—which a consumer might conclude means around the forehead and eyes. In the fine print under "Important Safety Considerations," Restylane's manufacturer warns that "the safety or effectiveness of treatment in areas other than nasolabial folds and lips...has not been established in controlled clinical studies." But that's in the fine print. No mention is made of potential blindness.

In their report, the eye doctors say that this side effect is rare. Still, it's curious that three such patients were recently seen at one single ophthalmology practice. In fact, digging deeper, we found reports of 44 additional cases of vision loss after filler injections, a significant number of which were in the glabella—the part of the forehead in between the eyebrows where cosmetic surgery patients try to get rid of their "scowl lines."

Self-defense: The authors of this report suggest that doctors who perform filler injection procedures should make patients aware of this potential complication. That's an understatement! Hopefully at some point in time, doctors will simply not inject cosmetic fillers where they are not proven to be safe. And hopefully patients will stop risking their eyesight for a few months of smoother skin.

Birth Control Pills Linked to Glaucoma

Shan C. Lin, MD, professor of clinical ophthalmology, and director, glaucoma service, University of California, San Francisco, and Ye Elaine Wang, MD candidate, Duke University School of Medicine, and glaucoma research fellow, UCSF whose research was presented at a meeting of the American Academy of Ophthalmology in New Orleans.

Were you ever on the Pill...or has a woman you love ever taken oral contraceptives? If so, you need to know about recent research that links a history of birth control pill use to an increased risk for glaucoma, a very serious eye disease.

Second only to cataracts, glaucoma is a leading cause of blindness. The condition, which is characterized by excessive pressure inside the eye, eventually can cause irreversible damage to the optic nerve. And it's very common, affecting upwards of two million adults in the US. Women are more than 50% more likely than men to develop this disease...so for a new study, researchers went looking for factors related to gender that could affect glaucoma risk.

The researchers drew upon data from the ongoing National Health and Nutrition Examination Survey, extracting information on 3,406 women age 40 and up. All the women completed questionnaires about their reproductive health, including number of pregnancies, ages at which their periods started and stopped, history of oral contraceptive use and history of hormone replacement therapy use. They also answered questions about their vision, including whether they had ever been told that they had glaucoma. After adjusting for age, general health conditions, socioeconomic status and other factors known to affect glaucoma risk, the researchers analyzed the data.

Their disturbing finding: Women who had used birth control pills for a total of three or more years had more than double

Better Treatment for Varicose Veins

Background: Foam injections and laser therapy are popular alternatives to surgery for treating varicose veins, a common condition in which veins in the legs weaken, swell and become twisted.

New finding: In a study of nearly 800 patients, all three procedures were found to be effective and safe, but laser therapy had the highest success rate and fewest complications.

Julie Brittenden, MD, professor of vascular surgery, University of Aberdeen, UK.

the risk for glaucoma compared with women who never used the Pill or who had stayed on it for less than three years. The increased risk was found with three or more years of cumulative use of the Pill, not just with continuous use.

There are still a lot of unanswered questions. For instance, the study did not look at whether the glaucoma risk associated with oral contraceptive use topped out at three years or whether women who used the Pill longer—say, for a total of five or 10 or 20 years—might be at even higher risk than those who used it for three years. Nor did the study analyze which type or which dose of birth control pills the women used—and given that birth control pills used to contain much higher doses of hormones than they do now, accounting for these variables might significantly affect the findings.

Former pill users, take note: This study does not prove that birth control pills cause glaucoma...and given the unanswered questions, more research clearly is needed. Still, the findings are disquieting enough that women with a history of using oral contraceptives for a total of three years or longer would be wise to mention this fact to their ophthalmologists and discuss whether they might need any extra glaucoma screening during their annual eye exams. This is particularly important for women who also have other glaucoma risk factors, such as African heritage, diabetes, heart disease, high blood pressure, hypothyroidism or retinal problems...a history of smoking, early menopause (prior to age 45) or long-term use of corticosteroids...a family history of glaucoma...and those who are age 60 or older.

Good news: If glaucoma is detected in time, treatment can reduce eye pressure before the optic nerve suffers permanent damage...safeguarding the precious ability to see.

How to Prevent Glaucoma Vision Loss Before It's Too Late

Harry A. Quigley, MD, A. Edward Maumenee Professor of Ophthalmology and director, Glaucoma Center of Excellence, Wilmer Eye Institute, Johns Hopkins University, Baltimore. Dr. Quigley is author of *Glaucoma: What Every Patient Should Know: A Guide from Dr. Harry Quigley.*

Imagine that, as you read this on your computer screen, the many pixels on the screen begin to stop working, a few at a time...not right in the center, but in clusters all around the screen. It happens slowly, eventually wiping out all but a tiny central spot...which eventually drops out, too. The screen is blank then.

That's a pretty close analogy of what happens when glaucoma runs its course. You'll start losing your peripheral vision first, one eye at a time, and you likely won't even realize that it's happening until much of the damage has been done. The damage is irreversible! But the process can be stopped with early detection and treatment.

Glaucoma is the second-leading cause of blindness in the world after cataracts, and it mostly affects people as they age past 60. The disease is characterized by dying ganglion nerve cells in the retina, the light-sensitive tissue at the back of the eye that catches the images we see. Once these cells die, they are never replaced, which makes early detection of glaucoma critical.

Among the many different types of glaucoma, the most common is open-angle glaucoma, caused by clogging of the eyes' drainage canals in people who have a wide angle between the iris and cornea. Besides older age, risk factors include genetic predisposition, nearsightedness, higher eye pressure, high and low blood pressure, diabetes an hypothyroidism.

Detection

The lack of symptoms is a major reason why glaucoma is often not detected early. And the idea that glaucoma always has something to do with high eye pressure is a prime reason why diagnosis is often missed by eye specialists during regular eye exams. Although high eye pressure is a hallmark of a condition called angle-closure glaucoma, it is not necessarily present in the more common open-angle glaucoma.

People who are over age 60 should have annual eye exams and anyone with a first-degree relative (parent, sibling or child) who has or had glaucoma should get annual exams, too. People younger than 60 should consider getting eye exams, including glaucoma screening, every two years.

To ensure that your exams are thorough enough to detect glaucoma, make sure that, besides having eye pressure measured, you receive a side vision test, which examines peripheral vision, or a visual field test, which examines both peripheral and central vision. The optic nerve head or optic disc (a part of the eye where ganglion cells enter the optic nerve) should also be examined by the eye specialist to evaluate the health of those ganglion cells.

Treatment

If glaucoma is detected, treatment can prevent further damage by restoring eye-fluid drainage and/or relieving eye pressure. This is accomplished by use of daily eye drops or a combination of eye drops and oral medication. Many different types of eye drops—some known as *prostaglandin analogs* (such as Xalatan, Lumigan and Travatan Z)...some *alpha agonists* (such as Alphagan P)...and some *carbonic anhydrase inhibitors* (such as Trusopt)—are prescribed, depending on glaucoma symptoms that need to be managed. Laser eye surgery or traditional types of eye surgery that relieve pressure and correct blocked drainage ducts are options for people who don't get adequate relief from eye drops or who experience allergy or severe side effects from medications—but these people still may need to continue using some form of medication after surgery until eye pressure and drainage aright themselves.

Side effects of eye drops can include change in color of iris and eyelid skin, stinging and burning of the eye, blurred vision and related problems. But most people who become lax about eye drop use don't do so because of side effects. They do so because they forget to use them, sabotaging their fight against glaucoma symptoms.

Although use of daily eye drops is the first-line treatment for glaucoma, the sad truth is that people don't remember to take their eye drops even though they may claim to use them every day. My colleagues and I conducted a study in which we electronically monitored people who were using eye drops for glaucoma management. We discovered that, under the best of circumstances, patients were taking their eye drops only 70% of the time. Of course, eye drops can't help relieve glaucoma unless they are consistently used. I advise that people using eyed rops set up a reminder system. For example, a person could set his/her cell-phone alarm to alert them when to use the drops.

As for alternative treatments for prevention of open-angle glaucoma beyond early detection and management, scientific evidence shows no association between glaucoma and a person's personal habits, such as diet, use of vitamins and supplements, alcohol consumption and caffeine intake. Altering these behaviors, unfortunately, will not decrease your chances of getting glaucoma or prevent it from getting worse. However, aerobic exercise (20 minutes four times a week) can increase blood flow and reduce eye pressure, which can keep glaucoma from worsening.

Where to Get Treatment

Optometrists can diagnose glaucoma and treat it with eye drops. Ophthalmologists can diagnose it and treat it with a wider range of therapies—eye drops as well as laser treatments and eye surgery. But whichever type of specialist you consult, make sure that he is up-to-date on how best to detect glaucoma during an eye exam. To find optometrists and ophthalmologists in your area who have specialized training in glaucoma diagnosis and treatment and have been given a seal of approval by glaucoma experts, visit the American Glaucoma Society website at *AmericanGlaucomaSociety.net*.

Prevent Glaucoma with a Folate Supplement

Study titled "A prospective study of folate, vitamin B-6, and vitamin B-12 intake in relation to exfoliation glaucoma or suspected exfoliation glaucoma," published in *JAMA Ophthalmology*.

Glaucoma is an insidious disease—literally happening before your very eyes undetected, having virtually no symptoms until, in a blink, you've got eye surgery on your plate and you may even be going blind. You may think that, nowadays, glaucoma is easily treatable, but one form of glaucoma, pseudoexfoliation glaucoma (called "PEX" or sometimes just exfoliation glaucoma) is much harder to fix than others. Research from Harvard Medical School, though, is showing that the more folate you get each day, the less likely PEX will develop.

Are You at Risk?

PEX is caused by pressurized buildup of debris that clogs the eye's ability to drain, and it can lead to cataract formation, destruction of the optic nerve and blindness. PEX can happen because it's in your genes or because your eyes have been exposed to too much of the sun's ultraviolet (UV) light. People who live in some northern parts of the world, such as Scandinavia (possibly because of genes) and higher altitudes (where the thin air encourages more UV-radiation exposure) are also more at risk for this eye disease. People with PEX also have high levels of an amino acid called homocysteine in their blood, tears and eye fluid. Because B vitamins can help keep homocysteine levels in check, some researchers thought that getting enough B vitamins was the key, but

the team from Harvard Medical School discovered that it's not quite that simple—it appears that you must get a certain B vitamin in a certain specific way.

Uncovering the Precise Nutritional Link

To get a clearer picture, the Harvard researchers analyzed information from about 120,000 people from two very large, long-term health study databases, the Nurses' Health Study and the Health Professionals Follow-up Study, with a specific focus on people who were 40 years old or older, were free of glaucoma at the start of the study, had had eye exams within a certain two-year period and had provided information about their dietary habits. They discovered that people who ultimately got PEX were deficient in one particular B vitamin, folate. They also found that, although the amount of folate gotten only from food had little impact on prevention of PEX, getting enough from a supplement made a big difference.

Folate Is an Eye-Saver

People with the highest intake of folate—at least 335 micrograms (mcg) per day for women and 434 mcg for men—from vitamin supplements had an 83% reduced risk of PEX compared with people who did not take such supplements. The good news is that any high-quality B complex vitamin supplement, which will generally contain 400 mcg of folate, together with a diet rich in green leafy vegetables, fortified whole grains, beans and peas and especially beef liver (if you have a taste for it) will supply you with enough folate to protect you from PEX. You can even find folate supplements that contain 800 mcg or more, but be aware that the daily tolerable upper limit of supplemental folate for adults, according to the Institute of Medicine, is 1,000 mcg. Also, be aware that folate supplements can interfere with the anticancer effectiveness of the drug methotrexate. Speak with your doctor if you take that drug. Folate supplements also aren't well absorbed in people taking antiepileptic drugs or *sulfasalazine* (Azulfidine, used to treat ulcerative colitis), so guidance about folate supplement dosage, in these instances, also should be discussed with a doctor.

We're increasingly being told by medical experts to ditch vitamin supplements and get our nutrients from whole foods. Although I think this is generally sound advice over pill-popping, even if those pills are vitamins, I also think it's important to pay heed to studies like this one that show that a supplement is exactly what's needed to stave off a serious condition. And sight-robbing glaucoma is serious enough in anyone's book!

Color Vision Changes As We Age

Marilyn Schneck, PhD, research scientist, Smith-Kettlewell Eye Research Institute, San Francisco and University of California, Berkeley. Her study was published in *Optometry and Vision Science*.

Do flowers seem less beautiful and rainbows less vibrant than they used to be? Do clothes you used to love seem a little more ho-hum? It's not that you're getting crabbier with age. Instead, it's likely that your color vision is changing.

That's right. A surprising proportion of seniors experience a marked decrease in the ability to perceive subtle differences in color. This doesn't just affect people's enjoyment of the visual world—it can affect their safety, too, especially since they often do not realize what's happening. *Here's what you should know...*

Two Tests for Aging Eyes

Earlier research suggested that the ability to discriminate among colors decreases with age, but those studies excluded people over age 70 and people who had eye problems normally associated with aging, such as cataracts—meaning that they ignored a significant portion of the population. To address that oversight, the new study included 865 adults who ranged in age from 58 to 102 years old...and the only people excluded were those with a known congenital color-vision deficiency (the red-green color blindness that about 8% of males and 0.5% of females are born with).

The researchers used two proven tests to screen for color-vision changes. Both tests require participants to arrange colors of very slight variations in a particular order. The number and type of errors made is translated into a "color confusion score." A perfect score is zero...a failing score is 30 or higher.

Here's how the study participants did...

•**Overall, 36% of people failed the first test, 21% failed the second test and 18% failed both tests**—much higher percentages than the "up to 8%" usually cited when talking about congenital red-green color blindness.

•**Across the board, failure rates increased markedly as the participants' ages rose.** For instance, on the Farnsworth D-15 test, less than 8% of people under age 65 failed...but more than one-quarter of those in their mid-to-late 70s failed...and nearly half of those age 90 and up failed.

•**The most common problem by far, accounting for nearly 80% of the abnormalities, was the blue-yellow defect, which makes it hard to distinguish between colors in the blue-yellow section of the spectrum.** For instance, blues are easily confused with blue-greens, especially pale ones...and for people with more severe problems, yellows may be confused with violets.

Explanation: This study was not designed to explain why people lose their ability to discern certain colors as they age. However, the researchers noted that most common age-related vision diseases, including macular degeneration, glaucoma and diabetic eye disease, all produce blue-yellow anomalies. Also, with age comes pupillary miosis (a decrease in the size of the pupil), which lets less light into the eye...and yellowing of the lens of the eye (associated with cataracts), which blocks the wavelengths that allow us to perceive blue correctly.

See for Yourself

Why is failing color vision a concern? People who have trouble distinguishing colors may have difficulty carrying out important everyday tasks—such as distinguishing between different-colored medications! And often people are unaware that their color vision has diminished, so they don't know that they need to be on guard against such hazards.

Online test: At your next eye checkup, ask your eye doctor to test you for color-discrimination problems. In the meantime, you can try this online test *www.color-blindness. com/color-arrangement-test*. The goal is to arrange the colored squares in order by dragging each square into a line, placing each one next to the color it's most similar to. If your score indicates diminished color vision, talk to your doctor about ways to compensate for problems this might cause—for instance, by carefully noting the size and shape (and not just the color) of your various medications, so you don't mix them up.

Secrets to Choosing the Best Glasses for You

Melvin Schrier, OD, FAAO, optometry consultant based in Rancho Palos Verdes, California. A fellow of the American Academy of Optometry and past president of the New York Academy of Optometry, he operated a private optometry practice in New York City for more than 40 years.

With all the lenses that are available today—from sophisticated progressives to drugstore readers—and an array of contacts and fashionable frames to choose from, you might think that selecting your eyewear has never been easier. The truth is, there now are so many choices out there—each with its own quirks and pitfalls—that you really need to know what you're doing to avoid making costly, potentially eye-damaging mistakes.

How to guard against the most common mistakes…

Mistake #1: Assuming that progressives are always the best choice. Those nifty lenses known as "progressives," which offer a continuum of clear vision from near to far (close-up, midrange and distance) within a single pair of glasses or contacts, may seem like the ideal solution for aging eyes. Unlike bifocals and trifocals, progressives have no line separating the different viewing zones.

But for many people, progressives are not all they're cracked up to be. Stationary objects may sometimes appear to be moving because the edges of the optical zones are somewhat blurred by design. This also can make driving tricky—for example, you must move your head to the right or left rather than glancing to the sides, where the edges will be blurred.

On top of that, progressives are more expensive than traditional bifocals and trifocals—about $400 and up versus about $200 to $300 for bifocals or trifocals, which have separate viewing zones separated by lines.

If your eye doctor agrees that progressives are a good choice for you, ask about lenses from manufacturers that are pulling out all the stops to try to address some of the common pitfalls.

Two progressive lenses you may want to discuss with your doctor…

• **Varilux S Series.** To help do away with blurry peripheral vision, these new lenses use a patented design that is intended to even out the magnification across the lens. For more information, go to *Varilux-S-Series. com.*

• **Shamir Golf glasses.** These progressive lenses are designed to provide sharp focus for the distances that are most important to golfers—for the scorecard in their hands… the ball at their feet when putting or teeing off…and the green in the distance. For more details, go to *ShamirLens.com.*

Mistake #2: Expecting one set of eyewear to do the trick. Even if you can get by with a pair of progressives, you may want to have more than one set of eyewear to get the best possible vision correction for different tasks.

For example, if you spend long hours in front of a desktop or laptop computer, you may need a prescription for single-vision glasses designed specifically for the distance between you and the screen. These glasses will help reduce eyestrain and fatigue, dry eyes and blurred vision.

Very helpful: Measure the distance from the bridge of your nose to your computer screen (laptop or desktop), and take this measurement to your eye exam. The American Optometric Association recommends that the computer screen be placed 20 to 28 inches from the user's eyes.

So-called "computer glasses" can even be made with lenses that selectively filter out harmful blue light, also known as high-energy visible (HEV) light. In the blue and violet part of the light spectrum, HEV is a particularly intense light wave that is emitted from electronic devices, including computers, tablets and smartphones. (Certain bands of blue light, such as blue-turquoise, are found in the sun's UV rays and are beneficial, aiding in color perception and vision sharpness.)

Studies published in the *Archives of Ophthalmology* show that chronic exposure to harmful blue light may damage the retina, the light-sensitive tissue of the eye, and may increase risk for eye disorders such as age-related macular degeneration and cataracts.

Single-vision eyeglasses designed specifically for computer work usually offer the best correction for heavy computer users. If you're over age 40, however, you may want to consider using bifocal computer glasses. This allows you to see the computer screen clearly and read written material on your desk.

For eyeglasses that are designed to block out harmful blue light and glare, you may want to talk to your eye doctor about the following high-quality lenses: Crizal Prevencia No-Glare blue-light lenses, *CrizalUSA.com.*

If you are a computer user and prefer progressives, ask your doctor about these well-crafted lenses: Zeiss Business and Gradual RD, *Vision.Zeiss.com*…and Seiko PCWide, *SeikoEyewear.com.*

Mistake #3: Opting for fashion over function. Lots of people accept less than excellent vision in exchange for chic eyewear, but this can set you up for trouble.

Examples: If the frames are too big for you, your eyes will not be optimally centered, which could cause visual distortion…if you favor the look of small frames, there may not be enough room for the bifocal or progressive lenses you need.

Either way, you are increasing your risk for blurry vision, headaches and neck pain.

Mistake #4: Not getting the right fit. No matter what your prescription and frames, your eyes should sit precisely in the center of the eyeglass (this may not be the center of the frame) to see clearly.

Progressive lenses have the least room for error. If they're off by even a millimeter, you may have trouble seeing at all three distances.

Important: A precise fit is something online retailers can't offer. Sure, purchasing glasses online may save you money, but this could also prevent you from having clear and comfortable vision.

Better approach: Get your exam from an eye-care professional (optometrist or ophthalmologist), and purchase your glasses there for easy follow-up in case there are any problems.

Also: There is no reason to accept thick, "Coke-bottle" type lenses these days. The technology now is available for even very strong prescriptions to be made in relatively thin lenses.

Mistake #5: Not getting double-checked. Many people never revisit their eye-care specialists even if they suspect there's a problem.

Good rule of thumb: It may take up to three days to get used to a new prescription and frames—but if you're uncomfortable after that time, go back to the eye-care doctor who gave you the prescription.

Sometimes all it takes is a simple adjustment to your frames. In many people, for example, one ear sits slightly higher than the other, so such an adjustment is needed.

Mistake #6: Getting hooked on drugstore readers. You can't beat the price! And these simple reading glasses do offer various levels of magnification.

However, because these readers provide identical magnification in both lenses, they're a viable option only for people who need the same level of vision correction in both eyes—something that rarely occurs.

Many adults have a condition known as anisometropia, in which the eyes require significantly different prescriptions. In fact, a new study has found that nearly one-third of people over age 75 have the condition.

If you have anisometropia and try to get by with drugstore readers, your vision will not be as clear as it would be if you wore prescription readers—not to mention the ill effect it will have on your ability to complete your weekly crossword puzzle!

Index